D1093237

Animal Health Diagnostic Laboratory
P. O. Box 30076   (517) 353-1683
Lansing, MI   48909

PRENTICE-HALL
FOUNDATIONS OF IMMUNOLOGY SERIES

EDITORS

Abraham G. Osler

*The Public Health Research Institute of the City of New York
and New York University School of Medicine*

Leon Weiss

The Johns Hopkins University School of Medicine

THE IMMUNOBIOLOGY OF TRANSPLANTATION
Rupert Billingham and Willys Silvers

THE CELLS AND TISSUES OF THE IMMUNE SYSTEM
Leon Weiss

COMPLEMENT: MECHANISMS AND FUNCTIONS
Abraham G. Osler

THE IMMUNE SYSTEM OF SECRETIONS
Thomas B. Tomasi, Jr.

COMPARATIVE IMMUNOLOGY
Edwin L. Cooper

THE IMMUNOBIOLOGY OF MAMMALIAN REPRODUCTION
Rupert Billingham and Alan E. Beer

RADIOIMMUNOASSAY OF BIOLOGICALLY ACTIVE COMPOUNDS
Charles W. Parker

COMPARATIVE IMMUNOLOGY

EDWIN L. COOPER

School of Medicine
University of California, Los Angeles

PRENTICE-HALL, INC., *Englewood Cliffs, New Jersey*

Library of Congress Cataloging in Publication Data

COOPER, EDWIN LOWELL,
   Comparative immunology.

   Includes bibliographies and index.
   1. Immunology, Comparative. I. Title.
   [DNLM: 1. Immunity. QW504 C776c]
QR181.C73   591.2'9   75-20200
ISBN 0-13-153429-7

PRENTICE-HALL INTERNATIONAL, INC., *London*
PRENTICE-HALL OF AUSTRALIA, PTY. LTD., *Sydney*
PRENTICE-HALL OF CANADA, LTD., *Toronto*
PRENTICE-HALL OF INDIA PRIVATE LIMITED, *New Delhi*
PRENTICE-HALL OF JAPAN, INC. *Tokyo*
PRENTICE-HALL OF SOUTHEAST ASIA (PTE.) LTD., *Singapore*

Acknowledgements

For initiation into the world of textbook writing I extend my appreciation to Dr. Howard Bern, Professor of Zoology, University of California, Berkeley, who in 1969, did the initial arranging with Prentice-Hall for the production of this text—the fruition of a dream. Writing was continued in earnest during a sabbatical (1970–71) in the laboratory of Professor Göran Möller, Immunobiology, Karolinska Institutet, Stockholm, Sweden, when I was the recipient of a Guggenheim Fellowship. I acknowledge the hospitality extended to me by Professor Möller and his wife, Erna, and wish to extend my gratitude to them for the generous space and the conveniences with which I was supplied for beginning this book and for doing experiments with earthworm coelomocytes.

Several colleagues read the first version, and confirmed that the project was worthwhile by providing additional encouragement. Among them I especially wish to mention: Doctors Phyllis Johnson, S. Krassner, W. Hildemann, H. Hilgard, R. Walford, G. Granger, M. Tripp, T. Humphreys, R. Goss, W. Hink, and P. Perlman. I owe a note of appreciation to Mrs. Maude Våglund and to my wife, Héléne, who typed early versions. To Mrs. Pamela Konrad I express gratitude for valuable editorial suggestions. For the final typing a note of deep appreciation is accorded Mrs. Lois Treichler Gehringer who, with patience and accuracy, provided those necessary clean pages for re-reading.

The author acknowledges the editors at Prentice-Hall who helped to begin the text, Mr. Edward Lugenbeel and Mr. Paul Feyen. A special note of appreciation is extended to Drs. Abraham Osler and Leon Weiss who included this book in the Immunobiology Series. Ms. Penelope Linskey assisted me greatly with production and to her I'm most appreciative.

I am especially indebted to Dr. Richard K. Wright, colleague, and fellow comparative immunologist who provided inestimable help by reading and by making valuable suggestions for clarity of the final version. The author acknowledges partial support for original research and the preparation of this book from a Guggenheim Fellowship, The National Science Foundation Research Grant GB17767, a Brown-Hazen Grant, a Grant HD09333-01 from the USPHS, a Fulbright Travel Award and Grants from The Swedish Medical Research Council, Swedish Cancer Society and Wallenberg Foundation to Professor Göran Möller.

Finally, I wish to express appreciation to colleagues and students who have persisted, despite some obstacles in approaching immunology from the comparative and the evolutionary viewpoint. For their help in providing illustrative material, I am grateful. For those colleagues unable to send material before publication, I apologize for this unintentional omission.

Foundations of Immunology Series

This series of monographs is intended to provide readers of diverse backgrounds with an authoritative and clear statement concerning significant aspects of immunology. Each volume represents an individual contribution by a distinguished scientist. As a series, they provide a comprehensive view of the field.

The editors have encouraged the individuality of each author in content and method of presentation. They have sought as the major objective of the series, that each monograph be comprehensible and of interest to a broad audience. The authors provide an authoritative treatment of important problems in major research areas, in which rapid development of new information requires an integrated and reliable evaluation. The series should therefore prove valuable to advanced college students, graduate students, medical students and house staff, practitioners of medicine, laboratory scientists, and teachers.

ABRAHAM G. OSLER
LEON WEISS

Contents

Preface

This is the first textbook to offer a comprehensive review of exciting advances in comparative immunology. This book presents an evolutionary approach to cellular and humoral immunity and reveals the immune system as ubiquitous, and necessary for all animals to survive. Many textbooks of immunology are available, but often they are oriented solely toward medicine or allied professions. This textbook of Comparative Immunology is a unique beginning text for those advanced undergraduate students of biology, zoology, and immunology who are interested in a more biologic or comparative approach to studies of immune competence.

The book will provide undergraduates with an overview of immune reactions— a possible stepping stone for graduate study in comparative immunology. Specialists, often with a mammalian orientation, can use the text as an introduction to a wealth of other vertebrates and invertebrates, sources of new and meaningful facts pertinent to immunology. Despite this orientation, the book would not be foreign to medical, dental and nursing students. Thus, Comparative Immunology is important for anyone who understands and appreciates the fundamental aspects of immunology and biology, and who can grasp significant breakthroughs in immunology when viewed in phylogenetic perspective.

The reader will quickly recognize many fruitful approaches to understanding immunity. To aid the reader, much illustrative material and many references to original works and reviews are presented. This expanding information reveals that analyses need not be restricted to rabbits or guinea pigs, since the invertebrates, fishes, amphibians, reptiles, and certainly birds, are excellent species for deciphering the basic mechanisms of immune reactions. It should be remembered that cellular immunity, undergoing rapid refinement and extended breadth, had deep historical roots in observations on invertebrate cellular immunity. For this reason a good deal of attention is devoted to specific cellular immunity in invertebrates. The apparent absence of circulating immunoglobulins, but the presence of a complicated and efficient humoral immune system, in invertebrates should offer fertile ground for speculating on the nature of those pressures which lead to the evolution of antibody synthesis in vertebrates.

This book begins by first introducing the concept of specific and nonspecific immunity. Animals preserve their unique individuality against infection and possible extinction by distinguishing between self and not-self. This introduction to immunity, its phylogeny, the nature of antigens, and phagocytosis comprise the first four chapters. The earliest beginnings of immune reactions, as best exemplified among the invertebrates, is presented in the next two chapters, which deal primarily with quasi-immunorecognition in certain phyla and graft rejection, primarily in earthworms. This reveals for the first time, anamnesis and memory after transplant rejection. In the following chapter, the cells, tissues and organs of the immune system are presented as the necessary machinery that animals must possess if the immune system is to function. Because transplantation immunology is an important subdiscipline, it is treated from both the ontogenetic and phylogenetic viewpoint in the subsequent three chapters, with emphasis on the vertebrates.

Invertebrate humoral immunity, a possible evolutionary precursor of vertebrate antibodies, is discussed in a separate chapter. Humoral immunity in invertebrates lacks specificity and memory; thus, it is unlike invertebrate and vertebrate cell mediated immunity and antibody synthesis in vertebrates. One chapter is devoted to antibody synthesis and another to the structure of vertebrate immunoglobulins, since herein lies the basis for immunologic specificity. Next, the activities of immune cells are presented, stressing those vertebrate cells that secrete antibody. Because clinicians are often interested in suppressing immunity a brief introduction to non-specific immunosuppression is included. The last chapter offers a brief summary and deals with the evolution of immunity by acknowledging the problem of antibody diversity and recognizing, but not defining, the evolutionary pressures that may have led to the development of immunity. To this end, this book clearly suggests that there is much more to be gained by including in our searches, the invertebrates, fishes, amphibians and reptiles.

EDWIN L. COOPER

Chapter 1

The Immune System

General

It is impossible for animals to live successfully without the full capacity to function in a variety of ways. Living beings are capable of eating, eliminating wastes, respiring, reproducing, and responding to diverse environmental stimuli. The executors of, these varied functions are the cells, tissues, and organs of the digestive, urinary, respiratory, reproductive, and nervous systems. The immune system is likewise an indispensable organ system. It too contains various cells, tissues, and organs that encompass and protect the whole organism against potentially harmful pathogens from the external environment. In fact, the immune system probably arose during evolution not only to defend an organism against external, but also against internal pathologic threats.

The present concept of immunity has changed considerably from its original definition. Literally, its earlier usage referred to exemption from military service or paying taxes. Now, an individual's immune status frees one from disease. One foundation for the science of immunology was laid when the microscope was discovered, making it possible to identify at least one group of microorganisms, the bacteria, that cause disease. Toward the end of the eighteenth century an English country physician, Edward Jenner, reported the first successful attempt to prevent a disease by immunization. His approach grew out of his observation of a naturally occurring phenomenon; dairy maids and farmers often became infected accidentally with cowpox and later seemed to be automatically protected against smallpox. Jenner deliberately inoculated a small boy with pus from a cowpox sore and found that the boy was immune to smallpox six weeks later. Through the use of various modifications of this method, the disease is now virtually eradicated.

A natural result of Jenner's work was the gradual elaboration of the germ theory of disease by Pasteur in France and Koch in Germany during the nineteenth century. Immunology as a science began after they demonstrated that antibacterial substances or factors in the blood of animals immunized against microorganisms ("germs"). Pasteur was successful in culturing many of these bacteria in his laboratory. As often happens in science, fruitful discoveries result from accidents. During one summer he cultured the bacteria that cause cholera in chickens. He found after returning from vacation that he had inadvertently left the cholera organisms in a dish on the laboratory shelf. Such bacteria, after exposure to heat and air, lost their ability to produce disease. However, chickens receiving these defective organisms were protected against freshly cultured cholera bacteria. These attenuated bacteria did not cause disease but conferred immunity, an observation that forms the principle for the development of vaccines.

The Machinery

The immune system, like all other organ systems, consists of several cell types; generally, lymphocytes, plasma cells, macrophages, and granulocytes are found in lymphoid and myeloid tissues and organs. They are often classified as reticuloendothelial (RE) cells and tissues, because of their association with the fibers of these organs. Furthermore macrophages, usually phagocytic, line sinusoids, another function of RE cells. Although the liver, parts of the nervous system, and the lungs of man contain macrophages and fibers making them technically part of the RE system, it is only those cells of a typical immune organ (e.g., the spleen) that participate in immune responses that result in antibody synthesis. Table 1-1 presents those parameters of various vertebrates that are considered indispensable when describing their immune systems. These parameters include cells, organs, and two measurable characteristics: antibody synthesis and allograft rejection. An expansion to include the invertebrates lists an impressive array of immunologic potentialities (Table 1-2).

Cellular vs. Humoral Immunity

The organs of the immune system are the thymus, spleen, lymph nodes, tonsils, Peyer's patches, appendix, and bone marrow. By means of the circulatory system the blood cells, which originate from the bone marrrow, communicate with every available space in the body. Only lymphocytes travel in lymphatic vessels. Indeed, one can readily distinguish between thin-walled lymphatics and comparably sized veins by examination of the contents; they are superficially similar in appearance. Erythrocytes or red blood cells are not found in lymphatic vessels. An animal's first line of defense is the integument, with additional surface reinforcement in the form of lymphocytes and plasma cells just beneath the epithelium. Not only is the external epithelium underlain by lymphocytes, but beneath any internal epithelium, especially at orifices, there is substantial reinforcement by aggregations of immune cells. Portions of the respiratory and digestive system are as equally vulnerable to pathogens as the more exposed integument.

The lymphoid organs and the bone marrow are important because they serve as sites for the genesis of lymphocytes and plasma cells. In these organs, the presence of small, medium and large lymphocytes and plasma cells can readily be demonstrated. Germinal centers in lymph nodules serve as sites for the differentiation of these cells. Monocytes, ubiquitous phagocytic cells of the blood (sometimes called circulating macrophages), apparently arise from the bone marrow.

Metchnikoff, a Russian biologist who worked at the Pasteur Institute in Paris during the latter half of the nineteenth century, clearly recognized the role of cells in effecting immune reactions (Metchnikoff, 1891). Phagocytosis, the process of ingesting foreign material, is an immune reaction that usually does not require the specificity that accompanies immunoglobulin or antibody synthesis. From the viewpoint of evo-

Table 1-1

Immunological parameters exhibited by vertebrate classes.

Class	Lympho-cytes	Plasma cells	Thymus	Spleen	Lymph nodes	Bursa	Anti-bodies	Allograft rejection
Tunicates*	+(?)	−	−	−	−	−	?	+(?)
Cyclostomes								
Lamprey	+	−	PRIM.	PRIM.	−	−	+	+
Hagfish	+	−	N.F.	N.F.	−	−	+	+
Elasmobranchs								
Primitive	+	−	+	+	−	−	+	+
Advanced	+	+	+	+	−	−	+	+
Holosteans								
Bowfin	+	+	+	+	−	−	+	+
Chondrosteans								
Paddlefish	+	+	+	+	−	−	+	+
Teleostei	+	+	+	+	−	−	+	+
Dipnoi	+	(+)	+	+	−	−	+	+
Amphibians								
Urodeles	+	+	+	+	−	−	+	+
Anurans	+	+	+	+	+(?)	−	+	+
Reptiles	+	+	+	+	+(?)	+(?)	+	+
Aves	+	+	+	+	+(?)	+	+	+
Mammals								
Prototheria	+	+	+	+	+(?)	+(Eq.)	+	+
Metatheria	+	+	+	+	+	+(Eq.)	+	+
Eutheria	+	+	+	+	+	+(Eq.)	+	+

*Tunicates represent a protochordate subphylum of the chordates. All other group headings represent classes of vertebrates.

PRIM = Primitive.

Eq = the presence of a lymphoid structure which serves an equivalent function is indicated.

(?) indicates that some question exists regarding the exact homology of the lymphoid cells or structures under consideration, although such structures have been described.

NF = not found.

(*From*: Marchalonis & Cone, AJEBAK **51** : 461 1973)

lution, phagocytosis is probably the oldest of immune responses, traceable even to the protozoans. Phagocytic cells are ubiquitous. To verify their presence, one need only inject an animal with carbon particles; shortly thereafter phagocytes are blackened, being heavily engorged with the ingested particles. Thus, phagocytosis can contribute significantly to an animal's resistance to infectious organisms. In fact, Metchnikoff's discovery of phagocytosis among invertebrates was extended to man,

Table 1-2

Comparative immunologic potentialities of invertebrates

Phylum[a] or Subphylum	Specialized leukocytic cells	Specific xenograft rejection	Specific allograft rejection	Trans- plantation immunologic memory	Inducible circulating "antiboides"[b]
Protozoa	No	Yes	No	No	No
Porifera	No	Yes	No	No	No
Coelenterata	?	Yes	Yes	?	No
Annelida	Yes	Yes	Yes	Yes	No (earthworms) Yes (sipunculids)
Mollusca	Yes	Yes	Yes	?	No (?)
Arthropoda	Yes	Yes & No	No (?)	?	Yes
Echinodermata	Yes	Yes	Yes	Yes	?
Tunicata	Yes	Yes	Yes	?	?

[a]Several phylums omitted because little or no data available.

[b]Mainly bactericidins and not completely specific. Vertebrate-type immunoglobulin antibodies have *not* been demonstrated in *any* invertebrate species.

(*From*: Hildemann and Reddy, Federation Proceedings, **32**: 2188 1973.)

thereby paving the way for reconciling the controversy concerning the importance of humoral immunity vs. cellular immunity.

Cellular immunity gives special credit for immune activity to cells of the immune system, whereas humoral immunity emphasizes the products of some cells. In most vertebrates there is at least integrated cellular and humoral immunity, which combines the activity of cells and their products, antibodies. For cells of the immune system to recognize *not-self*, they must bear recognition units. Such units, or receptors, are antibodies, which are found on the surface of lymphocytes, rendering them capable of detecting antigen. After sensitive lymphocytes select the proper antigen, they are in an advantageous position, capable of reproducing their kind and leaving their descendants ever ready for a second, faster reaction to the same antigen, should it be encountered.

Since the events in cell-mediated immune reactions have been deciphered through experimental procedures, we must now find the reason for the existence and the evolution of these reactions. Assuming that no animal, including man, will ever be grafted with foreign skin during the normal course of its life, what is the explanation for the existence of cell-mediated immunity? It is believed that the immune system, acting as an *immunologic surveillance system*, evolved to police the surfaces of all cells, so as to readily dispose of those cells that are antigenically changed and are therefore *not-self*. Such cells could become cancerous and thereby offer a real threat to survival of the organism.

CELLS OF THE IMMUNE SYSTEM

Lymphocytes

The *lymphocyte* occupies the center of most immunologic activity. In its mature state the lymphocyte is small, measuring only 7–9 μ, about the same size as a mammalian erythrocyte. In fact, measuring it against an erythrocyte in blood smears often quickly distinguishes the mature lymphocyte from its medium or large immature forms. According to earlier views, the small lymphocyte was an effete or terminal cell, finished with its functional activity. However, it was discovered that isolated samples of small lymphocytes could respond to mitogens by dedifferentiating, becoming large lymphocytes again and subsequently dividing. *Mitogens* are substances such as phytohemagglutinin (PHA), an extract of the plant *Phaseolus vulgaris*, which exert this remarkable effect on lymphocytes, causing them to show a burst of activity. The importance of PHA effects may not be readily apparent, but when PHA is administered to lymphocytes in culture it acts as a specific mitogen for glycoproteins of the cell surface. Specific mitogens are *antigens*, which trigger a response from lymphocytes.

The response of lymphocytes *in vivo* offers unequivocal proof for their role in one commonly described immune response, graft destruction. Actually, the newer, more popular *in vitro* approaches are a fundamental outgrowth of the observation of lymphocyte activities in two well-established *in vivo* experiments, namely, *adoptive transfer* and the *graft-versus-host (GVH) reaction*. Ordinarily an immunologically competent animal will destroy a graft through its host lymphocytes. However, if lymph node cells or spleen cells are transferred into a neonatal animal or into an adult rendered immunologically incompetent by lethal doses of irradiation, the host cannot reject the graft and the graft instead rejects the host. Animals being attacked by immunologically competent lymphocytes show a pronounced series of pathologic effects, both gross and microscopic. They lose weight, the lymphoid organs are severely depleted of lymphocytes, and death inevitably occurs. The experimentally induced *GVH reaction* is a model of how foreign cells might proliferate and attack an immunologically crippled animal. Such a model resembles how cancer may develop when cells with alien surface antigens proliferate in an immunologically crippled host.

Instead of the drastic effects of GVH reactions, quite the contrary can occur if lymphocytes are transferred between genetic strain combinations that do not differ. Lymphocytes that are made immune in strain A animals can be transferred into young F_1 hybrids, the result of two inbred strains, and can lodge in the new hosts. When tested for the state of immunity formerly induced in strain A, the new host is now found to be immune. Immunity has been *adoptively transferred*.

Stem Cells

Differentiated immunocytes must originate from some primitive source of *stem cells* thought to reside in the bone marrow (Fig. 1-1). Through a series of unknown influences, preceded by direct migration, stem cells are thought to be destined for "education" in two sites—either the thymus environment or, in mammals, the equivalent to the bursa of Fabricius of birds.

T and B Cells

Stem cells that pass through the thymic environment end up as *T cells* that effect cell-mediated type immune responses. Those that pass through an environment like the avian bursa of Fabricius become *B cells*, differentiate into plasma cells, and thus effect humoral type immune responses. The precise mammalian equivalent of the avian

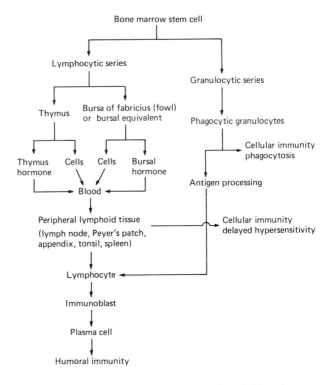

Fig. 1-1 The division of the immune response. A stem cell, probably in bone marrow, is the progenitor of granulocytes, which contribute to the immune response by phagocytosis and antigen processing. Cells of the lymphocytic series produce immunoglobulins if they are of the bursal dependent type, and the delayed hypersensitive response if they are of the thymus type. (*From:* Barrett, *Textbook of Immunology*, C. V. Mosby. Page 54.)

bursa of Fabricius is unknown, but perhaps it is the gut-associated lymphoid tissue (GALT), which includes the *appendix* and *Peyer's patches*. Indeed, these lymphoid aggregations are immunologically competent, and under appropriate circumstances their cells show immune reactivity.

ANTIGENS

Definition

To demonstrate that an individual has an immune system, several approaches can be taken. An experimental immunologist utilizes empirically some known soluble or particulate antigen, injects it, and waits for a host response. The host response is dependent upon many parameters. The route of immunization is important and the antigen dosage is crucial. Antigens constitute a multitude of chemical substances capable of stimulating an animal's immune system to produce antibody or to show cell-mediated immune reactions. Starting with the response to antigen and ending with the final product antibody, we can observe an amazing specificity. Specificity is apparent since the antibody, directed against a particular determinant of an antigenic molecule, will react only with this determinant or another of very similar structure. The antibody response to a given antigen is so exquisitely specific that even minor alterations in the determinant markedly alter the ability of the determinant to react with antibody. In other words A must react with A but not with A_1.

Kinds of Antigens

Antigens can be soluble or particulate. Soluble antigens are substances such as purified proteins (e.g., egg albumin). Foreign erythrocytes or bacteria are examples of particulate antigens that stimulate cells to evoke humoral immunity or antibody synthesis. Once antigen enters an animal it acts to set in motion a chain of events usually resulting in antibody synthesis. Depending upon the antigen, but generally after two weeks, antibody first appears in the serum, specifically in the gamma globulin portion. Even before this time there is pronounced activity in the antibody-forming cells and tissues, a time known as the *induction* or *latent* period. This is easily demonstrable by the intense uptake of isotope-labelled precursors into cell components such as DNA and protein. Direct histologic examination also reveals increased lymphocyte mitoses within such organs as the spleen and lymph nodes.

Examples of Antigen-Antibody Reactions

If the antigen is sheep erythrocytes (SRBC) for example, one can remove the spleen or lymph nodes, dissociate them into their component cells, and then mix them with more of the same (SRBC); those lymphocytes actively secreting antibody will readily form rosettes with the SRBC. Rosette-forming cells (RFC) occur as two main types: 1) those that produce antibody that remains surface bound (*cytophilic* antibody), or 2) those that *secrete* antibody. In the first, SRBC attach as single rows onto these cells; in the second, SRBC attach in multiple rows resembling a bunch of grapes.

Another convenient test demonstrates plaque-forming cells (PFC). If immune lymphocytes are mixed with SRBC in monolayers in agar (Jerne technique) or between two slides (Cunningham technique), along with *complement*, a heat-labile serum component, the mixture (lymphocytes + SRBC + complement) produces lysis. Lysis appears as plaques or clear spaces in the erythrocyte monolayer that can be easily counted.

SPECIFICITY AND MEMORY

Antibody Synthesis

Specificity and *memory* are inherent to humoral and cellular immune responses. Antigen administered for the first time initiates a *primary immune* response. Antibody in this case is at low levels, appears transient, and does not persist for long periods unless a second dose of antigen is administered. If this happens, in a short time, even after one day, there is a spectacular rise in antibody, faster and to a level higher than *primary* response antibody. This *secondary* response differs in another respect by remaining at a high level for a longer period (Fig. 1-2). Long-lasting immunity results from the antibody that remains after periodic boosters to such antigens as smallpox

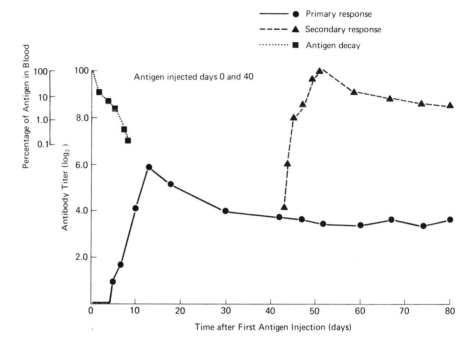

Fig. 1-2 The antigen decay (elimination) and primary and secondary immuncglobulin formation curves. The antigen elimination curve shows the three phases of equilibration, metabolic
elimination, and immune elimination, the latter beginning at about the fifth day. Circulating
immunoglobulins are not detectable until about the fifth day. Notice how the secondary immunoglobulin response following the readministration of antigen at the fortieth day reaches a very
high titer compared to the primary response. (*From:* Barrett, *Textbook of Immunology*, C. V.
Mosby, Page 41.)

or poliomyelitis virus; this provides protection against disease, although antibody
levels do decline. Memory to a specific antigen means that after antibody levels in the
primary response have declined, a subsequent encounter with that same antigen usually evokes an enhanced secondary (anamnestic) response. Thus the immune system
(which like the nervous system, possesses *memory* or *anamnesis*), with its specificity and
memory, ensures more rapid recall or elimination of antigen after a second encounter.
Memory resides in those long-lived lymphocytes capable of reproduction.

Transplantation Immunobiology

If a skin transplant is exchanged between two individuals of the same genus and
species (*allograft, not-self*; formerly *homograft*) this graft behaves initially as an *autograft* or *self* tissue. The allograft will heal and enjoy, so to speak, a brief period of
nourishment by the host, despite its status as *not-self*. Shortly after healing, the presence of the foreign graft's antigens causes the host's immune system to recognize
it, triggering the immune system. Later lymphocytes, and to some extent macrophages,
penetrate the graft and there effect destruction. The evidence is certain that lymphocytes cause graft destruction, but the histology of the process is static and offers only
circumstantial proof.

By some gross criterion such as feathers and hair pattern in birds and mammals, or pigment cell survival (earthworms, fishes, amphibians, reptiles) we are aware that a transplant is destroyed. It is only through *in vitro* approaches that we can surmise what may be happening *in vivo*. Regardless of what does occur at the cell level when a graft is destroyed, this form of immunity at the gross level possesses the same characteristics as the humoral immune response: *primary* and *secondary* responses and *specificity* and *memory*. A *first-set* transplant induces a primary immune response and if its destruction is followed by a *second-set* graft from the same donor as the first, it will be destroyed in a shorter time. A third, independent graft is destroyed at a completely different time from either the first or the second.

IMMUNOLOGIC TOLERANCE

The concept of *immunologic tolerance* has an interesting history, based on a comparative approach using animals other than man. Owen (1945) observed that in nonidentical, fraternal, dizygotic cattle twins, the placentae often fuse, causing an exchange of blood. Fraternal twins are of different (but still related) antigenic composition, and do not arise from the same egg and sperm as are identical or maternal twins. Lack of placental fusion can be confirmed by exchanging skin allografts between fraternal twin siblings. The graft's different antigenic composition is recognized by the host's immune system. Identical twins, nature's own "inbred animals," accept mutually exchanged syngeneic or isogeneic transplants.

With placental fusion, fraternal cattle twins are mutually tolerant of allografts exchanged between them. Since these twins are exposed to mutually foreign antigens *in utero*, each of the developing immune systems "learns" to tolerate those antigens of it's fellow sib. Sir Mac Farlane Burnet (Burnet and Fenner 1949) realized the consequences of nature's "trick" and predicted that if one confronted a mammalian fetus with a foreign antigen when its immune system is "learning," tolerance to the new antigen could be included within its immunologic educational experience. It was Sir Peter Medawar and his colleagues (Billingham, et al. 1953) in Great Britain who simulated the condition observed by Owen in nature, confirmed the predictions of Burnet, and produced in the laboratory *acquired immunologic tolerance*. Although tolerance to a wide variety of external antigens can be induced, an animal should always accept its own *self* antigens during this crucial period in it's immunologic development. Lack of development of tolerance to *self* antigens unfortunately can lead to *auto-immunity*, a paradoxical disease state that results from an animal reacting against its own self antigens.

ANTIBODIES

Antibodies are proteins of known molecular weight and structure. Several classes of antibodies or immunoglobulins are found in vertebrates. The most primitive of vertebrates, the cyclostome fishes, possess immunoglobulin type IgM, the only antibody these fish synthesize regardless of the type of soluble or particulate antigen employed. The genetic machinery of cyclostomes at this evolutionary level is programmed only for the synthesis of this particular immunoglobulin molecule. By contrast, at the other end of the vertebrate spectrum, placental mammals (including man) possess at least five types of immunoglobulins. In addition to IgM, there is IgG, IgE, IgA, and IgD. All invertebrates are equipped with nonspecific hemagglutinins, hemolysins, and bactericidins whose actions mimic that of antibody.

IMMUNOSUPPRESSION

When an animal is confronted with an antigen, this acts as a trigger that causes cells of the immune system to differentiate in a certain direction and sequester the provoking antigen. Briefly, this is what happens under normal experimental conditions, and it is assumed that most of these events occur naturally. It is often desirable to suppress, rather than induce, an immune response. This is of clinical importance, for example, where an individual is to be a recipient of a transplant from an histoincompatible donor. At this point, host-donor matching is limited and must be supplemented by immunotherapy designed to suppress the host's immune response. Suppression is usually accomplished by chemical and physical means, incidentally employing the same drugs often used in cancer chemotherapy; both cancer and immune cells are actively dividing. These drugs are usually antimetabolites, which interfere with nucleic acid or protein synthesis, thereby suppressing the immune response. Irradiation at some appropriate dose also effectively suppresses the immune response. The procedure is obviously delicate. The challenge, using either of the two approaches, is to balance the dosages effectively so that the immune system is suppressed, while at the same time the recipient is still capable of defending itself against environmental pathogens. Immunity is an essential physiologic state; however, it can be inactivated, paradoxically, for man's temporary advantage.

EVOLUTION OF IMMUNITY

Immunology is no longer a discipline that encompasses the thoughts and expertise of classical microbiologists only. Immunology is now a broad field, ranging from simple phagocytosis in invertebrates to antibody syntheses in all vertebrates (Cooper, 1974). No longer is immunology concerned primarily with the practical consequences of antigen entrance into the body; it now also encompasses plausible approaches to the problem of diversity. One immediate theoretical and practical byproduct is a consideration of how the immune system recognizes cancer, leading to the proposition that the immune system developed phylogenetically as a defense against abnormally differentiated cells.

Modern immunology is not unattractive to biologists because of its past clinical orientation. It is a pure, fundamental science, prepared to answer evolutionary questions about cell differentiation and recognition, which are, separately and together, enigmas that have challenged the intellectual and technical expertise of many investigators. As nearly as we can piece together the bits of immunology information gathered from studies of various animal groups, the adaptive immune response can be traced back in evolutionary history some 400 million years to the Paleozoic Era. According to current thinking, the origins of the immune system should be extended to the most ancient period of that era, the Cambrian, which includes the invertebrates where, indeed, immune responses are demonstrable by present-day criteria. Thus the immune system is as old as the oldest invertebrates and as young as man.

BIBLIOGRAPHY

Billingham, R. E., Brent, L., and Medawar, P. B. 1953 Actively acquired tolerance of foreign cells. Nature (London) **172**: 603.

Burnet, F. M. and Fenner, F. 1949. The Production of Antibodies 2nd Ed. New York: Macmillan.

Cooper, E. L. [ed.] 1974. Invertebrate immunology. In *Contemporary topics in immunobiology*, vol. 4. New York: Plenum Press.

Hildemann, W. H., and Reddy, A. L. 1973. Phylogeny of immune responsiveness: marine invertebrates. *Fed. Proc.* **32**: 2188.

Marchalonis, J. J. and Cone, R. E. 1973. The phylogenetic emergence of vertebrate immunity. Australian J. Exptl. Biol. Med. Sci. **51**: 461.

Metchnikoff, E. 1968. *Lectures on the Comparative Pathology of Inflammation* (Edition of 1891 Monograph.) New York: Dover Publications, Inc.

Owen, R. D. 1945. Immunogenetic consequences of vascular anastomoses between bovine twins. Science **102**: 400.

Chapter 2

Phylogeny of the Immune Response

A STATEMENT ON PHYLOGENY

It is necessary in the study of comparative immunology to know something of the place of all animals within the broad taxonomic scheme as recently reviewed by Marchalonis and Cone (1973). There are two major groups of animals: the invertebrates and the vertebrates, as illustrated in Fig. 2-1a and Fig. 2-1b. The Protozoa are one-celled animals represented by several classes, at least one of which, the Sarcodina (amoebae), is important for this exposition. The Porifera, or sponges, are likewise of interest because of their scavenging cells, the archeocytes, the earliest known primitive macrophages. Also, sponges occupy a crucial position, since they represent the first multicellular animal group. They exhibit characteristics of the progenitors of immunity, i.e., mechanisms for sorting of *self* and *not-self* components.

At the level of the coelenterates advanced invertebrate lines diverged. The chordate line, to which vertebrates belong, consists of animals characterized by the deuterostomate pattern of embryogenesis. In such a pattern, the blastula possesses two separate openings that become the mouth and anus. Echinoderms such as the sea stars share this trait with vertebrates. Thus, to study the evolution of immunity through this line of invertebrates may have a direct bearing on how the vertebrate immune system evolved. By contrast, most other invertebrates belong to a group referred to as the *protostomates*. During blastogenesis it is the blastopore alone that splits to form the mouth and the anus of either an adult or larval form, depending on the animal species. It could be argued therefore that to study the phylogenetic origins of the vertebrate immune system through the invertebrate line beginning with the annelids is without relevance. However, this argument loses validity if we accept the biologist's view of every other functional system: knowledge of all immune systems is important in order to explain a phenomenon vital to living creatures. It should also be pointed out that the greatest amount of existing data on invertebrate cell-mediated and humoral immunity is derived from the study of groups splitting off from the annelid line (Bang, 1967; Hildemann and Cooper, 1970; Cooper, 1974a,b; Duprat, et al., 1970), and cell-mediated immunity in this line of invertebrates possesses striking resemblances to that found among the vertebrates. However, invertebrate humoral immunity does not as yet fit into the established criteria for vertebrate antibody synthesis. Investigators may be devising the wrong experiments to deal with invertebrate humoral immunity.

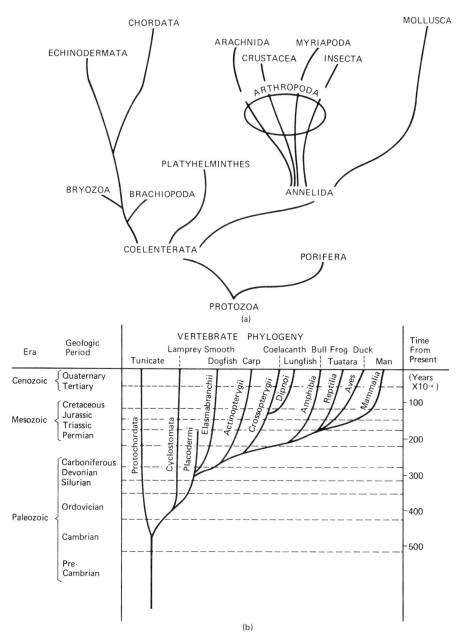

Fig. 2-1 Phylogeny of the animal kingdom. (a) Phylogeny of invertebrates. (b) Phylogeny of vertebrates. (*From:* Marchalonis & Cone, AJEBAK, **51**: 461 1973.)

For our purposes, the phylum Chordata has one important subphylum, the Vertebrata. Vertebrates possess a dorsal hollow nerve cord, a notochord, and, at some stage during their life histories, pharyngeal gill slits. The earliest vertebrates were the ostracoderms, a group of fish-like forms that lacked jaws and paired fins and had a single dorsal nostril. Apparently these arose during the Ordovician period some 400 million years ago. Although the ostracoderms are extinct, their nearest living relatives are the present day hagfish and lamprey, jawless cyclostome fishes. According to Moffett (1966) they apparently descended from two different ostracoderm types. Still, their immune systems are comparable. True jaws first appeared among the placoderms, extinct fish that arose during the Devonian period. The cartilaginous fishes (chondricthyes) and the bony fishes (osteichthyes) arose from different placoderm lines during the Devonian period. The crossopterygians were ancestral to the amphibians; the nearest living relative is the lungfish, order Dipnoi. The cotylosaurs were the stem reptiles that arose from the labyrinthodont amphibians, according to Romer (1962), or from the microsaur amphibians, according to Vaughn (1962), during the Carboniferous period. From the stem reptiles there emerged two forms, the thecodonts and the therapsids, which gave rise to the birds and mammals. We can only surmise, based on the data gained from existing animals, that immune response patterns developed phylogenetically. Certainly the fossil record can tell us nothing about a functioning immune system.

THE CONCEPT OF IMMUNOEVOLUTION

According to a recent interpretation by Hildemann and Reddy (1973) there are three major phylogenetic levels of immuno-evolution: quasi-immunorecognition, primordial cell-mediated immunity, and integrated cell-mediated and humoral antibody immunity (Tables 2-1, 2-2). They refer to all three levels as types of surveillance systems. Quasi-immunorecognition, characteristic of both invertebrates and verte-

Table 2-1

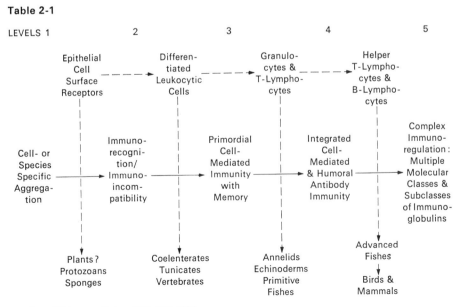

From Hildemann Nature **250**: 116 1974

Table 2-2

Three major phylogenetic levels of immunoevolution

Type of surveillance system	Occurrence	Phylums or classes identified	Experimental evidence
1) *Quasi-immunorecognition*	Invertebrates and vertebrates	Coelenterates Tunicates Mammals	Allograft incompatibility Allogeneic incompatibility MLC reactions
2) *Primordial cell-mediated immunity*	Advanced invertebrates Vertebrates?	Annelids Echinoderms	Allograft incompatibility with specific memory
3) *Integrated cell-mediated and humoral antibody immunity*	All vertebrates	Fishes Amphibians Reptiles Birds Mammals	Very extensive

From: Hildemann and Reddy, Federation Proceedings, **32**: 2192 1973.

brates, may be found specifically among the coelenterates (cnidarians), the tunicates, and mammals, evidenced in broad terms as allogeneic incompatibilities. The second major step, exemplified by advanced invertebrates such as annelids and echinoderms, is likewise demonstrable as allograft incompatibility; however, specific immunity with a memory component of short duration can be shown at this level. Finally, only the vertebrates—fishes, amphibians, reptiles, birds, and mammals—possess integrated cell-mediated and humoral antibody immunity.

Quasi-immunorecognition is demonstrable when *self*, *not-self* recognition occurs after allogeneic or xenogeneic encounters between cells and tissues. Such responses are not purely biochemical (e.g., enzyme substrate incompatibilities) since allografts and xenografts heal in and experience a brief period of normal viability before destruction. This is not typically immunological as defined by vertebrate criteria since there is an apparent lack of memory. However, Hildemann and Reddy (1973) assert that

> to call these systems "nonimmunological" seems unjustified because the mechanism of specific recognition and subsequent incompatibility are unknown. Among [primitive] invertebrates, soft tissue cells in general might be capable of quasi-immunorecognition—a function increasingly assumed by more specialized leukocytes in [advanced] animals. To the extent that the integrity of the body is being specifically defended, use of the immunoprefix is justified.

Primordial cell mediated immunity, the second major level of immuno-evolution, is found first among the coelomate invertebrates, notably the annelids and echinoderms. Their coelomic cavities are filled and monitored by a complex group of coelomocytes that sequester any insulting foreign material. The most striking feature of their surveillance system is immunologic memory and specificity.

Certainly the highest level of immuno-evolution is integrated cell-mediated and humoral antibody immunity. This level of immunity incorporates the two earlier types of surveillance systems; it is increasingly complex and now includes T and B cell type immunites. T cells execute cell-mediated immunity that removes tissue graft antigens, and it is suspected that T lymphocytes do the policing of cancerous cells. We assume that the T cell is phylogenetically the oldest immune cell. B cell immunity involves the synthesis of antibody, an event apparently restricted to vertebrates. The two are integrated by way of antibody, the recognition unit or receptor on the surface of lymphocytes. Finally the ubiquitous macrophage represents still another cell type that is crucial to immunity; its origin can be traced, undoubtedly, to the amoeboid activities of protozoans.

PROGENITORS OF IMMUNOCYTES

Receptor molecules of vertebrate immune cells are antibodies that remain bound to the cell's surface. There may be invertebrate cells that bear receptor molecules; however their nature is unknown. Invertebrate immunocyte receptors may be related to the common agglutinins in the coelomic fluid wherein coelomocytes are suspended. The coelomic fluid, therefore, with its coelomic cells is like vertebrate blood carrying certain immune cells.

Many immunologists believe that invertebrate coelomocytes are the evolutionary precursor of all known vertebrate immunocytes; see for example the scheme outlined by Burnet in Fig. 2-2. All known immunocytes of vertebrates originated from an invertebrate precursor cell that recognized and reacted to antigen. However, unlike vertebrate lymphoid cells, surface receptors of invertebrate immunologically competent cells may not be numerous, so that the invertebrate is incapable of responding

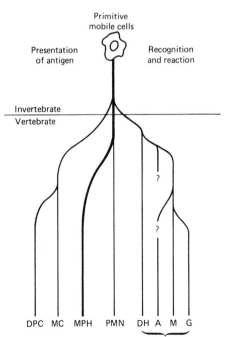

Fig. 2-2 Diagram suggesting the evolution of the mammalian immune system from the haemocyte or primitive mobile cell of the invertebrate. MPH, Macrophage; MC, monocyte; DPC, dendritic phagocytic cell of lymphoid follicles; PMN, polymorphonuclear leucocyte; DH, Immunocytes mediating delayed hypersensitivity and homograft rejection (thymus-dependent); A, M, G, immunocytes differentiated to produce the immunoglobulins shown (GALT-dependent). (*From:* Burnet, *Nature,* **218**: 426 1968.)

to a wide variety of antigens. This limited number of receptors may result in limited specific recognitions and subsequent limited memory responses for invertebrates.

In the absence of demonstrable antibodies or immunoglobulins in those invertebrates studied to date, we remain uncertain about how specificity and perhaps ultimately memory are mediated. Nevertheless, it is tempting to envision the possibility that the complex structure of immunoglobulins is the result of evolution, and that, in some group of invertebrates, molecular configurations with (obvious) resemblances to the vertebrate immunoglobulin molecule may be found, using proper research techniques. Alternatively, the agglutinins as substances unique to the invertebrates may fulfill this role of invertebrate immunocyte recognition units.

To explain how the invertebrate coelomocyte may be both an immunologically competent cell and a precursor of vertebrate immunocytes, Burnet (1968) offers some cogent and incisive comments:

> Among the globulins present in the surface membrane of wandering cells there may well have been protoantibodies. Two developments are required to convert this to an adaptive immune system. The first is an increased flexibility on the part of somatic genome (coupled) with coding for the pattern of these protoglobulins. This conceivably arose as a phase of changing patterns or mechanisms of differentiation. Its function was (a) to provide a means of greater diversification of pattern and, (b) to associate this diversification with an increasingly absolute phenotypic restriction. In this way, there would be an increasing number of foreign patterns that could be recognized and a concentration on a few cells of high ability to deal with any one specific pattern of foreignness. The second requirement is that contact of foreign pattern antigenic determinant with recognition globulin combining site should in appropriate conditions allow proliferation of the haemocytes concerned with retention of its specific character throughout the descendant clone. This, at the cellular level, is the essential feature which makes an immune system adaptive.

We might begin a search for the existence of protoglobulin molecules in the fluid that bathes the coelom or hemocoel of most advanced invertebrates. This fluid is like vertebrate blood in that it contains both granular and nongranular leukocytes. In other words, a situation analogous to the vertebrate condition does exist, awaiting analysis using methods well worked out for vertebrates. This then supports more precisely the possible existance of a recognition unit, but it does not pinpoint a source of such units. Certainly it seems probable that the producers of recognition units would be coelomocytes or hemocytes.

Although Medawar (1963) formulated the term *immunologically competent cell* to define the mammalian immunocyte, it is also applicable to the invertebrate cell that may be capable of synthesizing what are, for now, unknown humoral substances. Furthermore, both invertebrate and vertebrate leukocytes are responsible for the destruction of foreign soluble or particulate cell or tissue antigens. According to Medawar, the immunologically competent cell makes the necessary distinction between the capability of immunological behavior and actual immunological performance. It may hold an evolutionary clue to the differences between invertebrates and vertebrates regarding immunity. This is an important distinction, since this cell is capable of, but not involved in, immunological performance. In embryological terms antigen is to an immunologically competent cell what inducer is to a competent cell, for both antigens and inducers commit cells to a path of differentiation determined by the cell's genetic capability. Presumably the incompetent cell has no potential for exercising immunologic reactions.

We now have leukocytes (coelomocyte, hemocyte, lymphocyte, plasma cell) that produce unknown substance x, retaining it on the cell surface or releasing it into the blood or coelomic cavity; cells then stand ready to recognize and sequester an antigen. According to Sir MacFarlane Burnet (1968) (see Fig. 2-2),

> there is at least a limited capacity to recognize foreignness in the haemocytes of invertebrates. There are also proteins in invertebrate body fluids which have pseudo-immunological capacities, and can, for example, agglutinate mammalian red cells . . . What recognition of foreignness there is in invertebrates is a function of wandering phagocytic cells that are . . . in some sense ancestral to the immunocyte, polymorpho-nuclear and macrophage of the vertebrates (Fig. 2-2).

Thus, we have the most primitive representations of immune cells capable of recognizing (how?) antigen and reacting (how?) to that antigen. It is also possible that antibody genes that produce proteins that react with *self* have not yet evolved in simple organisms. Invertebrates might produce natural "antibodies" and release them into the body fluids as molecules having random specificities and no special affinity for their leucocytes. To prevent destruction of *self*, the organism quickly absorbs any molecules that react against self components, so that they never reach deleterious proportions. Only molecules with *not-self* affinities remain in abundance in the fluids.

According to Boyden (1960), two types of cells enable the invertebrate to recognize *self* and *not-self*:

> One . . . produces and liberates into the body fluids molecules which have [differing affinities but] also [an] affinity for the phagocyte surface [in common]. Subsequently, those molecules in which the randomly determined specificity is complementary to self-components are soon "neutralized" and [disappear] from the body fluids. The other [molecules] continue to circulate in the fluid until absorbed by [leukocytes] by virtue of their second and constant affinity for the [leukocyte] surface. Thus the [leukocytes] become coated with molecules complementary for many different "determinant groups" other than those occurring on self-components.

Invertebrate immunologists would do well to follow the burgeoning efforts to characterize the vertebrate lymphocyte surface components responsible for effecting recognition. A concerted effort would undoubtedly lead to concepts based on facts obtained after comparisons of both animal groups.

COMPARISON OF VERTEBRATE AND INVERTEBRATE IMMUNE RESPONSES

Though vertebrate immunity results from an animal's production of antibodies against a foreign antigen, the invertebrate response seems to be entirely dependent upon the synthesis of other types of macromolecules that may be associated with cell surfaces, but are definitely known to be released into fluids. As neither immunoglobulins such as those of vertebrates nor portions of immunoglobulin molecules have been demonstrated in invertebrates, it has been difficult to account for or define the specificity of invertebrate immune responses. However, the limited specificity that invertebrates possess may be a result of other types of large molecules. Perhaps enzymes act as surface receptors; if so, a search for the possible existence of these components seems warranted.

Invertebrates do possess cells that mediate immunity. Thus, invertebrate recognition molecules may be cell-bound or, possibly, released from cells into the fluids as molecular components or subunits of vertebrate immunoglobulins. Existing theories of vertebrate immunity are applicable to invertebrates because cells engage in immune reactions. Invertebrate animals possess a mixture of cells similar to vertebrate blood cells. In fact, their coeloms are really quite comparable to vertebrate bone marrow (where it exists) in that they possess analogous leukocytic types. In many invertebrates there is minimal leukocyte centralization into discrete organs similar to the vertebrate thymus, spleen, and lymph nodes. There are some exceptions, notably the *Octopus* white body described recently by Cowden and Curtis (1974). We thus have the cells and the compartment from which they are generated. More characterizations of the invertebrate coelomocyte and its function remain to be determined.

Despite their simpler organization and body plan, invertebrates still exibit reactions equivalent to vertebrate cellular responses. With increasing taxonomic and anatomic complexity, which seem to parallel immune response complexity, isolated invertebrate cells can, like those of vertebrates, exhibit characteristic immune reactions. The two are compared in Fig. 2-3. As can be seen, the major difference rests upon the degree of specificity of invertebrate and vertebrate immune responses to foreign antigens. Furthermore, new information since the formulation of this figure renders invalid the statement that nonspecific reactions exist. As we will see later, there are instances of specificity quite easily demonstrable in certain invertebrates.

With regard to phagocytosis and immunity, Boyden (1963) proposes that both defense and food-getting among the less differentiated invertebrates are reactions governed by cell surface receptors. In the phylogenetic progression of species, food-processing cells become different from defense or antigen processing cells. There is a progressive evolution of cells concomitant with this specialization. In other words, although a single-cell amoeba combines in one act both defense and nutrition, the metazoan's phagocytes are involved with defense and other cells cope with nutrition. Single-cell protozoans such as amoebae, as well as some simple metazoans, recognize foreign matter; it is phagocytosed by means of surface factors for defense, but nutrition is also satisfied in the process. The phagocytes of simple metazoans are probably coated with molecules having structures that are complementary to both food and bacterial components. More advanced organisms possess a larger number of different receptor molecules having various steric configurations. They are thus able to distinguish among a much wider range of microorganisms and between a defense and a nutrition response.

THE INVERTEBRATE IMMUNOCYTE AND HYPOTHETICAL SPECIFICITY MOLECULE

An explanation for both the invertebrate's ability to manufacture substances that neutralize foreign antigens and its specific recognition of *self, not-self* components is an hypothetical specificity molecule (HSM), which may be a primordial analogue

Immunological Defense Mechanisms

Invertebrates	Vetebrates
Mainly "unspecific" = directed against common, widespread receptors (for instance, terminal carbohydrate structures)	"Specific" = directed against individual, highly specific receptors, "Unspecific" response also possible (Virus-inhibitors)

Defense System

Naturally occurring (preexisting)	Naturally occurring (preexisting)
Noninducible (exceptions)	Stimulated by immunogens
No booster effect	Booster effect
No stimulation	Immunological memory

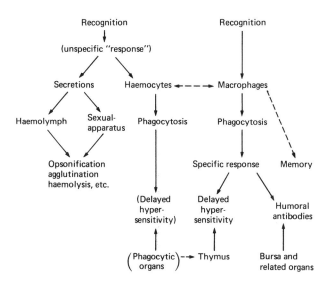

Fig. 2-3 Immunological defense mechanism in invertebrates and vertebrates. The unspecific mechanisms in vertebrates (lysozymes—which occur in invertebrates too—interferon etc.) are not all mentioned in this connection, although there may be some resemblances and parallels to the secretions of the invertebrates. (*From:* Uhlenbruck et al., Z. fur Immunitat. Allergie und klin. Immunol., **139**: 486 1970.)

to antibody. The first step in the production of HSM must almost certainly consist of antigen uptake by a particular kind of invertebrate immunologically competent cell. This cell is probably coated with receptors for a number of foreign molecules or antigens that are apparently unrelated to immunoglobulins, but may be related instead to other large specific molecules, e.g., enzymes. One possible explanation for an invertebrate's inability to respond immunologically to its own proteins is that the HSM cells possess no receptors for *self* components. This absence of *self* receptors can, in turn, be accounted for by supposing either that antigen receptors are produced elsewhere and then neutralized before they reach the HSM cell by the invertebrate's own components, or that they are produced by the immature HSM cell itself before its full maturation.

SPECIFICITY AND ANAMNESIS

To determine whether the immune reactions of invertebrates are comparable to those of vertebrates, investigators must deal with two parameters of the immune reaction: specificity and anamnesis. Inherent in specificity and memory is a faster and heightened response to a second immunization by the same antigen as the first. Furthermore, memory depends upon specificity. Readying the immune system with a first antigenic challenge induces a state of memory such that a second challenge with the same antigen requires less time for the response to appear.

As in the nervous system, environmental stimuli must be perceived, so also in the immune system there must be a way to perceive antigens. There must be receptor cells sensitive to antigenic stimulation. We require, then, cells that can recognize and are equipped with recognition units. Moreover, these cells must be capable of reproducing themselves. Thus, recognition cells capable of infinite numbers of reproductions, each of which bears recognition units, insure specificity and memory. Countless numbers of antigens can be received and acted upon and the information recorded permanently within their progeny.

In the past, this search among the invertebrates has often been futile because of conceptual or technical deterrents. For example, Hilgard (1970) experienced in dealing with both mammals and invertebrates in immunology research, believed that there is "little or no phylogenetic relationship between vertebrate and invertebrate immune responses, for invertebrate receptor molecules which combine specifically with antigens rarely have been demonstrated, and in invertebrates there is often no increased or accelerated response to antigen as a result of prior contact with the same antigen" (Table 2-3). In spite of his criticism, Hilgard, et al. (1967) hoped to detect receptor

Table 2-3

Hypothetical model of an invertebrate immune system

Characteristics	Expected consequences
Cells produce specific receptor molecules (antibody).	Specificity of responses can be demonstrated.
Receptor molecules usually remain cell-bound.	No circulating antibody.
Contact with antigen does not cause any permanent alteration in the cell population which produces receptors.	No increased response to antigen after first response has been completed.
Antigen may induce increased production of receptor molecules, but increased production ends when free antigen is no longer available for combination with receptors.	An augmentation of specific responsiveness to antigen can be demonstrated only during an ongoing response to that antigen.

(From Hilgard, Transplantation Proceedings, **2**: 240 1970.)

molecules in the sea urchin that might combine specifically with antigen, but might not be found in increased numbers in immunized animals. On the basis of *in vivo* injections with various proteins, he and his colleagues found that not all of the receptor molecules reacted to each protein. Their results suggest that the receptor molecules involved in the uptake of these different proteins do indeed have different specificities.

As Hilgard points out, the sea urchin coelomocyte response, like the vertebrate immune response, discriminates between foreign proteins. Certainly the ability of the sea urchin's coelomocytes to respond to small amounts of foreign protein has protective value, for it enables them to respond significantly to pathogens or microorganisms that could otherwise gain entrance by cracking or breaking the sea urchin's tough outer covering. Inherent in these observations, and predictable in all animals, is the capacity to distinguish *self* and *not-self*. Moreover, there is a strong suggestion of immunologic specificity.

We still search for memory as a characteristic of various animal immune responses. According to Talmage (1957) immunologic memory can "be both positive and negative, so that the first injection of antigen may either increase or decrease the subsequent response to the same antigen." Later Talmage (1970) also noted that

> *immunologic memory is much more stable than that of the permease system of bacteria and may last for years . . . The two most striking features of the immune response, its universality and negative memory, must have developed together in evolution because of the biologic requirements of survival. The ability of an organism to make an almost unlimited variety of proteins could not have developed without the capacity to selectively repress the production of those which are self-destructive.*

Assuming that all animals, unicellular or multicellular invertebrates or complex vertebrates, can recognize antigens (distinction between *self, not-self*) we are left then with the need to search for ways to reveal the two other parameters: specificity and memory.

BIBLIOGRAPHY

Bang, F. B., [ed.] 1967. Symposium on defense reactions in invertebrates. *Fed. Proc.*, **26**: 1664.

Boyden, S. V. 1960. Antibody production. *Nature* **185**: 724.

——. 1963. Cellular recognition of foreign matter. *Int. Rev. Exptl. Pathol.*, **2**: 311.

Burnet, F. M. 1968. Evolution of the immune process in vertebrates. *Nature* **218**: 426.

Cooper, E. L. 1974a. Symposium on Invertebrate Transplantation. *AAAS* (unpublished).

——. [ed.] 1974b. Invertebrate Immunology. In *Contemporary Topics in Immunobiology*, Vol. 4, New York: Plenum Press.

Cowden, R. R., and Curtis, S. K. 1974. The octopus white body: an ultrastructural survey. In *Contemporary in Immunobiology*, ed. E. L. Cooper, vol. 4, p. 77. New York: Plenum Press.

Duprat, P., Du Pasquier, L., and Valembois, P. 1970. Colloque sur les réactions immunitaires chez les invertébrés. Arcachon: Laboratoire de Zoologie (Université de Bordeaux).

Hildemann, W. H., and Cooper, E. L., [eds.] 1970. Phylogeny of transplantation reactions. *Trans. Proc.* **2**: 179.

Hildemann, W. H., and Reddy, A. L. 1973. Phylogeny of immune responsiveness: marine invertebrates. *Fed. Proc.* **32**: 2188.

Hilgard, H. R. 1970. Studies of protein uptake by echinoderm cells: their possible significance in relation to the phylogeny of immune responses. *Transpl. Proc.* **2**: 240.

Hilgard, H. R., Hinds, W. E., and Phillips, J. H. 1967. The specificity of uptake of foreign proteins by coelomocytes of the purple sea urchin. *Comp. Biochem. Physiol.* **23**: 814.

Marchalonis, J. J., and Cone, R. E. 1973. The phylogenetic emergence of vertebrate immunity. Aust. J. Exper. *Biol. Med. Sci.* **51**: 461.

Medawar, P. B. 1963. *Introduction: Definition of the Immunologically Competent Cell in Ciba Foundation Study Group No. 16: The Immunologically Competent Cell, It's Nature and Origin.* London: J. & A. Churchill Ltd.

Moffett, J. W. 1966. The general biology of the cyclostomes with special reference to the lamprey. In *Phylogeny of Immunity*, [eds.] R. T. Smith, P. A. Miescher, and R. A. Good. Gainesville, Florida: Univer. of Florida Press.

Romer, A. S. 1962. *The Vertebrate Body.* Philadelphia: W. B. Saunders.

Talmage, D. W. 1957. Allergy and immunology. *Ann. Rev. Med.* **8**: 239.

———. 1969. The nature of the immunological response. In *Immunology and Development*, [eds.] M. Adinolfi and J. Humphreys. London: Spastics International Medical Publications in Association with William Heinemann Medical Books, Ltd.

Vaughn, P. P. 1962. The paleozoic microsaurus as close relatives of reptiles again. *Am. Midl. Nat.* **67**: 79.

Chapter 3

Nature of Antigens

INTRODUCTION TO ANTIGENS, HAPTENS, AND ANTIGENIC SPECIFICITY

Definition of Antigens

Antigens, ordinarily defined, are any foreign protein or polysaccharide that induce the formation of and react specifically with antibodies. Such a definition is restrictive however, if the entire animal kingdom is considered; all animals do not possess cells capable of synthesizing antibody. However, every animal is endowed with cells capable of recognizing foreignness, distinguishing between *self* and *not-self*, and eliminating alien material. That a foreign insult such as bacteria is banished is all that should happen, if we judge the value of antigen elimination to animal survival on teleological grounds. Antibody need not be the end result. Although the ability to synthesize antibody may be considered advanced and complex, the invertebrate's method of handling antigen apparently does not involve antibody. Thus, whether an antigen or foreign material is sequestered by an invertebrate's phagocytic cell or any of its several nonantibody humoral components (e.g. lysins, bactericidins, agglutinins) is important. Antigen elimination in an invertebrate is as efficient as that in a vertebrate, which inactivates antigen by its phagocytic cells, and in addition synthesizes antibody.

We can now provide two definitions. *Antigens*, or the property of *antigenicity*, refer to the characteristics of molecules that allow them to interact with *antibodies*. *Immunogens* with the property of *immunogenecity* refer to the characteristics of molecules that elicit the production of specific antibodies. According to Chadwick (1967), *insect immunogen* is a suggested term that can be applied to insects, since the final product is not antibody (see Chapter 11). The remarkable difference between vertebrates and invertebrates lies in the fact that vertebrate antibody specificity is strict, whereas substances from invertebrates are quite often not specific.

Several variables profoundly affect antigenicity and immunogenicity. These are: choice of animal species, age of the animal, nature of the antigen (i.e., whether it is soluble or particulate), amount or dosage of antigen, whether it is combined with adjuvant, and, if so, the route of antigen administration. Whatever is antigenic in vertebrates is likewise antigenic in invertebrates. They both recognize foreignness and antigen is sequestered.

Haptens

In addition to naturally occurring antigens, which are often complex molecules, there are well-defined, simple chemical substances incapable by themselves of inducing an immune response; these are termed *haptens*. However, an immune response can be induced by a hapten if it is attached to a carrier molecule such as a protein, e.g., albumin. The hapten molecule acts as a determinant of antigenic specificity, referred to as the *antigenic determinant*. Haptens are important to understanding antigenicity, the mechanisms of antibody synthesis, and the structure of antibody molecules. It is only after a hapten combines with a protein carrier that the two, then known as *hapten-carrier complex*, can interact with immunologically competent cells, permitting antibody induction that is then hapten specific.

Simple haptens include many small but natural molecules such as polynucleotides, oligosaccharides, certain steroids, peptides, as well as other types of simple compounds such as picryl chloride and formaldehyde; the latter two can cause sensitization when injected, applied to the skin, or even inhaled. Haptens are any substances which do not elicit antibody formation alone, i.e., are not immunogenic but are capable of reacting with antibodies synthesized against a complete immunogenic molecule. Haptens readily form complexes with host proteins in the skin or with plasma proteins, resulting in the formation of artificial antigens. Simple haptens produce no visible antigen-antibody reactions after interaction with antibody. They must be coupled with a protein, an indirect method for demonstrating their activity.

An example of Landsteiner's classic demonstration of hapten specificity as revealed by its activity is diagrammed in Table 3-1. Landsteiner first described the serological

Table 3-1

The contribution of acidic radicals to serologic specificity*

	Antisera versus			
Antigen conjugated with	NH$_2$ (Aniline)	NH$_2$ / COOH (PABA)	NH$_2$ / SO$_3$H (PASA)	NH$_2$ / ASO$_3$H$_2$ (PAAA)
Aniline	+++	—	—	—
PABA	—	+++±	—	—
PASA	—	—	+++±	—
PAAA	—	—	—	+++±

*From Landsteiner, K.: The specificity of serologic reactions, revised edition, New York, 1962, Harvard University Press, Cambridge Massachusetts.

specificity of different azo-proteins by attaching different artificial haptens such as arsanilic acid and p-aminobenzoic acid to various protein molecules. When the three isomers of aminobenzene sulphonic acid (ortho, meta, and para) were diazotized and coupled to a protein (horse serum protein) he could then produce antibodies against such hapten-carrier complexes in rabbits. Rabbit antisera against these complexes are specific and can distinguish among the three isomers. Thus antibody mixed with the hapten (hapten-carrier complex) evokes a visible reaction (precipitate). For example, antibodies to the protein containing the meta azobenzene sulphonate group give good precipitates with a different carrier protein bearing the meta isomer. However, poor precipitates are formed with the other two isomers.

Antigenic Specificity

An important aspect of antigens is their specificity. Each antigen is different from every other, causing it to react specifically with the antibody that it induces. Antigenic specificity is based on the configuration of antigenic determinants. The size of an antigenic determinant is minute in relation to the size of the entire antigen molecule, a specific, limited portion that induces antibody formation. Antibody, once induced, also reacts with that portion, the antigenic determinant site or epitope. Valence of antigen refers to the number of antigenic determinants per molecule of antigen, or the number of antibody molecules with which the antigen can combine.

The total valence of an antigen molecule is the sum of the functional and non-functional (hidden) valence sites. The functional valence is equal to at least two and may be proportional to the molecular weight of the antigen. There is one valence site for each molecular weight (MW) of 10,000. Therefore, those molecules with greater than 10,000 MW would be expected to have more than one valence site. Functional valence sites occur on the outer surface of the antigen molecule. These can be measured by determining the number of antibody molecules that attach to the antigen. After an antigen is degraded by hydrolysis, the resulting products induce antibody synthesis. This is not to suggest however that soluble antigens are not antigenic; antigens can be soluble or particulate.

THE REACTIONS OF ANTIGEN WITH ANTIBODY

Most techniques used to demonstrate antigen-antibody reactions involve reacting putatively immune serum with antigen. Whatever the test situation, there is a characteristic reaction between antigen and antibody. For example, if a soluble antigen such as bovine serum albumin (BSA) is used, the resulting antibodies that react with BSA lead to precipitation and are termed *precipitins*. The presence of antibodies in the serum is affected by an appropriate immunization schedule and the control of other variables, (e.g., dose, route). Alternatively, antigen can be reacted directly with immunocompetent cells demonstrating the earliest antibody prior to its appearance in the serum. Reactions of this kind usually involve antigen adherance, particularly that of bacteria or erythrocytes to the immunocompetent cells in question. To complete the mixture, complement, a thermolabile component of guinea pig serum, must be added. *Lysis* then occurs by means of antibodies known either as *bacteriolysins* or *hemolysins*, depending upon the antigen.

TYPES OF ANTIGENS

Antigens and Antibody Synthesis

An animal may respond differently to a variety of antigens. For example, hamsters produce antibody whose presence, amount, and persistence in the serum appear to be markedly influenced by the antigen used for immunization (Fugmann and Sigel, 1968). Hamsters immunized with influenza virus or sheep erythrocytes show 19S antibody in significant amounts only during the early phases of immunization; however, in the case of sheep erythrocytes, hemolytic activity associated with the 19S antibody predominates at all times. No 19S antibody was found after immunization with bovine γ-globulin, but there were two different populations of 7S antibodies with different electric charges after immunization with sheep erythrocytes, influenza virus, and bovine γ-globulin. Thus, different kinds of antigens affect the resulting kinds of antibody.

Species-Specific Antigens

Closely related antigens are detectable by the immune system. The concept in immunology of species specificity is derived from the work of Nuttall (1904). He injected serum as antigen from one animal into another and produced antibodies. Thus, animals can be distinguished from each other by means of precipitation reactions. In other words, the more closely related are two individual animal species, the less likely there will be strong reactions between the two antisera directed against their respective antigens (serums). For example, serum of animal X injected into a rabbit will induce antibodies (precipitins) that should react strongly with precipitins induced against the serum from individual X. However, species specificity is often not absolute. Thus, kinship can be shown to exist even between different species. In fact, cross-reactions based on phylogenetic relationship are demonstrable and can be used as another means of classifying various species (Boyden, 1942), an alternative to conventional methods of taxonomy.

Although such species-specifiic determinants occur in the serum, tissue cells of the body also possess antigens that characterize a species. These antigens are distributed widely; they occur in all or most animal tissues and certainly provide the specificities to which a host can react after tissue transplants are performed between genetically disparate donors and hosts. Contrary to this rule, however, there is a remarkable tissue specificity that can even transcend species specificity, especially when embryonic cell surface antigens are considered. If cells of one histiotypic type are mixed after prior dissociation with the same type of cells derived from different species, (e.g., mouse liver and chicken liver) they regularly aggregate again. However, if cells of two different histiotypes from the same animal are mixed (kidney and liver for example), these cells are not attracted to each other and end up forming isolated and separate aggregates.

To test whether certain organs or tissues are related because of their antigenic composition, one can inject extracts of tissues into a rabbit, which then develops antibodies (Bonstein and Rose, 1971). Rabbit antisera to tissue antigens can be completely absorbed with human serum to remove any cross-reactivity between tissue antigens and antigens in human serum. For example, one can prepare crude extracts of human liver, tracheal mucosa, oesophagus, and stomach with Freund's complete adjuvant and inject it into rabbits. Because of common antigens between tissues and human serum, one can obtain cross-reactions between the antigenic extracts and the antisera or similar cross-reactivities between serum and these extracts (Fig. 3-1). Antisera to human trachea extract show lines of identity to extracts of human trachea, spleen, bladder, and liver. Another antiserum to human trachea (e.g., 14) produces

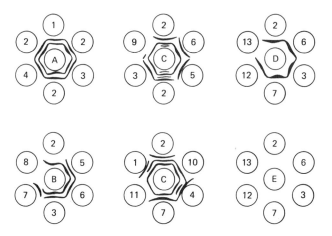

Fig. 3-1 Ouchterlony test with human organ extracts. Well 1, bladder; 2, trachea; 3, liver; 4, splean; 5, lung; 6, oesophagus; 7, kidney; 8, pooled NHS; 9, skeletal muscle; 10, thyroid; 11, ovary; 12, stomach; 13, pooled NHS. Well A, antiserum 20 absorbed with NHS; B, antiserum 26 absorbed with NHS; C, antiserum 14 absorbed with NHS; D, antiserum 24 absorbed with NHS; E, antiserum 24 absorbed with NHS and kidney extract. (*From:* Bonstein & Rose, *Clin. Exper. Immunol.,* **8**: 291 1971.)

two or three lines of identity with oesophagus, lung, liver, bladder, thyroid, spleen, and kidney; with skeletal muscle and ovary, only one line appears. Antiserum to oesophagus extract precipitates one or two antigens of trachea, lung, oesophagus, liver, and kidney. In testing for the lack of true species specificity when rhesus monkey extracts were used, (Fig. 3-2) an antiserum 20 produces at least one line with monkey esophagus, liver, spleen, stomach, jejunum, kidney, and lung, but there were no reactions with monkey muscle. It is important that no reactions are found to occur when antisera to human tissue extracts are tested with organ extracts derived from horses, sheep, cattle, and pigs; this observation supports the theory of the kinship of certain monkey and human antigens.

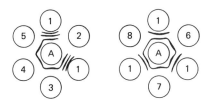

Fig. 3-2 Ouchterlony test. Well 1, human trachea; 2, monkey muscle; 3, monkey lung; 4, monkey jejunum; 5, monkey stomach; 6, monkey kidney; 7, monkey liver; 8, monkey oesophagus. Well A, antiserum 20 (anti-trachea) absorbed with NHS. (*From:* Bonstein & Rose, *Clin. Exper. Immunol.,* **8**: 291 1971.)

Genetic Control of Allotypes

A host animal such as a rabbit can be injected with sera from two animals of the same or even different genera and species. This induces antisera of one or two distinct types. However, Oudin (1956) showed that serum proteins of one individual can induce the formation of precipitating antibodies in others of the same species. In other words, sera contain antigens that evoke antibodies in another animal after immunization even if the host is of the same genus and species as the donor of the serum. The isoantibodies formed can thus characterize serum protein specificities within a species that are genetically controlled. The term *allotype* defines a serum protein specificity (Dray and Young 1958) existing within a species. The capacity develops early in ontogeny and is not restricted to mammalian organisms. In bullfrog tadpoles, Cooper, et al. (1964) succeeded in producing alloantibodies to serum from adult bullfrogs.

The Mendelian basis for antibody or immunoglobulin allotypes has been established for several species. In rabbits, three alleles at each of two loci (*a* and *b*) have been described (Dray et al. 1962). In mice, allotypes of at least three multiple allelic systems have been demonstrated (Lieberman and Dray 1964; Warner and Herzenberg 1967). Allotypic specificities occur in chickens, pigs, and cattle (Skalba 1964; Rasmusen 1965; Rapacz et al. 1968).

Eight immunoglobulin allotypic specificities have been identified in fowl by isoimmunization; genetic control is by means of codominant genes at three genetic loci (David et al. 1969). Aal and Aa2 are controlled as codominants at the *a* locus, Ab1 and Ab2 at the *b* locus, and Ac1, Ac2, Ac3, and Ac4 at the *c* locus. Column chromatography, ultracentrifugation, and immunoelectrophoresis reveal these specificities at the *a* locus corresponding to the immunoblobulin G molecule with a sedimentation coefficient of 7S.

Erythrocyte Isoantigens

In addition to the presence of numerous antigens on various whole organs and tissues, blood, literally a tissue that flows, contains multiple kinds of cells that also possess antigens. The red cells or erythrocytes are widely employed as experimental antigens, and the relationship between various individuals is measured by reacting erythrocytes, usually with homologous sera. The whole system of blood transfusion involves the interaction of allogeneic human serums and erythrocytes. Incompatibilities are possible without proper matching. White cells or leukocytes also possess antigens, and there is incresed experimentation designed to reveal individuality by testing homologous sera against leukocytes. This forms the basis for matching donors and hosts for organ transplants, currently a technique of clinical importance.

Antibodies that clump erythrocytes or bacteria are termed *agglutinins*. If the serum from one individual of a given species agglutinates the erythrocytes of another, the serum contains antibodies directed against the erythrocyte antigens. Knowledge of erythrocyte antigens and corresponding antiserums in individuals forms the basis for the ABO blood grouping system in humans. Such an immunogenetic approach can be studied from a phylogenetic viewpoint (Hildemann 1969).

During the 1950's there was a surge of interest in immunogenetic studies of marine fishes, particularly in Japan and the United States. Such work had a twofold purpose: one for pure science and the other for the identification of subpopulations of economically important teleosts such as tuna, Atlantic herring, Pacific sardines, and Pacific salmon by quantitative studies of erythrocyte antigen frequencies. Individual differences in erythrocyte antigens have been detected in many fishes. Even among elasmobranchs, largely because of intensive work by Sindermann (Sindermann and Honey, 1962), there is genetic information about blood-group antigens of the spiny dogfish, *Squalus acanthius*. The S-system has been proposed for their blood-group system. Like sharks, skates are ideal for immunogenetic studies. One can demonstrate discrete isoantibody systems within their own species as well as high titers of natural heteroagglutinins for the erythrocyte antigens of other animal species.

The methods for demonstrating hemagglutinins to erythrocyte antigens merit consideration. The winter skate, *Raja ocellata*, can be obtained from the Western North Atlantic ocean; it is bled from the heart and serum is obtained, after which it is refrigerated. Cross-matching tests are performed with undiluted serum previously inactivated for 30 minutes at 50°C to destroy complement; this is absolutely necessary to prevent the lysis of erythrocytes by complement. Cross reactions between different skate sera and erythrocytes are then tested by tube agglutination. To remove agglutinins before valid testing, skate sera are absorbed with skate erythrocytes by the addition of undiluted serum from one skate to washed erythrocytes of another skate in 1:1 proportions. Skates possess a blood-group system as evidenced by cross matches of sera and cells. The system contains two erythrocyte antigens tentatively labeled SK_a and SK_b, and their corresponding specific serum isoagglutinins anti-SK_a and anti-SK_b, which are stable throughout the year. In addition to isoagglutinins, sera of certain individual skates contain natural heteroagglutinins for Atlantic herring, *Clupea harengus*, and human type O erythrocytes. In contrast to isoagglutinins, heteroagglutinins do show seasonal variation. They increase in the spring and exceed the previous autumn level by June (Fig. 3-3). Heteroagglutinins directed against herring erythrocyte antigens distinguish individual variations just as if antisera had been prepared experimentally.

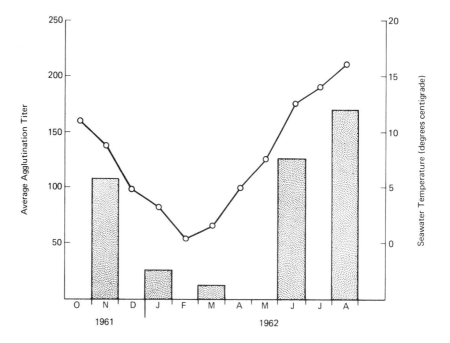

Fig. 3-3 Monthly mean seawater temperatures (solid line) and average skate serum heteroagglutinin titers (bars) when tested against human type O erythrocytes. (*From:* Sindermann & Honey, *Copeia*, March **26**: 139 1964.)

Transplantation Antigens

Transplantation antigens, determined by various histocompatibility genes, can be solubilized and thus can provide chemical markers of biologic individuality (Kahan and Reisfeld 1969). Transplantation antigens induce allograft immunity, humoral alloantibodies, and cutaneous hypersensitivity reactions. In relation to allograft destruction, if one injects 1.3×10^{-10} mole of water-soluble purified guinea pig transplantation antigen into a host prior to transplantation, this treatment hastens allograft rejection. By contrast, prolonged graft survival is obtained if a prospective host is treated with high doses of antigen prepared by homogenization or sonication of cells combined with treatment using immunosuppressive agents.

Transplantation antigens develop early in ontogeny and are generally present on all cell surfaces. Lymphoid tissue contains the greatest amount of extractable antigen; kidney, lung, adrenal, and liver tissue have moderate amounts; and the brain, placenta and muscle are poorer sources. The strongest antigenic determinants are intimately associated with the cell surface membrane from which they can be solubilized by chemical fractionation, using a variety of approaches. A second major technique involves exposing cells to ultrasound; this liberates water-soluble transplantation antigens from cells of various organs. Low frequency sound releases patent antigens, but high frequency generators liberate small quantities of less active material.

For antigen activity the presence of a polypeptide is necessary, as is easily confirmed by showing irreversible destruction of antigenic activity after exposure to conditions that cause denaturation: 50% urea, 90% phenol, aqueous alcohol, heat, and pH values of less than 4 and greater than 9. Furthermore, the proteolytic enzyme pronase degrades antigenic material to an inactive, lower molecular weight substance. As marker substances for cell membrane physiology in general, transplantation antigens are valuable.

HOST AND EXTERNAL INFLUENCES ON ANTIGENS

Genetic Constitution of the Responding Animal

There is much evidence that the immune response is genetically controlled (Benacerraf 1974). Thus, all facets of the immune response, including events of the inductive phase such as antigen recognition and phagocytosis, are influenced by an animal's genetic constitution. Whereas substance X is antigenic in one animal, it may not be so in animals of a different species. Single genes are known to profoundly affect the response to various immunogens with limited ranges of antigenic determinants. For example, the multichain synthetic polypeptide antigen, poly (tyr, glu) poly-DL-ala–polylys (T, G)-A–L) is genetically controlled by the locus Ir-1 that is closely linked to the H-2 locus on the ninth chromosome in mice. The H-2 locus controls histocompatibility in mice. As another example, in guinea pigs, the ability of poly-L-lysine to function as a macromolecular carrier for the 2, 4-dinitrophynl (DNP) group as a hapten depends upon a single gene.

Rathbun and Hildemann (1970) found that antibody synthesis is substantially regulated by products of alleles of the H-2 locus. They studied antibody responses to the 2, 4, 6-trinitrophenyl hapten (TNP) conjugated to mouse serum albumin (MSA)

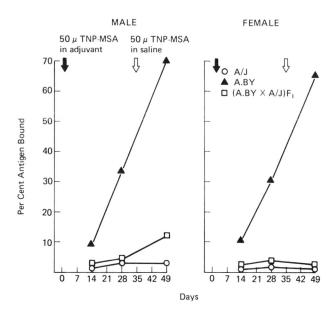

Fig. 3-4 Comparative antigen-binding capacity (ABC) assays of individual sera from A/J, A.By and (A.BY × A/J)F_1 mice as a function of per cent of antigen (TNP-BSA) bound and the time after immunization. (*From:* Rathbun & Hildemann, *J. Immunol.,* **105**: 98 1970.)

in each of five mouse strains representing congenic strains that differ at the H-2 and H-3 loci; their respective F_1 and F_2 progeny were also studied. These are: pair 1, A/Jax (H-2^a) and A.BY (H-2^b); pair 2, B10.A (H-2^a) and C57BL/10 (H-2^6); and pair 3, C57BL/10 (H-3^a) and B10.Lp-a (H-3^b) and the F_1 and F_2 progeny of (C57BL/10

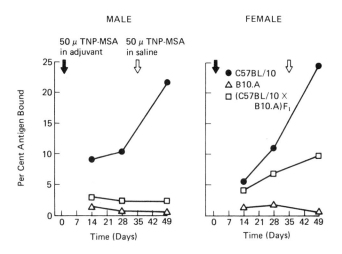

Fig. 3-5 Comparative ABC assays on sera from B10.A, C57BL/10 and (C57BL/10 × B10.A)F_1 mice as a function of per cent of antigen (TNP-BSA) bound and the time after immunization. (*From:* Rathbun & Hildemann, *J. Immunol.,* **105**: 98 1970.)

× B10.A) and (A.BY × A/Jax) hybrid crosses. Antibody responses were measured by a sensitive test for antigen-binding capacity after individual serial bleedings. It is interesting to see the comparative results after immunizing A/Jax, A.BY, and (A.BY × A/Jax)F_1 with 50 μg TNP_{11}-MSA in complete Freund's adjuvant followed, five weeks later by 50 μg in saline. Both sexes of the A/BY (H-2^b) strain gave significantly higher antibody responses to TNP-MSA than did either the strain's H-2 disparate congenic partner A/Jax (H-2^a) or its (A.BY × A/Jax) F_1 progeny (Fig. 3-4). Furthermore, strain C57 BL/10 also carries the H-2^b allele, resulting in an increased response to TNP when compared to either its congenic partner B10.A (H-2^a) or the C57 BL/10 × B10.A F_1 progeny. F_1 females gave significantly higher responses than males, but no such sex differences were found with (A.BY × A/Jax) F_1's (Fig. 3-5).

With regard to another antigen, sheep erythrocytes, both A/Jax (H-2^a) and B10.A (H-2^a) mice give significantly higher responses at the peak period of four days after immunization with 5 × 10^6 SRBC than did their respective H-2 disparate congenic partners A.BY (H-2^b) and C57BL/10 (H-2^b). Strain C57BL/10 (H-2^b, H-3^a) and its H-3 disparate partner B10.LP-a (H-2^b, H-3^b) give similar responses to SRBC (Fig. 3-6). The H-2^a allele is associated with high antibody responses when SRBC are used as antigen in contrast to the low responsiveness found toward the TNP hapten. Antibody responses to at least two antigens, one of which has been chemically defined, is genetically controlled particularly by the H-2 locus, but the mechanism of gene action associated with this complex locus is unclear.

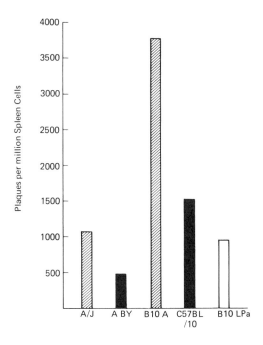

Fig. 3-6 Comparative hemolysin responses of several strains of mice in plaques/10 × 10^6 spleen cells at 4 days after immunization with sheep red cells. (*From:* Rathbun & Hildemann, *J. Immunol.,* **105**: 98 1970.)

Adjuvants

Certain soluble substances are not immunogenic when administered alone in saline to animals. It is therefore necessary to combine them with other substances that somehow increase the immunogenicity leading to more effective antibody synthesis. These substances are known as *adjuvants* (e.g., *Freund's incomplete* and *complete adjuvant*) and alum gels. When any of these adjuvants is combined with a soluble antigen, the resulting antibody concentration increases in the serum in significant amounts when compared to the antibody evoked by antigen that is administered alone to an animal.

A typical immunization involving a soluble antigen (e.g., BSA) and adjuvant is done in the following way. The antigen (in aqueous phase) and complete Freund's adjuvant (an oily mixture) are mixed vigorously to form a water-in-oil emulsion. Water droplets (the antigen) are surrounded by a continuous oil phase containing tubercle bacilli (the adjuvant). Mixing is ideally done in a double syringe, forcing the two substances together and creating a frothy mixture. Antigen-adjuvant emulsion is injected subcutaneously in an experimental animal, and after its injection the mixture forms a granuloma that stimulates the activity of macrophages and lymphocytes. Because of the persistence of such granulomas, certain adjuvants are not encouraged for use in man. Instead, in humans immunized with diphtheria and tetanus toxoids for example, certain aluminum compounds are recommended.

It is not entirely clear how adjuvants promote increased antibody synthesis. The antigen-adjuvant-induced granulomatous depots allow small quantities of antigen to leak slowly into and make contact with cells of the immune system. An extended explanation suggests that this mixture is very attractive to macrophages, resulting in greater phagocytosis. As a more immunological explanation, granulomatous sites attract competent lymphocytes and plasma cells, causing more efficient contact between cells and leaking antigen. Any one or a combination of these three explanations—persistence of antigen, more efficient inflammatory response, or earlier priming of immunologically competent cells—may explain why it is important to use adjuvant in conjunction with certain soluble antigens for more effective immunization.

Rowlands (1970) studied the effect of Freund's complete adjuvant on the opossum's immune response. Opossums were immunized with 5 μg of bacteriophage f2 suspended in either Freund's complete adjuvant or in saline. Serum was collected from each group of opossums at 7, 14, 21, 28, and 35 days after an initial injection of antigen. A second antigen injection was given immediately after the last bleeding for the primary response; thereafter, serum was collected at 7, 14, 21, and 28 days for the secondary response (Fig. 3-7a, b). Both primary and secondary responses to bacteriophage f2 are similar if the opossums are given antigen in adjuvant or antigen in saline. Antibodies are detected in both groups after seven days, and peak immune responses occur by 14 days for the primary response. However, final antibody levels of the primary response are greater if the antigen is given in adjuvant than when combined with saline. Apparently in the opossum, a marsupial mammal, this antigen and adjuvant produce a difference in the secondary response.

In comparison, the response of a rabbit (a placental mammal) differs from that of opossums even at a lower dose of antigen (0.5 μg of bacteriophage f2) plus adjuvant (Fig. 3-7 c, d). Neutralizing antibodies are present in the serum of both types of mammalian species at seven days, but they reach higher levels more rapidly in rabbits

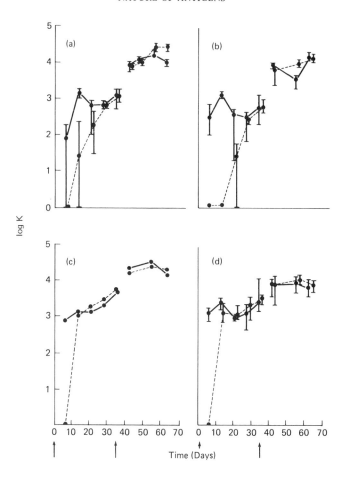

Fig. 3-7 Antibody responses in oppossums (a and b) and rabbits (c and d) given 5 ug of bacteriophage f2 in Freund's complete adjuvant (a and c) or in saline (b and d). Antibody expressed as $\log_{10}$ of the neutralization constant K. Solid curves, antibody activity without reduction; broken curves, antibody activity after reduction with 2-ME. (*From:* Rowlands, *Immunology,* **18**: 149 1970.)

than in opossums. Furthermore, there is an early conversion from mercaptoethanol-sensitive (19S, IgM) to mercaptoethanol-resistant antibodies (7S, IgG) in rabbits, unlike the slower conversion in opossums. Freund's complete adjuvant combined with phage antigen enhances the immune response more in rabbits than in opossums.

Antigen Dosage and Route of Administration

Regardless of the antigen type, be it soluble, particulate, or cellular, the dosage for each experiment is important. However, it is largely empirical and must be determined for each antigen, especially if the antigen is used for the first time in a new animal. If soluble antigens are combined with an adjuvant and the mixture is injected subcutaneously, bleeding can be done after a primary injection of antigen following an appropriate period to test for antibody. Alternatively, one could allow the animal

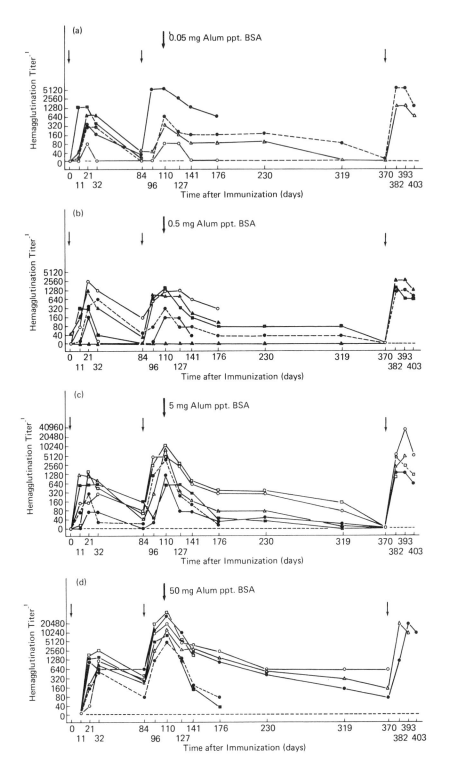

Fig. 3-8 Kinetics of antibody response of gar immunized with bovine serum albumin, alum precipitated. ((a) 0.05 mg, (b) 0.5 mg, (c) 5.0 mg, (d) 50 mg.) (*From:* Bradshaw et al, *J. Immunol.,* **103**: 496 1969.)

to rest, administer a second intraperitoneal injection of the antigen without adjuvant, and follow this shortly thereafter by a bleeding to test for antibody. It is impossible to describe all the varying dosages and how these could be matched with various routes; such decisions depend upon the investigator.

If we were to vary the antigen dosage and route with adjuvant (alum precipitated) what would be the response of an animal? A primitive holostean fish for example is advantageous for any study particularly aimed at understanding the responses of varying animal species to antigen. Bradshaw et al. (1969), used several antigens and looked for differences in responses to several dosages. The antibody response to BSA-AP (bovine serum albumin, alum precipitated) was studied in four groups of gar that had been immunized at 0.05, 0.5, 5, and 50 mg/ml on days 0, 84, and 370. All fish respond to BSA-AP with the production of antibodies that are demonstrable by passive hemagglutination (Figs. 3-8a, b, c, and d). For the passive hemagglutination test the putative antiserum is reacted with erythrocytes to which the soluble antigen has been attached by chemical methods. When antibody reacts with the antigen attached to the red cells, agglutination results.

There was a noticeable dose effect in this experiment. Most fish had antibodies on day 11 following injection of 5 mg, whereas few of them had antibodies at this time after injection of 0.05 mg. It is interesting that fish receiving the largest dose, 50 mg, had no demonstrable antibodies until day 21; in some, the maximal titer was not reached until day 32. Even though the primary response is delayed, efficient priming by antigen probably occurred, since all fish in this group showed a rise in titer 12 days after the secondary stimulation. By contrast, fish that received smaller doses for the primary immunization had a more variable response upon secondary injection; the inductive period required 12–26 days. The maximal titers were reached by day 26. Thus, the amount of antibody is related to the antigen dose. Soluble BSA is a poor antigen in the gar, yielding negative results, but its immunogenicity is greatly increased by adjuvant and precipitation with alum, thus rendering BSA a particulate antigen.

Age and Species

Adult Responses to Four Types of Viral Antigens

Sigel and Clem (1965) studied the response of elasmobranch and teleost fishes to viral antigens. The two species of elasmobranchs include the lemon shark; *Negaprion brevirostris* Poey; the nurse shark, *Ginglymostoma cirratum* Bonnaterre; one teleost, the margate *Haemulon album* Cuvier; and the gar, *Lepisosteus platyrhincus* DeKay, a holostean fish. The following viruses were used: PR8, human influenza type A; AZ/Equi/Miami/63, the prototype strain of North American equine influenza type A; and Sendai, mouse parainfluenza virus.

Lemon sharks do produce antibodies to PR8 virus antigen administered in 4 ml doses divided among four subcutaneous sites. The initial series of immunizations consisted of five weekly injections of the antigen (measured from 5,000 to 10,000 hemagglutinating (HA) units per ml). An anamnestic response could not be elicited. Furthermore, the response is not dependent on the administration of live virus since formalinized PR8 virus also elicits antibody formation. Actually the rate of antibody production appears to be similar to that obtained with live virus, but the peak levels are lower. The responses to equine influenza virus, human influenza virus, and murine parainfluenza virus Sendai were all very similar.

Response of Infant Sharks to Antigen

Sigel and Clem (1965) tested whether the absence of a secondary response depends upon the age of the animal when antigen is administered. They injected a single 4 ml dose of PR8 virus into lemon sharks and adult nurse sharks, and a single 0.4 ml dose into infant nurse sharks delivered two days previously by Cesarean section. The results show that most sharks synthesize significant antibody titers of 1:160–1:640. Peaks are reached by 23 days in the adult, by 30 days in newborn nurse sharks, and by 39 days in lemon sharks. However, there was no secondary response, suggesting that age is important for realizing the full potential for antibody synthesis.

Species Variability

Studies of fishes illustrate how different species respond to antigen. The margate and the gar, a teleost and a holostean fish respectively, were immunized with a variety of procedures and schedules using PR8 as antigen. In margates, there appears to be a dose effect, since repeated injections of 2 ml produced higher titers than did a single injection of 2 ml (A) or two injections of 0.5 ml (B). The maximum titer is attained in 10 days in most instances. In this respect the margate is apparently more efficient than the lemon and nurse shark. Gars, more primitive phylogenetically than the margate, produce antibodies efficiently. Following a single injection, peak titers were obtained in 10 days or less. With regard to time and immunization requirements, this specie appears to be more responsive than either the shark or the margate.

SUMMARY

Antigens are any foreign material to which an animal will respond. All animals sequester antigen and, depending on numerous variables, the manner of antigen riddance is different for each. These variables include whether the antigen is soluble, particulate, or cellular. The species, age, and probably the sex also influence the response. Other factors that greatly affect antigenicity and its resulting antibody are the amount of antigen, its route of administration, and whether it is combined with an adjuvant.

BIBLIOGRAPHY

Benacerraf, B. 1974. The genetic mechanisms that control the immune response and antigenic recognition. *Ann. Immunol. (Inst. Past.)* **125**: 143.

Bonstein, H. S., and Rose, N. R. 1971. Species-specific tissue antigens. *Clin. Exp. Immunol.* **8**: 291.

Boyden, A. 1942. Systemic serology: A critical appreciation. *Physiol. Zool.* **15**: 109.

Bradshaw, C. M., Clem, L. W., and Sigel, M. M. 1969. Immunologic and immunochemical studies on the gar, *Lepisosteus platyrhincus*. I. Immune responses and characterization of antibody. *J. Immunol.* **103**: 496.

Chadwick, J. S. 1967. Serological responses of insects. Fed. Proc. **6**: 1675.

Cooper, E. L., Pinkerton, W., and Hildemann, W. H. 1964. Serum antibody synthesis in larvae of the bullfrog, *Rana catesbeiana. Biol. Bull.* **127**: 232.

David, C. S., Kaeberle, M. L., and Nordskag, A. W. 1969. Genetic control of immunoglobulin allotypes in the fowl. *Biochem. Genetics* **3**: 197.

Dray, S., and Young, G. O. 1958. Differences in the antigenic components of sera of individual rabbits as shown by induced isoprecipitins. *J. Immunol.* **81**: 142.

Fugmann, R. A., and Sigel, M. M., 1968. Immunologic and immunochemical studies in the hamster. I. The role of the antigen in eliciting IgG- and IgM-associated antibodies. *J. Immunol.* **100**: 1101.

Hildemann, W. H. 1969. *Immunogenetics*. San Francisco: Holden-Day.

Kahan, B. D., and Reisfeld, R. A., 1969. Transplantation antigens. *Science.* **164**: 514.

Lieberman, R., and Dray, S., 1964. Five allelic genes at the Asa locus which control gamma globulin allotypic specificities in mice. *J. Immunol.* **93**: 584.

Nuttall, G. H. F. 1904. *Blood immunity and Blood relationships*. Cambridge: University Press.

Oudin, J. 1956. The "allotypy" of certain protein antigens of serum. Compt. Rend. Acad. Sci. (Paris) **242**: 2606.

Rapacz, J., Korda, N. and Stone, W. H. 1968. Serum antigens of Cattle. I. Immunogenetics of a macroglobulin allotype. Genetics. **58**: 387.

Rasmussen, B. A. 1965. Isoantigens of gamma globulin in pigs. *Science* **148**: 1742.

Rathbun, W. E., and Hildemann, W. H. 1970. Genetic control of the antibody response to simple haptens in congenic strains of mice. *J. Immunol.* **105**: 98.

Rowlands, D. T., Jr. 1970. The immune response of adult opossums (*Didelphis virginiana*) to the bacteriophage f2. *Immunol.* **18**: 149.

Sigel, M. M., and Clem, L. W. 1965. Antibody response of fish to viral antigens. *Ann. N. Y. Acad. Sci.* **126**: 662.

Sindermann, C. J., and Honey, K. A. 1964. Serum hemagglutinins of the winter skate, *Raja ocellata* Mitchill, from the Western north Atlantic ocean. *Copeia* **1**: 139.

Skalba, D. 1964. Allotypes of hen serum proteins. Nature **200**: 894.

Warner, N. L., and Herzenberg, L. A. 1967. Immunoglobulin isoantigens (allotypes) in the mouse. IV. Allotypic specificities common to two distinct immunoglobulin classes. *J. Immunol.* **99**: 675.

Chapter 4

Phagocytosis

INTRODUCTION

To seek to understand the phylogeny of specific and nonspecific host defense mechanisms is an intriguing pursuit. Vertebrates depend to a great extent on immunoglobulins or antibodies to effect their specific immune reactions. Invertebrates do not have specific substances in their hemolymphs that are comparable to vertebrate antibodies structurally. Both invertebrates and vertebrates do possess, however, comparable nonspecific host defense responses executed primarily by phagocytes. During evolution, phagocytosis may have acquired some degree of specificity. Specific cell surface receptors are bound to vertebrate macrophages and granulocytes, but the presence of receptors in multicellular invertebrates requires clarification.

Whatever invertebrates possess as an analogue to vertebrate immunoglobulin, it enables them to rapidly dispose of particulate pathogens and has, thus, been of distinct survival value. The vast majority of invertebrates, and certainly all vertebrates, are multicellular species where functional differentiation of cells prevails. Some cells are responsible for nutrition, while others are phagocytic and participate, therefore, in defense or immune reactions. The protozoans are the one and only unicellular taxonomic group in the animal kingdom. Thus, in the protozoan we have a single cell that possesses in a single unit all the necessary equipment for all of its vital physiologic processes; of relevance here are phagocytosis and digestion. Whether the amoeba engulfs foreign material for food or defense is academic. Phagocytosis is peculiar to all animal species and results in antigen clearance. Disposition of antigen by phagocytosis may precede specific immunity or defense, but this depends upon where one observes phagocytosis in the phylogenetic scale.

History of Cellular Immunity

The foundation for the theory of cellular immunity rests on Metchnikoff's (1892) early work with phagocytosis in invertebrates. Only recently, however, has there been an attempt to connect his observations with studies of vertebrate immunologic competence (Cooper, 1974). The invertebrate phagocytic cell, coelomocyte, or hemocyte or, simply, the invertebrate blood cell, mediates the invertebrate's immune response and is thus functionally similar to vertebrate leukocytes. There is a striking similarity between the structure of invertebrate and vertebrate leukocytes. Among the melange of cells found in the coeloms or hemocoels of all coelomate invertebrates and, indeed, in the blood and peritoneal exudates of vertebrates, are other functional cell types such as lymphocytes.

Blood cells of invertebrates are hemocytes because they circulate in the vascular system or they occupy the hemocoel; often they are called coelomocytes because they occupy the coelom, which in this case is separate from the blood. Coelomocytes are leukocytes except in *Glycera* for example, a marine annelid that possesses erythrocytes among its coelomocytes. Thus, the terminology is often confusing; clarity demands more functional definitions. *Leukocyte* is a general term for all white cells of invertebrates and vertebrates; *erythrocytes* are the red blood cells. Invertebrate and vertebrate leukocytes are mainly classified by morphological criteria, although functional definitions are emerging. There is still no generalized scheme applicable to the many types of leukocytes of invertebrates as there is for vertebrate leukocytes; still, vertebrate hematologists often disagree among themselves. Vertebrate leukocytes consist of from one to three different sized lymphocytes, monocytes, plasma cells, and three types of granulocytes, usually neutrophils, eosinophils, and basophils. All are important to the immune system and some participate in nonspecific phagocytosis. Phagocytosis, antigen metabolism, and subsequent multiplication of immune cells such as lymphocytes are crucial for an animal's response to foreign material. Phagocytosis and a related phenomenon, pinocytosis, imply cell engulfment of some material; antigen metabolism means antigen breakdown accompanied by its final sequestration. Multiplications of immune cells may occur in coelomate invertebrates as a result of antigen stimulation and it is known to be common in vertebrates.

Origin of Cell Receptors

The invertebrate immunologically competent cell, sometimes called a *wandering cell*, is the evolutionary precursor of vertebrate immunocytes, as it, too, is capable of recognizing and reacting with antigen. To do this it must presumably possess a receptor or antigen recognizing unit. Drawing an analogy between the immune system and the nervous system makes it easy to envision the existence of receptor cells. With regard to the sense organs, the eyes, ears, nose, and tongue all possess receptor cells that receive stimuli of various kinds and later trigger responses. All animals exhibit immune responses of some form, for recognition exists throughout the animal kingdom. Antigen must be and is eliminated after it has been recognized as *not-self*.

Probably cell surface receptors are responsible for the initial recognition events in an invertebrate's immune reaction just as they are for a vertebrate. Receptors may have originated on animal cell surfaces in order to detect food sources, but eventually evolved to provide animals with a system of defense against foreign antigens. Boyden (1960) for example, hypothesizes that such receptors play a role in the protozoan's feeding and defense. He notes that:

> *If a suspension of* [Entamoeba hartmonella] *is mixed with certain flagellated bacteria, the* . . . [bacteria eventually clump] *on the surfaces* [and afterwards are phagocytosed]. *Apparently,* . . . [attachment] *is due to the presence on* [Entamoeba] *of molecules which have an affinity for components of the* [bacterial] *flagella.*

Some protozoans, including *Entamoeba hartmonella*, synthesize their own receptor molecules. However, receptors are no longer produced when *Entamoeba* reaches

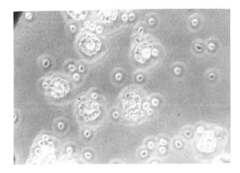

Fig. 4-1 Sheep-erythrocyte rosettes around mouse peritoneal cells mediated by macrophage-cytophilic antibodies. (Phase-contrast; ×3,700.) (*From*: Tizard, *Bacteriol. Rev.*, **35**: 364, 1972.)

maturity and is able to phagocytose. If we are to account for the differentiation of the capacity to distinguish between *self* and *not-self*, we may begin with the proto-zoans.

Alternatively, two phylogenetically distant phagocytes may possess features that are common to all cell membranes and that underlie every animal's ability to recognize *not-self*. In their studies on the wax moth, Rabinovitch and De Stefano (1970) discovered that hemocytes ingest a broader range of particles *in vivo* than they do *in vitro*. This may be due to recognition factors found in the hemolymph. Such unidentified factors, often referred to as *opsonins*, render particles more susceptible to phagocytosis. However, even modified or damaged erythrocytes interact *in vitro*

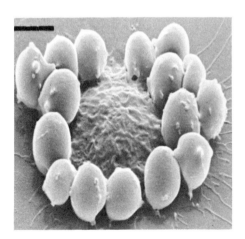

Fig. 4-2 E. A. Rosette. Note that the ring of sphered distorted erythrocytes is attached to the periphery of the body of the cell and that cyto-plasmic projections extend some distance beyond that point. All photographs are of air dried pre-parations. The bar indicates a distance of 5 um in all figures. (Through the author's permission (Tizard)—Unpublished.)

with either insect or mouse phagocytes suggesting that any altered antigenic surface aids in recognition. Untreated sheep erythrocytes are often not phagocytosed, but after fixation in formalin most of them are phagocytosed. In fact, certain of these hemocytes show erythrocytes attached to their surfaces (prior to phagocytosis) before forming rosettes. Rosette-forming cells may not be uncommon in invertebrates, but in vertebrates where they have been studied more extensively their significance is better known. In vertebrates, rosette-forming cells possess receptors that recognize antigen such as erythrocytes and bind them to their surfaces (Figs. 4-1, 4-2, 4-3.)

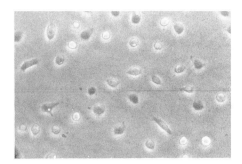

Fig. 4-3 Mouse peritoneal cells exposed to sheep erythrocytes in the absence of macrophage-cytophilic antibody. (Phase-contrast; ×2,500.) (*From*: Tizard, *Bacteriol. Rev.*, **35**: 365, 1972.)

Opsonins

Opsonins are substances, usually antibody, in the serum that coat particulate antigens such as bacteria and promote phagocytosis. Oyster blood agglutinates the erythrocytes of several vertebrate species. We assume that it contains an opsonin and that it specifically exerts an opsonic effect on, for example, rabbit blood cells *in vitro*. Furthermore, it seems to influence the rate of phagocytosis and the final disposal of foreign erythrocytes after injection into oysters. According to McDade and Tripp (1967), oyster hemolymph opsonizes foreign material through the presence of a hemagglutinin, an important component of the oyster's humoral immune system. It is not unlikely that the hemagglutinins are indeed primitive precursors of antibody molecules, possessing therefore the capacity of combining with diverse naturally

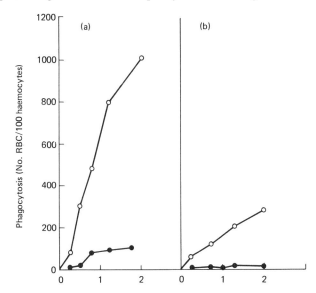

Fig. 4-4 Phagocytosis of sheep erythrocytes by haemocytes of: A. immune, or B. normal crayfish.

    ○——○ Erythrocytes pretreated with crayfish serum.
    ●——● Erythrocytes pretreated with saline.

It is evident from these results that haemocytes from the immune crayfish show far greater phagocytic activity than normal haemocytes. However, it is also apparent that this increased activity can only be demonstrated if the particle has been opsonized. (*From*: McKay & Jenkin, AJEBAK, **48**: 599, 1970.)

occurring antigens. The hemagglutinin provides a recognition factor (perhaps a receptor), and it serves as a functional, not structural, natural "antibody," rendering the oyster capable of distinghishing between *self* and *not-self*.

There is substantial evidence for the presence of hemagglutinins in all coelomate invertebrates. To demonstrate hamagglutinins in another mollusc, Pauley et al. (1971) pretreated chicken erythrocytes with normal or heated serum from the California sea hare, *Aplysia californica*. Phagocytosis increases in normal serum, evidently due to opsonic factors whose activity can be destroyed by heating. McKay and Jenkin (1970) believe that opsonins are present in the crayfish, an arthropod. Hemocytes from crayfish immunized with four weekly doses of endotoxin show far greater phagocytic activity than hemocytes from nonimmunized crayfish. This increased activity occurs, however, only if the particle has previously been opsonized, as Fig. 4-4 reveals. Thus heightened resistance against antigen may, in part, involve an increased activity of immune hemocytes due to prior opsonization. Tyson and Jenkin (1973) have recently demonstrated that the removal of bacteria from the circulation of the fresh water crayfish, *Parachaeraps bicarinatus*, follows an exponential curve as in vertebrates and is dependent on the presence of opsonic factors in the hemolymph. In fact, lysates from hemocytes opsonize just like the hemolymph. Undoubtedly, much information will be gained in understanding immunoglobulin precursor molecules in evolution once the opsonins are characterized, especially those that occur among the invertebrates.

The Role of Enzymes

As components of phagocytic cells, enzymes are important in the destruction of antigens in both invertebrates and vertebrates and are involved in the defense mechanisms of both vertebrate and invertebrate phagocytic cells. In invertebrates, enzymes are the only large molecules that are presently recognized as being crucial in the destruction of foreign matter. It therefore seems likely that enzymes are of prime importance to the invertebrate's immune system, since there is no evidence of antibody synthesis. Many similarities exist between antibodies and inductive enzymes (Table 4-1). Both are relatively large protein molecules synthesized *de novo* but not by protein precursors. Both have a more or less specific affinity for the substrate or the antigen with which they react and by which they are induced. Finally, anamnesis or memory capabilities are associated with both enzymes and antibodies. Monod (1959) has compared antibody formation in vertebrate cells with adaptive enzyme production. He suggests that antigen is captured by a specific permease on the cell surface and subsequently, as the cell produces more of the same permease, its capacity for taking up that specific antigen greatly increases. Not only does increased antigen uptake result in further production of permease and of antibody, but it also stimulates cell division.

Degradative enzymes play a role in the phagocytic processes of invertebrates. According to Tripp (1966), oyster hemolymph contains degradative enzymes that have characteristics common with those of the enzymes produced by vertebrate immunocompetent cells. He found that lysozyme in oyster hemolymph can destroy the bacteria *Micrococcus lysodeikticus*; it simultaneously releases amino acids and reducing sugars. Although the exact function of lysozyme in oysters and in other

Table 4-1

Comparison of Enzymes and Antibodies

Property	Enzymes	Antibodies
Phylogenetic distribution	Uniquitous; made by all cells	A late evolutionary acquisition; made only in vertebrates (and in certain cells of the lymphatic system)
Structure	Proteins with variable chemical and physical properties; an enzyme of a given specificity and from any particular organism is homogeneous; many have been crystallized	A group of closely related proteins having a common multichain structure with the chains held together by —SS— bonds. Molecules of a given specificity are heterogeneous in structure and function
Constitutive	Yes	"Natural" antibodies?
Inducible	Often	Yes
Function	Specific reversible binding of ligands* with breaking and forming covalent bonds	Specific reversible binding of ligands* without breaking or forming covalent bonds
Reaction with ligands*	Wide range of affinities; populations of enzyme molecules of a given specificity are uniform in affinity for their ligand	Wide range of affinities; but populations of antibody molecules of the same specificity are usually heterogeneous in affinity for their ligand
Affinity	Usually measured kinetically	Usually measured with reactants at equilibrium (because the reactions are so fast)
Number of specific ligand-binding sites per molecule	Different in different enzymes, depending on number of polypeptide chains per molecule; usually one site per chain	2 per molecule of the most prevalent type (NW **4r** 150,000); each site is formed by a pair of chains (a light plus a heavy chain)
Inducers	Primarily small molecules	Usually macromolecules, especially proteins and conjugated proteins

*Ligand = substrate or coenzyme in case of enzymes, and antigen or hapten in case of antibodies.
From: Eisen, H. N., 1974. Immunology (An introduction to molecular and cellular principles of the immune responses). Harper and Row Hagerstown Maryland pp. 352–624.

invertebrates is unknown, lysozyme may destroy phagocytized particles in vertebrates. Conceivably then, lysozyme is directly linked to the oyster's defense or immune system.

PHAGOCYTOSIS IN INVERTEBRATES

The Single Cells: Protozoa

The simplicity of unicellular protozoan organisms makes phagocytosis a combined defense and food-getting mechanism. Phagocytosis in the amoeba serves both as a protection against potentially fatal organisms and as a means of acquiring food. As the amoeba never eats its own or another amoeba's pseudopodia, it must recognize *self* components; this observation confirms the amoeba's capacity for some degree of specific discrimination, which presages the specificity of discriminating between *self* and *not-self*. It is problematic how an amoeba would confront a dissected piece of itself.

Reynolds (1924) studied the shelled amoeba *Arcella polypora*, especially its capacity to distinguish its own protoplasm from that of another amoeba. If the pseudopods are severed from one individual, they are readily reincorporated upon subsequent contact with that same individual. Furthermore, in some instances these fragments are also readily incorporated into different individuals; in others, contact is followed by the immediate shattering of the protoplasms into beadlike masses. Obviously this is a reaction that expresses incompatibility. The behavior of different clones is determined by the length of time they can be separated experimentally. For example, those descended from a single individual but separated in different environments develop incompatible descendants in periods as short as a week. This incompatibility can be reversed in about one week by returning individuals to a common culture dish for further multiplication together.

The electron micrographs of Korn and Weisman (1967) have revealed specificity of protozoan phagocytic reactions. Apparently the initial stimulus to each phase of phagocytosis in amoebae is physical rather than chemical. *Acanthamoeba* ingests various sizes of latex beads by a bead-to-surface attachment that precedes ingestion. Since size was the only variable, this initial attachment is probably a mechanical event.

According to Hirshon (1969), ciliates such as *Paramecium bursaria* ingest a variety of particles by reactions that differ from the amoeba's; however they may show greater specificity. Phagocytosis by paramecia discriminates among different types of particles that are of similar size when such particles are present in approximately equal concentrations. This kind of discrimination is distinct from the amoeba's, which is apparently not even specific with regard to particle size.

The First Multicellular Animals: Porifera

The phagocytic response in sponges is of particular importance. Sponges are the first diploblastic metazoan species with evidence of cellular differentiation and specialization. Thus, one would expect that special food-getting cells would be distinct from other cells. According to Cheng et al. (1968), the marine demonspongid, *Terpios zeteki*, has five types of free parenchymal cells in the mesoglea (an antecedent to mesoderm) that enable it to phagocytose foreign particles. Archaeocytes and collencytes, for example, can phagocytose India ink, carmine particles, and human erythrocytes. The archaeocytes can also accomodate foreign cells slightly larger than themselves by hypertrophy. Thus the archaeocyte can be considered the first distinct phagocytic cell. Collencytes and archaeocytes are forerunners of immune recognition; they arrange irregularly, though without complete capsule formation, on the surfaces of experimentally transplanted xenogeneic muscle implants. The sponges thus lend support to the concept that the invertebrate's specific recognition of *self* and *not-self* components is an evolutionary precursor of similar vertebrate-type reactions. Clearly sponge phagocytes exhibit responses that resemble those of advanced animals.

The Coelomate Animals
Annelida

The phylum Annelida includes segmented worms that, like other coelomate invertebrates, have numerous differentiated cells in the coelomic cavity. Largely because of his and other work on the earthworm, Valembois (1974) believes that cellular immunity is not entirely accidental in coelomate animals. In all coelomate animals there are either granular or nongranular mononuclear leukocytes. Phagocytosis is but one of the functions of these cells. According to Liebman (1942), earthworms possess two morphologically and physiologically distinct types of coelomocytes: the eleocytes and the leukocytes. Both eleocytes and leukocytes originate from the peritoneal endothelium, which according to some definitions qualifies them for membership in the reticuloendothelial system, a term in the past usually reserved for vertebrates. The eleocytes are trephocytes or chloragogue cells, are frequently found free in the coelomic fluid. Actually, chloragogue cells do not normally seem to multiply in the body cavity, as mitotic figures are absent. Chloragogen cells are not phagocytic but are a part of the tissue superimposed on the intestine. The so-called lymph glands, sites of coelomocyte origin, are embedded within it. Chloragogen cells are not involved in defense but function in nutrition, since they contain nutritive granules. Leukocytes are mainly the amoebocytes or functional phagocytes that eliminate dead cells, foreign substances, and the degradation products eliminated by eleocytes. Earthworm coelomocytes can phagocytose several varieties of inert particles except fat within a few minutes, both *in vitro* and *in vivo*. The larger basophilic coelomocytes phagocytose living and dead spermatozoa of related and unrelated species, as well as mammalian erythrocytes. Living spermatozoa from worms of the same species are, however, not phagocytosed; this suggests the absence of strong antigenic differences within a given genus and species. Despite the research done on the role of coelomocytes in transplantation immunity, there is still no information, in modern terms, on the activities of those coelomocytes that are phagocytes.

Mollusca
   General reactions

The molluscs also occupy an important position in the evolution of immune mechanisms (Feng, 1967). At this phylogenetic stage, the capacity to distinguish *self* and *not-self* is certainly evident. The molluscs, like the annelids, undoubtedly represent one of the earliest phylogenetic groups with evidence of cellular immunity. Molluscs possess amoeboid phagocytes with a high degree of specialization that allows a variety of foreign substances to be sequestered (Stuart, 1968). Small particles in tissues and blood sinuses are phagocytosed and then either carried through epithelia to the exterior or degraded intracellularly. Masses of amoebocytes also respond to foreign material by infiltrating a lesion until it is walled off entirely by an epithelial layer.

Using the electron microscope, Nakahara and Bevelander (1967) studied the ingestion of particulate matter in two bivalves from Bermuda, *Isognomon alatus* and *Pinctada radiata*. Twenty four hours after the introduction of colloidal thorium dioxide (thorotrast) into the pallial space, thorotrast micelles appear on its surface, on the outer surface of the microvilli, in small pinocytotic vesicles between the bases of the microvilli, in vacuoles undergoing coalescence, and in the lysosomes. Evidently, both the surface epithelia and the amoebocytes participate in the mollusc's removal of particulate matter. Tripp's pioneer work (1961) on phagocytic mechanisms *in vivo* has been extended to similar, but perhaps more easily controlled, *in vitro* conditions. Foreign particles and red blood cells are phagocytosed and degraded by the oyster *Crassostrea* as quickly *in vitro* as they are *in vivo*. The rates at which

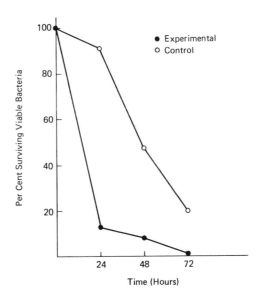

Fig. 4-5 Viable bacteria (*Escherichia coli*) in oyster phagocytes after phagocytosis had stopped. Experimental cultures contained bacteria, oyster cells, and medium; controlled cultures contained bacteria and medium. (*From*: Tripp & Kent, *In Vitro*, **3**: 129, 1970.)

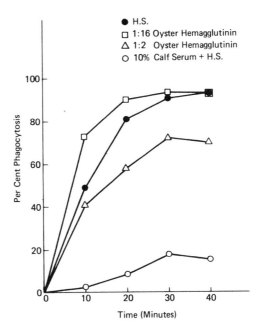

Fig. 4-6 Effect of medium on phagocytosis of human red blood cells by oyster phagocytes *in Vitro*. %phagocytosis = proportion of phagocytes containing one or more red blood cells at various times; H.S. = handling solution; 1:2 and 1:16 oyster hemagglutinin = oyster hemolymph diluted 1:2 and 1:16 with handling solution; 10% calf serum + H.S. = calf serum diluted to a final concentration of 10% with H.S. (*From*: Tripp & Kent, *In Vitro*, **3**: 129, 1967.)

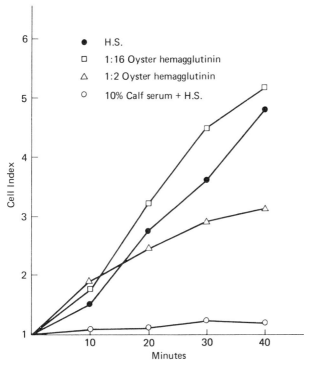

Fig. 4-7 Effect of medium on numbers of human red blood cells phagocytosed by oyster phagocytes *in Vitro*. The cell index represents the average number of red blood cells per phagocyte based on counts of at least 100 positive individual phagocytes. (*From:* Tripp & Kent, *In Vitro*, **3**: 129, 1967.)

bacteria are phagocytosed and digested intracellularly *in vitro* are comparable to those measured *in vivo*, as Figs. 4-5, 4-6, and 4-7 clearly reveal.

In the Australian clam *Tridacna maxima*, a bivalve of the Great Barrier Reef, Peter and Eve Reade (1972) noted some interesting distributions of carbon after phagocytosis. This large marine clam possesses circulating phagocytic hemocytes or macrophages which phagocytose particles introduced into the vascular system after a few hours. Later the phagocytes, engorged with carbon, collect in the digestive organs. From there they migrate across epithelial surfaces into various lumina, where they are effectively outside the animal; thus, trapping, digestion, and removal of *not-self* are handled efficiently. Within two minutes after injecting carbon into the adductor muscle, the gills change color; formerly white they appear grey. This coloration progresses so that by the end of ten minutes the gills are uniformly blackened, although blackening is not exclusive for the gills, since it encompasses the thin inner mantle membranes and muscles as well. Microscopic observations reveal that after two minutes many of the vessels, especially in the kidney, are occluded by carbon. Carbon also spreads to encompass the digestive diverticulum of the alimentary mass, where hemocytes that contain carbon appear extremely engorged.

Fixed and Circulatory Cells

Understanding discrimination by phagocytic cells is at the core of understanding the phylogeny of immune mechanisms. Molluscs and arthropods have been particul-

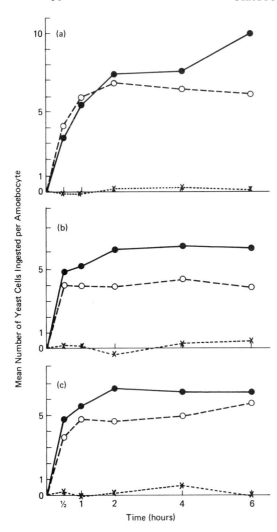

Fig. 4-8 The rate and extend of phagocytosis of yeast by snail amoebocytes, ●. Yeast in normal serum; ×, yeast in absorbed serum; ○, opsonized yeast in absorbed serum. (*From*: Prowse & Tait, Immunology, **17**: 437, 1969.)

arly useful in providing information that strengthens the concept of equivalent mechanisms occurring in the invertebrates and the vertebrates. Prowse and Tait (1969) studied phagocytosis of foreign particles by amoebocytes of the land snail *Helix aspersa*. An opsonin occurs in *Helix* serum. It exerts an effect by adsorption onto foreign particles. In fact, in the absence of this factor, phagocytosis does not occur, as is best shown by the curves depicting the rate and extent of phagocytosis of yeast by snail amoebocytes (Fig. 4-8). This represents probably the first successful demonstration of some degree of specificity by humoral components in molluscan immunity.

The extent of phagocytosis of both formalized yeast cells and SRBC is compared when each is suspended in snail serum absorbed with either yeast cells or SRBC. In other words, the recognition units found in hemolymph to one cell should be removed by absorption preventing cross reactivity. That this did indeed occur is evident from the fact that there was significant phagocytosis of the yeast or of the SRBC in a medium containing serum absorbed with either of the foreign particles. Foreign particles are phagocytosed in normal serum and in serum absorbed with the heterologous particle. In fact, there is no significant difference between the extent of phagocytosis of yeast cells in normal serum and in serum absorbed with sheep erythrocytes. This is equally true of SRBC in normal serum and in serum absorbed with yeast. The results from such an experiment are strongly suggestive of some degree of specificity and they tend to support the argument in favor of primitive ancestral immune responses among the invertebrates.

Like the Australian clam *Tridacna maxima*, the Australian chiton has been important to studies of phagocytosis, notably because of fine structure approaches and attempts to link molluscan phagocytic cells with comparable vertebrate macrophages. By using carbon and colloidal gold as labels, it has been shown that the chiton *Liolophura* possesses both fixed and circulating phagocytic cells. The observations regarding the distribution of fixed and circulating hemocytes of invertebrates are variable, as they are in vertebrates. In the fresh water crayfish *Parachaeraps bicarinatus*, the garden snail *Helix pomatia*, and in the octopus *Eledone cirrosa*, fixed cells are intimately associated with the vascular system and are primarily responsible for the removal of injected carbon. In the oyster *Crassostrea virginica* and the pulmonate gastropod *Australorbis glabratus*, circulating amoebocytes alone appear to be responsible for phagocytosis.

Fixed phagocytic cells, like circulating hemocytes, concentrate phagocytosed material within intracytoplasmic vacuoles. Fixed phagocytic cells possess long cytoplasmic processes, vesicles, and rough endoplasmic reticulum; these cells are often closely associated with collagen fibers and therefore resemble fibroblasts. Figure 4-9 shows the distribution of ferritin granules and bacteria within cytoplasmic vacuoles of fixed cells that also contain lysosome bodies crucial to particle digestion. Bacteria are seen within a hemocyte of the gill lumen. Phagocytic cells are especially abundant in the gills and foot, both being highly vascularized connective tissue. Twenty-four hours after the injection of carbon, colloidal gold, or heat-killed *Staphylococcus*

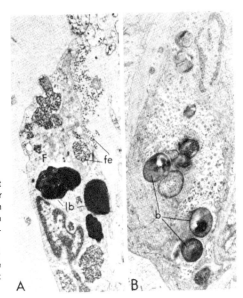

Fig. 4-9A Ferritin granules (fe) are present intra and extracellularly in the gill 24 h after injection. Intracellularly, they occur within cytoplasmic vacuoles of a fixed cell (F) which also has dark lysosome-like bodies (lb). (Magnification × *13,500*.)

Fig. 4-9B After 24 h a number of bacteria (b) have been phagocytosed by a haemocyte in the gill lumen. (Magnification × *17,900*.) (*From*: Killby et al., AJEBAK, **51** : 373, 1973.)

aureus, labelled cells occur in the gill lamellae. Fixed phagocytic cells predominate although some labelled circulating cells are also obvious. Fixed cells are greatly flattened and sometimes difficult to discern except by means of recognizable phagocytosed material.

The chiton's foot consists almost entirely of muscle and connective tissue. There is no well-developed circulatory system; thus the hemolymph percolates through numerous ill-defined channels and spaces, certainly reminiscent of the meshes in vertebrate lymphoid organs. The foot possesses a ventral region consisting of muscle fibers and irregular channels or lacunae. At twenty-four hours, carbon or colloidal gold appears in fixed cells, cells that attach to the "walls" of the lacunae, and that resemble, morphologically, fixed cells found in gill lamellae. Labelled hemocytes also occur within the lacunae. The dorsal portion of the foot is less compact and more spongy in appearance. The most conspicuous accumulations of connective tissue

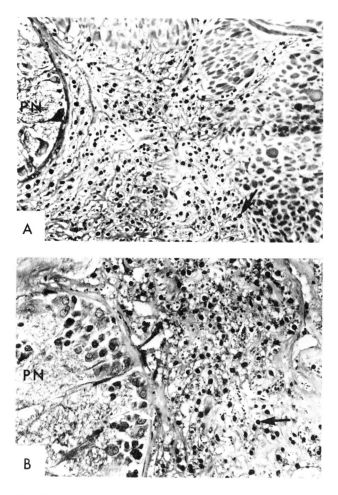

Fig. 4-10A Photomontage of transverse sections of *Liolophura* foot showing neuropedal connective tissue.
Fig. 4-10B 24 h following carbon injection. (Magnification × *260.*) (Black arrows indicate dark bodies of globular cells. White arrows indicate carbon; PN pedal nerv).
(*From*: Crichton et al., AJEBAK, **51** : 357, 1973.)

surround and support the paired pedal nerves. Twenty-four hours after injecting carbon, large numbers of labelled cells appear in the neuropedal connective tissue and other similar accumulations throughout the dorsal foot musculature (Fig. 4-10).

There is suggestive evidence that chiton cells do indeed discriminate specifically between *self* and *not-self*. For example, twelve hours following the injection of rhodamine-labelled BSA, large accumulations of specific (orange) fluorescence occur within fixed cells in the neuropedal connective tissue (Fig. 4-11A). By contrast, there is relatively little specific fluorescence in the same cells twelve hours after the injection of rhodamine-labelled haemolymph protein (Fig. 4-11B). The only fluorescence is autofluorescent (yellow green) in the dark bodies of globular cells, and residual studies of fluorescence confirm selective removal. Approximately 84% of the labelled

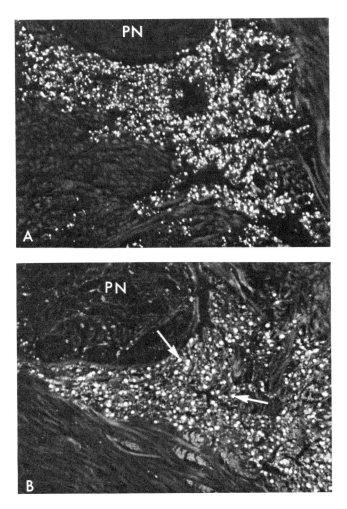

Fig. 4-11 Transverse section through the neuropedal connective tissue 12 h after the injection of:
A Rhodamine-labelled BSA. (Magnification × *260*.)
B Rhodamine-labelled *Liolophura* haemolymph protein. (Magnification × *260*). (White arrows indicate autofluorescent dark bodies of globular cells; PN pedal nerve). (*From*: Crichton et al., AJEBAK, **51** : 357, 1973.)

BSA, but only 10% of the labelled hemolymph, is eliminated during the interval from one to twelve hours post-injection. Specificity is suggested by these studies of selective phagocytosis.

Within the chiton's normal hemolymph, numerous free floating cells or hemocytes occur; there is a mean value of 7.2×10^6 per ml/population. Hemocytes are profoundly affected by temperature and are inactive and round at $0°C$. Raising the temperature causes hemocytes to assume a typical amoeboid appearance as they adhere to and spread over glass. The nuclei are variable in shape, depending on their position in the cell and the direction of cell movement. The cytoplasm stains weakly basophilic without visible inclusions, but vacuoles are obvious; these may be attributable to the presence of nonstainable glycogen, or else it is not unlikely that they represent vacuoles that participate in the destruction of phagocytosed material. Hemocytes often show parallel arrays of rough endoplasmic reticulum and prominent deposits of glycogen-like particles. This is best seen in Fig. 4-12 that details the hemocyte's

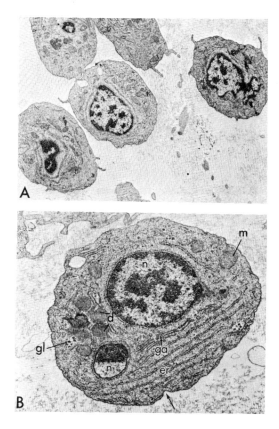

Fig. 4-12A Low power electron micrograph of cells in the haemolymph. The cells are uniformly compact and rounded with short pseudopodia. (Magnification × *7,600.*)

Fig. 4-12B A single haemocyte has pinocytotic invaginations at its surface (*see* arrow). Note the presence of mitochondria (m), dense bodies (d), a golgi apparatus (ga), glycogen-like particles (gl) and parallel arrays of rough endoplasmic reticulum (er). In this section two nuclear areas (n) are visible. (Magnification × *18,500.*) (*From*: Killby et al., AJEBAK, **51** : 373, 1973.)

fine structure. If different animals are used, the size distribution profiles of hemocyte populations appear similar. There are some variations, but each hemocyte sample constitutes a single uniformly distributed cell population. The mean volume is approximately 250 cubic microns, which corresponds to a spherical particle with a diameter of 7.8 microns (Fig. 4-13).

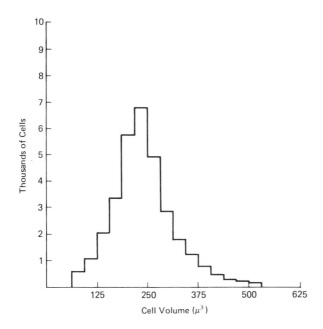

Fig. 4-13 Coulter counter size distribution profile of a population of normal *Liolophura* hemocytes. (*From*: Crichton et al., AJEBAK, **51**: 357, 1973.)

Arthropoda
  General considerations

The arthropods, historically and even now, have often been the sole animals used for intensive studies of phagocytosis and inflammation. Some early important observations were made by Cameron (1934), using lepidoptera larvae or caterpillars. Like most arthropods, caterpillars, despite their developmental immaturity, possess an effective phagocytic system composed of four main blood cell types: lymphocytes, other leukocytes, spherule or pericardial cells, and certain cells of the fat body. Lymphocytes and leukocytes are the most active, as they take up foreign particles, cells, and bacteria introduced into the body cavity. Though the number of lymphocytes increases rapidly during phagocytosis, it returns to normal once foreign substances are removed from the circulating hemolymph. Although the spherule cells are not actively phagocytic, the pericardial cells phagocytose certain bacteria, especially acid-fast organisms. These remain in the pericardial cells throughout metamorphosis and can, in fact, be isolated from the adult organism. Phagocytosis of foreign particles in caterpillars commences at once and results either in the obvious ingestion of particles by blood cells within a short time, or encapsulation of the foreign particles that are later stored in the pericardial cells.

During the phagocytic response foreign particles are picked up, engulfed, or digested by individual hemocytes. Thus an animal's phagocytic capacity can be defined as the maximum volume of phagocytosed particles or the number of circulating cells that contain foreign particles. Wittig (1966) injected commercial carbon ink into the armyworm *Pseudaletia unipuncta*; this results in phagocytosis of small ink particles, but larger particles are only surrounded by clusters of cells. According to Wittig, the phagocytic response denotes the total number of hemocyte reactions to small foreign particles in the hemocoel.

Phase-contrast microscopy allows the study of living cells. Jones identified several categories of hemocytes during various phases of insect life cycles; these include the genera *Galleria*, *Rhodnius*, and *Sarcophaga*. Within the population there are nondividing and dividing prohemocytes, nonvacuolated and vacuolated plasmatocytes, intact and quickly lysing granular hemocytes, oenocytoids with and without special cytoplasmic inclusions, adipohemocytes and fat body cells, and granulocytophagus cells.

Injecting foreign material such as bacteria or foreign erythrocytes into *Rhodnius* enables analysis of any subsequent changes in cell populations that may reflect primordial specific immunologic activity. The hemocytes of *Galleria* larvae, for example, phagocytose different concentrations of Chinese ink, latex, starch, *Sarcina lutae*, *Staphyloccocus spidermidis*, and sheep erythrocytes by forming vacuoles around such particles. Phagocytosis also occurs in dividing cells, plasmatocytes, and adipohemocytes (Werner and Jones, 1969). The phagocytic response however is lowest after injections of suspensions of sheep erythrocytes, latex, and starch.

Somewhat like the wax moth *Galleria mellonella*, the cockroach *Periplaneta americana* rapidly clears it's hemocoel of injected suspensions of foreign particles. The particles are phagocytosed by hemocytes, particularly the plasmatocytes and adipohemocytes. Hemocytes digest unfixed (without formalin) sheep erythrocytes or deposit them in cellular aggregates scattered among the tissues of the hemocoel; this also happens with yeasts, polyhedral bodies, carmine, carbon, and Sudan stain particles. All aggregates except those formed in response to viral polyhedra later become transformed into a melanized nodule; melanization is a very common feature among several of the known insect immune reactions. Contrary to the situation in *Blaberus craniffer*, another cockroach, three species of bacteria are not cleared effectively from the hemocoel of *Periplaneta americana*, although the hemolymph shows lytic activity against one, *Bacillus thuringiensis*. After twenty-four hours the hemocoel is greatly bloated, due partially to increased hemocyte numbers, even in the absence of noticeable mitosis. Increase in hemocytes is certainly reminiscent of the induction of peritoneal exudates in vertebrates, producing a melange of leukocytes.

Scott's (1971) work is important in dealing with cockroach hemocytes as possible functional ancestors of vertebrate phagocytic cells. Through observations using hemocyte monolayers he established a firm link between invertebrate and vertebrate blood cell characteristics, particularly with regard to their surface properties. Hemocyte monolayers consist almost entirely of plasmatocytes, the chief type of phagocytic cell; they, like mammalian macrophages, ingest neutral red and adhere to glass. Plasmatocytes spread on glass and thereby assume various shapes characterized chiefly by the formation of numerous filamentous pseudopodia. The cytoplasm is basophilic, granular, and riddled with vacuoles. After hemocytes are exposed to either sheep or chicken erythrocytes in medium 199 (a mammalian medium) the erythrocytes adhere avidly to the hemocyte surfaces, forming rosettes, a reaction similar to that of mammalian macrophages that bear cytophilic antibody when they are exposed to erythrocytes. Due to the large size of chicken erythrocytes, phagocytosis almost never occurs, even after five hours.

The importance of cell surfaces is revealed by enzyme studies. Assuming that a receptor site for sheep erythrocytes exists on the hemocyte surface, hemocyte mono-layers are treated with various enzymes and reactive chemicals. Pretreatment with trypsin almost completely inhibits the adherence of sheep erythrocytes without reducing the uptake of neutral red, an indicator of viability. Rosette cell formation is not restored after treating hemocytes with undiluted hemolymph, suggesting that trypsin changes the hemocyte receptors for an opsonic humoral component. Rather than reduce adherence, lipase treatment causes slight enhancement. Lecithinase-c reduces neutral red uptake and phagocytosis of sheep erythrocytes, due to impairment of the hemocyte membrane. The reducing agent 2-mercaptoethanol partially deters red cell adherence at 50 mM, but it is completely abolished at 200 mM when neutral red uptake is barely inhibited. When hemocytes are treated with sodium nitrate, an oxidizing agent, neutral red uptake and erythrocyte adherence are hampered at 50 mM. Iodacetamide, which reacts with sulphydryl groups, does not reduce erythrocyte adherence at 0.01 mM; it apparently does not affect the receptor site. The hemag-glutinin in cockroach hemolymph does not opsonize sheep erythrocytes. To test further for the existence of receptors, rabbit antisheep erythrocyte serum can be prepared; it is cytophilic for mouse, guinea pig, and rabbit macrophages. If cock-roach hemocytes are passively treated with rabbit antisheep erythrocyte serum there is a marked increase in adherent erythrocytes. In other words the antiserum binds to the hemocytes, and in turn the erythrocytes to the antiserum. This does not occur when erythrocytes, presensitized with antiserum, are added to hemocytes. Apparently the concentration of antiserum is crucial; with presensitization, more dilute serum is employed than when the hemocytes are sensitized passively. Thus, cockroach hemocytes lack a receptor site for cytophilic and noncytophilic components of mammalian immune serum, which is, incidentally, cytophilic for mammalian macrophages.

Physiological events are accompanied by metabolic changes. For these events to occur, there must be nutrition followed by utilization of energy and elimination of waste. This applies with equal force to invertebrate and vertebrate leukocytes. Anderson et al. (1973a, b) find interesting comparisons between the hemocytes of the cock-roach *Blaberus craniifer* and polymorphonuclear leukocytes (PMN), or neutrophils, of mammals. Phagocytizing cockroach hemocytes differ basically from mammalian PMN in that oxygen consumption is not stimulated. Particle ingestion stimulates normal human PMN oxygen consumption more than fivefold, but this respiratory increment is minimal or lacking in cockroach hemocytes. In mammalian cells, phago-cytosis is a process that requires energy, dependent on the glycolytic pathway. Simi-larly, glycolysis accompanies phagocytosis by cockroach hemocytes. Glycolysis can be inhibited in hemocytes by antimetabolities such as arsenite, iodoacetate, and fluoride; this leads to a decreased bacterial killing capacity as measured by inhibiting hemocyte engulfment of *Staphylococcus aureus*. Cyanide does not affect either bacte-ricidal activity or bacterial phagocytosis. Thus, energy to drive the phagocytic response in both the cockroach hemocyte and the vertebrate neutrophil is derived from glycoly-sis. However, the hexose monophosphate pathway activity of roach hemocytes, unlike mammalian cells, is not stimulated by phagocytosis. One characteristic of mammalian PMN is the reduction of nitroblue tetrazolium, but this is absent from the hemocytes of *Blaberus craniifer*. Finally, cockroach hemocytes utilize systems other than the myeloperoxidase—H_2O_2—halide system characteristic of mammalian cells.

Hemocytes of *Blaberus craniifer* may be different from the hemocytes of other arthropods. In short-term cell cultures, they can phagocytose and destroy *Staphylococcus aureus*, *Staphylococcus albus*, *Staphylococcus faecalis*, *Serratia marcescens*, and *Proteus mirabilis*. Whereas the phagocytes alone are responsible for bactericidal activity, the medium, the hemolymph, and cell products elaborated during incubations are not bactericidal. Unlike most molluscs, crustaceans, and representative vertebrates, no humoral opsonic factors seem to be required for, or even facilitate, bacterial phagocytosis *in vitro* by *Blaberus* cells, since washed hemocyte monolayers in hemolymph-free medium are capable of phagocytosing bacteria. In fact, to add hemolymph concentrated by ultrafiltration to bacteria opsonizes them but does not lead to more efficient killing. Unlike some of the previously mentioned pathogens, hemocytes will phagocytose, but will not kill, *Pseudomonas aeruginosa*, *Escherichia coli*, *Salmonella typhosa*, and *Diplococcus pneumoniae*, suggesting that bactericidal capacity and pathogenicity are not necessarily correlated. Pathogenicity may be due to bacterial strain, dose, and intracellular survival of ingested bacteria.

Molluscs, Arthropods, and Vertebrates Compared

Clams, unlike other invertebrates or vertebrates, apparently possess no system of fixed phagocytic cells. Instead they rely on circulating hemocytes to dispose of foreign particles, a situation like that of the oyster, *Crassostrea virginica*, and two species of sandy-beach snails, *Bullia laevissima* and *Bullia digitalis*. It is interesting that the migration route of engorged macrophages after phagocytosis is via the heart wall and the renopericardial canal to the kidney, and then through the nephropore into the mantle cavity. The situation is different for the freshwater crayfish *Parachaeraps bicarinatus*, an arthropod. It possesses a system of fixed phagocytic cells associated with the interlobular vessels of the digestive diverticulum where particles are stored for long periods; they also have phagocytic cells capable of movement. It is not unlikely that differing animal groups solve the problem of phagocytosis and clearance in one or two major ways; for example, by monitoring the whole system through migrating cells or by fixed cells that do not move. The former condition (i.e., circulating hemocytes in molluscs) is reminiscent of vertebrate monocytes that circulate in the blood, but the latter (i.e. fixed cells of crayfish) brings to mind the fixed vertebrate phagocytic depots such as those encountered in the spleen, lymph nodes, and bone marrow.

The Vertebrate Ancestors: Echinoderms and Protochordates
The Echinodermata

As echinoderms represent one of the more advanced invertebrate groups, their phagocytic response to foreign antigens is important to the study of the evolution of immune responsiveness. Whether or not echinoderm cells respond by specific synthesis of an inactivating substance similar to antibody remains unknown. The nature of the coelomocytes of echinoderms has been examined frequently. Ohuye (1934) studied the reaction of the holothurid *Caudina chilensis* to trypan blue and carmine dyes. The leukocytes, specifically the amoebocytes, ingest these dyes, but the cells that are red and those referred to as *crystal corpuscles* do not.

Johnson (1969a,b) characterized the coelomocytes of the echinoid echinoderms, using the red sea urchin *Strongylocentrotus franciscanus* and the purple sea urchin *Strongylocentrotus purpuratus*. She describes phagocytic leukocytes, vibratile cells, red spherule cells, and colorless spherule cells. The phagocytic leukocytes are bladder amoebocytes that flatten and form syncytia on contact with surfaces. Within culture fluids they form permanent aggregations, and presumably *in vivo* they are involved in cellular clotting. One of the two types of spherule-bearing cells contains echinochrome, a red napthoquinone pigment. Vibratile cells are PAS positive and, therefore, stain strongly for acid mucopolysaccharides, which appear in the coelomic fluid under certain conditions of stress. Both spherule-cell types exhibit either basophilic or acidophilic staining properties. They also possess chemical properties similar to those of vertebrate mast cells and other connective tissue cells.

Sea urchin leukocytes respond to gram-negative bacteria by: early regression of leukocytes from the bacterial area; walling off of bacteria into leukocyte clots; congregation of red spherule cells in *palisades* on the edges of leukocyte clots and encapsulation of masses of bacteria by leukocytes and red spherule cells. The pigment echinochrome is released in the presence of bacteria; motile species of bacteria become immobile in the presence of red spherule cells. Gram negative species are seldom phagocytized, but are usually disposed of by lysis or by killing. Curiously, two of the six gram-negative species, including an insect pathogen, cause a slight reaction, but three evoke an immediate and marked response from the coelomocytes.

The Protochordata

Tunicates are primitive chordates classified taxonomically in the phylum Chordata with the vertebrates. Phagocytosis occurs in the tunicates in two sites: the neural gland and the blood vascular system (Freeman, 1970). The gland is located to one side of the siphon, which brings food particles into the feeding apparatus; thus the siphon is in a functionally advantageous position. It is connected to the cavity where food is collected by a ciliated tube. Particles introduced into tunicates through the siphons are later found in phagocytes of the neural gland. Apparently no studies exist on the function of phagocytes from the tunicate's blood vascular system. During certain periods in the life cycle of some ascidians, phagocytes play an especially important role. For example, when zooids are resorbed by regression, leaving a stolon in place of the colony, there is a dramatic increase in the number of phagocytes. Presumably they are involved in digesting away colonial structures.

Phagocytic cells have been identified in several species of tunicates. Smith (1970) studied the blood cells and tunic of the solitary ascidian *Halocynthia aurantium* (Pallas), commonly called the *sea peach* because of its coloration and general shape. There are four morphological blood cell types: the mature morula cells, dispersed vesicular cells, stem cells, and stem cells with acidophilic vacuoles or granules. A fourth, the hyaline amoebocyte, is a phagocyte.

According to Anderson (1971), *Molgula manhattensis* possesses several blood cell types in the circulating blood. These are *vanadocytes, signet ring cells,* and *amoebocytes.* Glass fragments inserted into branchial sac tissue are encapsulated most actively by vanadocytes or cells derived from vanadocytes. The capsules are composed of multilayers of vanadocytes, monolayers of cells derived from vanadocyte aggregates, and strands of tunicin produced by vanadocytes. Injected carmine and trypan blue are ingested by phagocytes.

Brown and Davies (1971) utilized *Ciona intestinalis,* a cosmopolitan tunicate, to study the elimination of thorium dioxide from the body fluids by means of radiographs, sections, and samples of body fluid. Particles are phagocytosed by granular amoebocytes, green cells, and nephrocytes. They are then eliminated via the intestine and the vas deferens, while other particles appear to lodge in the test. Elimination from the body fluids is complete some nine days after injection. *Ciona* resembles certain molluscs somewhat in that it possesses several methods for elimination of foreign-particle.

In addition to phagocytosis, Wright (1974) also found that the serum of *Ciona intestinalis* contains a low titer natural agglutinin for a variety of erythrocytes that may play a role in phagocytosis. After primary injections of 8.5×10^3 human erythrocytes or 7.0×10^2 duck erythrocytes into the tunic tissues or perivisceral cavity, the erythrocytes are agglutinated and cleared by phagocytosis within twenty-four hours. Encapsulation occurs if higher concentrations of human or duck erythrocytes are injected into the tunic tissues. The serum agglutinin levels decrease concomitant with clearance or encapsulation and then return to normal within twenty-four hours. Despite their taxonomic position, Wright believes that tunicate internal defense mechanisms are still more closely allied to invertebrates than to vertebrates. However, studies by Fuke and Sugai (1972) using two species of solitary ascidians, *Styela plicata* (Lesueur) and *Halocynthia hilgendorfi* f. ritteri (Oka), are interpreted differently. Although both ascidians possess a natural hemagglutinin in the coelomic fluid that aggregates some mammalian erythrocytes, these hemagglutinins have no apparent opsonic effect; however, they may play a role in the adherence of cell-to-cell and cell-to-glass surface.

PHAGOCYTOSIS IN VERTEBRATES

Introduction

Phagocytosis is not a unique process in the animal kingdom, peculiar to any one group. All animals, beginning with unicellular protozoans, are capable of engulfing foreign material. From the protozoans through and including all advanced metazoans we finally encounter vertebrates, where phagocytosis by blood monocytes, neutrophils, and tissue macrophages is not always a secondary event in immunity. There is no need to assume that plasma cells and lymphocytes, executing specific immune reactions usually involving antibody, are the prime executors of immunity. In fact, phagocytosis is a major host defense mechanism in vertebrates and invertebrates. It evolved progressively with few drastic changes.

The vertebrate reticuloendothelial system (RES), like any of the other organ systems, consists of several types of interrelated cells, fibers, and their various products. The cells and organs of the immune system that are part of the RES are the thymus, spleen, bone marrow, lymph nodes, Peyer's patches, appendix, tonsils, and even the lungs, liver, and the microglia of the nervous system. Most of the organs of the RES possess the capacity for phagocytosis and also have stromal fibers with strong affinities for silver stains. The blood bathes an entire organism and in so doing renders it exposed to a great array of functional qualities of the immune and reticuloendothelial systems. In any organ system it is possible to deal with the characteristics of any one or a number of its component cells; in the RES we shall deal with the macrophages and to some extent certain granular leukocytes, the phagocytic cells.

The entire RES originates from embryonic mesenchyme. In birds and mammals, the blood islands of the yolk sac, derived from mesoderm and then mesenchyme, are the first sites of hematopoiesis. From the blood islands, stem cells migrate to the yolk sac and then into the circulation, and subsequently colonize and proliferate in various organs of the immune system. The presence of stem cells such as those in the yolk sac are readily demonstrable since such cells are capable of repopulating systems damaged by irradiation and, in so doing, provide the progenitor cells for granulocytes and macrophages.

In adult mice a bone marrow precursor of the monocyte-macrophage cell line exists. It is the promonocyte characterized by the presence of abundant phase-dense granules, absence of peroxidase, avid phagocytosis, and a surface receptor, the immunoglobulin type IgG. With regard to the IgG receptor, these macrophages, derived originally from yolk sac, are identical to peritoneal macrophages. In the mouse embryo the fetal yolk sac is the site of macrophage precursor origin; the yolk sac also seems to be involved, in the production of immunoglobulin-producing cells as well as granulocytes or neutophils, basophils, and eosinophils. Macrophage progenitors in the yolk sac and the promonocyte in the marrow undergo parallel differentiation that culminates in the monocyte and perhaps the mature macrophage. It still remains academic whether these two cells interchange states of being dependent upon their location in the body at any given time.

Although it provides lymphocytes and plasma cells, the RES is primarily important because of its phagocytic activity. Macrophages are ubiquitous and can be obtained from lymphoid organs such as lymph nodes and spleen. Yet the peritoneal cavity is also a rich source of macrophages, easily obtained by douching, especially after an inflammatory irritation. Even the lung possesses a rather typical cell, the alveolar phagocytic cell, that is capable of phagocytosis; in fact, there are reports of antibody synthesis by lung and by liver tissue. Where the peritoneal cells arise is controversial, but the relative ease of obtaining them suggests that they are attached to loose connective tissue and organ viscera and can be released after an inflammatory insult. There are reports of antibody synthesis by cells of the peritoneal cavity, and the presence of lymphocytes and plasma cells at least argues for the required machinery for antibody synthesis. Macrophages from the peritoneal cavity are incapable of antibody synthesis to sheep erythrocytes (SRBC) when tested by the Jerne plaque method. Still, macrophages are capable of forming rosettes, presumably because of cell-bound or cytophilic antibody that has an affinity for macrophage receptors. It may emerge that lymphocytes and plasma cells are not the only cells of the immune system capable of synthesizing antibody.

Teleost Fishes: Role of Temperature

The immune response is divisible into several stages, each with distinct characteristics, and each of which must be successfully executed if the immune state is to
be induced. The two extremes of such a chain of events are represented initially by
the first encounter with an antigen and almost immediately thereafter by antigen
trapping. Usually the end result is antibody synthesis. At various points in this process
different regulatory events may be operative. This is especially true in *all* vertebrates.
Poikilothermic vertebrates, i.e., fishes, amphibians, and reptiles, and also invertebrates,
are animals whose body temperatures mirror that of the external environment. In
fact, all physiological responses, including the immune response, are profoundly
affected by temperature; thus without rigid controls, the results will be varied under
experimental conditions. Higher temperatures will hasten responses, whereas lower
temperatures create the opposite effect. Phagocytosis and other events of the immune
system are affected by temperature.

Avtalion et al. (1973) breaks the immune response down into several categories,
one of which is the important event phagocytosis (Fig. 4-14). Using a teleost fish,
the carp, that is maintained at various temperatures, he concludes that phagocytosis
precedes the temperature-sensitive events of the immune response; it is not inhibited

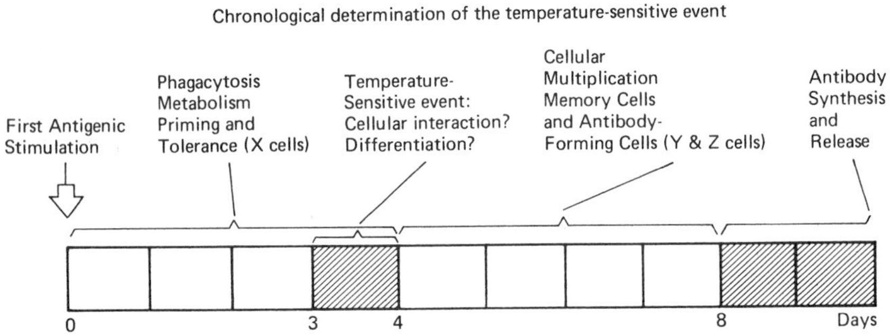

Chronological determination of the temperature-sensitive event

Fig. 4-14   (*From*: Avtalion et al., *Current Topics in Microbiology and Immunology*, **61** :
1, 1973.)

completely at low temperatures, but it does occur at a slower rate. Witness, for example, the clearance and phagocytosis of living *Staphylococcus aureus* by carp cells
(Fig. 4-15a,b). The clearance curves are different depending on whether the temperature is 12°C or 30°C. Within the blood, clearance is confined to large (macrophage) and small (microphage) phagocytic cells. Although regulation of phagocytosis
seems well defined, the effects of temperature on other events such as cellular multiplication and eventual antibody synthesis are still controversial.

A Hibernating Mammal

Vertebrate phagocytosis is greatly enhanced by the presence of heat-labile components in vertebrate serum known as *opsonins*. Since the turn of the century, it was
known that fresh serum and divalent cations such as Ca^{++} and Mg^{++} enhance particle
ingestion by mammalian phagocytes. During phagocytosis the phagocyte spreads

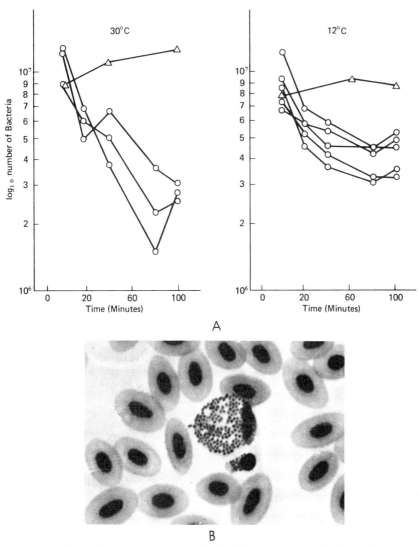

A

B

Fig. 4-15A *In Vitro* clearance of bacteria (*Staphylococcus aureus*) from blood of carp at 12°C and 30°C.

Fig. 4-15B Cellular uptake of staphylococcus aureus by a macrophage and a microphage. Δ, control. (*From*: Avtalion, et al., *Current Topics in Microbiology and Immunology*, **61**: 1, 1973.)

over the surfaces of particles and maintains intimate contact with them during engulfment. Since phagocytosis requires energy expenditure and contractile activity dependent upon hydrolysis of ATP, the particles to be phagocytosed may elicit spreading by acting on a contractile mechanism; opsonins and divalent cations stimulate this process. According to Stossel (1973), mammalian phagocytes can be activated by certain proteins bound to particles by divalent cations. Magnesium and calcium bound to albumin particles stimulate the rate of particle ingestion by human leukocytes and rabbit alveolar macrophages.

In many respects hibernating mammals, and perhaps birds in a state of torpor, may be in a situation analogous to poikilothermic vertebrates and invertebrates in that they too can regularly experience temperature extremes. Hibernating ground squirrels, *Citellus citellus*, do not produce demonstrable antibodies against heterologous erythrocytes as long as they hibernate for approximately 40 days. This condition changes after arousal however, when formerly hibernating squirrels now produce demonstrable agglutinins that spontaneously reach normal levels after one week.

The entire immune response is divisible into stages, and Jaroslaw and Smith (1961) believe that events of the latent period, namely induction, maturation, and proliferation, can occur during hibernation. With specific reference to phagocytosis, they found that amounts of circulating antigen are unaltered during hibernation. Taken several steps further, it was discovered that hibernating squirrels produce secondary hemolysin response to sheep erythrocytes if they had hibernated for 28 to 56 days but were aroused for 25 days between the first and second antigen injections. In spite of this clear observation, the precise events that occur during antibody synthesis, and that are most vulnerable to hibernation, are unclear. For example, considering the first event, is phagocytosis by the RES affected, and if so, what are the conditions that can later alter antibody synthesis?

Certain rodents, such as ground squirrels, that regularly hibernate are not exclusive. Franceschi and colleagues (1972) provide interesting information on hibernation, the RES, and immune responses in the north Italian hedgehog, *Erinaceus europaeus*, L. Awake or hibernating (maintained at 4°C ± 1°C in the dark with no food) hedgehogs show no significant difference in clearance rates of colloidal carbon from the blood after intravenous injection. It is peculiar, and indeed different from most animals, that hedgehogs, whether awake or hibernating, are unable to form antibody to SRBC, even after a second injection. A reverse situation occurs when rat erythrocytes (RRBC) are used as antigen; both primary and secondary responses can be elicited. Hibernating hedgehogs show no detectable levels of antibody to RRBC even after a second injection, and, since phagocytosis seems normal, other phases of the immune response may be vulnerable.

The liver's phagocytic cells, the von Kuppfer cells, are normal with regard to clearance of colloidal carbon. Thus, phagocytosis is not impaired, whether the hedgehogs are hibernating or aroused. This is interesting since the liver, not considered to be of much importance to specific immune reactions primarily involving antibody, is still capable of carrying out phagocytosis, the nonspecific immune response. Thus, facing the most adverse conditions, e.g., temperature extremes, mammals are at least protected by the capacity to phagocytose foreign particles (Fig. 4-16). This occurs even if antibody synthesis is retarded. Quite the contrary occurs, however, in the spleen, a major site of antibody synthesis and phagocytosis. Although the precise explanation is unclear, phagocytosis here is somewhat inhibited in hibernating hedgehogs (Figs. 4-17, 4-18, 4-19, and 4-20). In addition to malfunctioning splenic macrophages revealed by impaired phagocytosis, lymphoid nodules are reduced and appear smaller in size. This results in a pronounced absence of white pulp where mature lymphocytes and plasma cells are generated. The thymus is involuted, the bone marrow is less active, the lymph nodes contain brownish deposits, and the total number of leukocytes is markedly decreased—all characteristics that reflect the impaired antibody response. Phagocytosis is slower in hibernating mammals, particularly in the spleen whose main function is that of antibody synthesis.

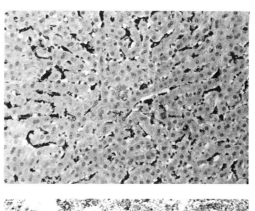

Fig. 4-16 Section of a liver from a hibernating hedgehog injected i.v. with carbon. There is no observable difference in carbon phagocytosis between this group and the control awake animals. Free carbon in the sinusoids is not observable. H. and E., (×270). (*From*: Franceschi et al., *J. Exp. Zool.*, **180**: 105, 1972.)

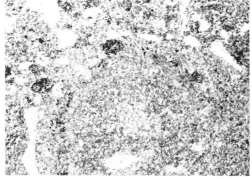

Fig. 4-17 Section of a spleen from a control awake hedgehog injected i.v. with carbon. Note the uptake of the carbon particles by the cells of the Schweigger-Seidel sheaths. Carbon-loaded macrophages may be seen also at the periphery of the lymphatic nodule. H. and E., (×250). (*From*: Franceschi et al., *J. Exp. Zool.*, **180**: 105, 1972.)

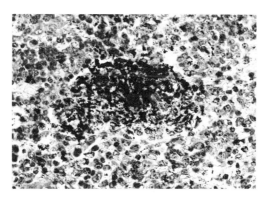

Fig. 4-18 Higher magnification of Fig. 4-17 showing a carbon-loaded Schweigger-Seidel sheath. H. and E., (×580). (*From*: Franceschi et al., *J. Exp. Zool.*, **180**: 105, 1972.)

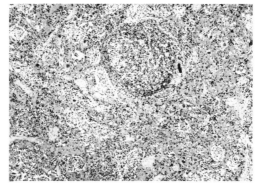

Fig. 4-19 Section of a spleen from a hibernating hedgehog injected i.v. with carbon. Note the absence of carbon phagocytosis. The Schweigger-Seidel sheaths do not contain carbon at all. By contrast, the carbon is inside the central vessel of a pericapillary sheath. H. and E., (×98). (*From*: Franceschi et al., *J. Exp. Zool.*, **180**: 105, 1972.)

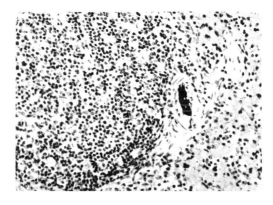

Fig. 4-20 Higher magnification of Fig. 4-19. Note the complete absence of phagocytosis around the lymphatic nodule. H. and E., (×*270*). (*From*: Franceschi et al., *J. Exp. Zool.*, **180**: 105, 1972.)

SUMMARY

Metchnikoff's classic observation of phagocytosis in *Daphnia*, a fresh water crustacean, during the latter half of the nineteenth century, underlined the importance of phagocytic reactions in invertebrate defense and provided a conceptual model for recognizing analogous phagocytic processes by macrophages and granulocytes of vertebrates. Phagocytosis, concomitant antigen processing, and even degradation by leukocytes other than lymphocytes are the only means of immunity in invertebrates; they are largely nonspecific reactions not involving antibody. These are necessary prerequisites to antibody synthesis among vertebrates; they still remain as vestiges of nonspecific and even specific immunity among vertebrates. Protozoans are single cells that digest and defend at the same time. In most metazoans, however, digestion of food is carried out by cells of the digestive system; other cells, those of the RES, remove foreign, potentially pathogenic material. Though this chapter is a cursory account, it should be clear that phagocytosis and its accompanying events were evolutionary precursors of acquired cellular immunity characterized later by specificity, memory, and integration with antibody synthesis. Invertebrate phagocytic cells, even the amoeba, are ancestors of vertebrate macrophages; invertebrate granular cells are, in turn, ancestors of vertebrate granulocytes, which are also involved in phagocytosis and immunity. At the level of the sponges (Porifera), the phagocytic cell as a discrete entity first appears. Later, with the evolution of the coelom, with its fluid and blood cells, an interdependence evolved between the cells and fluid. Hemagglutinins probably act as opsonins facilitating phagocytosis in invertebrates. In so doing, these invertebrate hemolymph components are not unlike immunoglobulin or other serum components of vertebrates in the protection their activities afford the invertebrates.

BIBLIOGRAPHY

Anderson, R. S. 1971. Cellular responses to foreign bodies in the tunicate *Molgula manhattensis* (DeKay). *Biol. Bull.* **141**: 91.

Anderson, R. S., Holmes, B., and Good, R. A. 1973a. Comparative biochemistry of phago-cytizing insect hemocytes. *Comp. Biochem. Physiol.* **46B**: 595.

———. 1973b. In vitro bactericidal capacity of *Blaberus craniffer* hemocytes. *J. Invert. Pathol.* **22**: 127.

Avtalion, R. A., Wojdani, A., Malik, Z., Shahrabani, R., and Duczyminer, M. 1973. Influ-ence of environmental temperature on the immune response in fish. *Curr. Topics in Microb. and Immunol.* **61**: 1.

Boyden, S. V. 1960. Antibody production. Nature **185**: 724.

Brown, A. C., and Davies, A. B. 1971. The fate of thorium dioxide introduced into the body cavity of *Ciona intestinalis* (Tunicata). *J. Invert. Pathol.* **18**: 276.

Cameron, G. R. 1934. Inflammation in the caterpillars of Lepidoptera. *J. Path. and Bact.* **38**: 441.

Cheng, T. C., Yee, H. W. F., Rifkin, E., and Kramer, M. D. 1968. Studies on the internal defense mechanisms of sponges. III. Cellular reactions *Terpios zeteki* to implanted heterologous biological materials. *J. Invert. Path.* **12**: 29.

Cooper, E. L. 1974. Invertebrate immunology. In *Contemporary Topics In Immunobiology*. ed. E. L. Cooper, vol. 4. New York: Plenum Press.

Feng, S. Y. 1967. Responses of molluscs to foreign bodies, with special reference to the oyster. *Fed. Proc.* **26**: 1685.

Franceschi, C., Forconi, G., Perocco, P., Di Marco, A. T., and Prodi, G. 1972. Reticulo-endothelial system activity and antibody formation in hibernating hedgehogs (*Erinaceus europaeus*). *J. Exp. Zool.* **180**: 105.

Freeman, G. 1970. The reticuloendothelial system of tunicates. *J. Ret. Soc.* **7**: 183.

Fuke, M. T., and Sugai, T. 1972. Studies on the naturally occurring hemagglutinin in the coelomic fluid of an ascidian. *Biol. Bull.* **143**: 140.

Hirshon, J. B. 1969. The response of *Paramecium bursaria* to potential endocellular symbionts. *Biol. Bull.* **136**: 33.

Jaroslaw, B. N. and Smith, D. E. 1961. Antigen disappearance in hibernating ground squirrels. Science **134**: 734.

Johnson, P. T. 1969a. The coelomic elements of sea urchins (*Strongylocentrotus*). II. Cytoche-mistry of the coelomocytes. *Histochemie* **17**: 213.

———. 1969b. The coelomic elements of sea urchins (*Strongylocentrotus*). III. In vitro reac-tion to bacteria. *J. Invert. Path.* **13**: 42.

Korn, E. D., and Weisman, R. A. 1967. Phagocytosis of latex beads by *Acanthamoeba*. II. Electron microscopic study of the initial events. *J. Cell. Biol.* **34**: 219.

Liebmann, E. 1942. The coelomocytes of *Lumbricidae*. *J. Morphol* **71**: 221.

McDade, J. E., and Tripp, M. R. 1967. Mechanism of agglutination of red blood cells by oyster hemolymph. *J. Invert. Pathol.* **9**: 523.

McKay, D., and Jenkin, C. R. 1970. Immunity in the invertebrates. The role of serum factors in phagocytosis of erythrocytes by haemocytes of the fresh-water crayfish (*Para-chaeraps bicarinatus*). *Aus. J. Exp. Biol. Med. Sci.* **48**: 139.

Metchinkoff, E. 1892. *Pathologic Comparee de l'Inflammation*. Masson, Paris.

Monod, J. 1959. Antibodies and induced enzymes. Cellular and Humoral Aspects of the Hypersensitive States, ed. H. S. Lawrence, pp. 628–45. New York: Hoeber Harber.

Nakahara, H. and Bevelander G., 1967. Ingestion of particulate matter by the outer surface cells of the mollusc mantle. *J. Morph.* **122**: 139.

Ohuye, T. 1934. On the coelomic corpuscles in the body fluid of some invertebrates. I. Reaction of the leucocytes of a holothurid, *Caudina chilensis* (J. Müller) to vital dyes. *Hatai Sci. Report Tohoku Imp. Univ. 4th Ser.* (Biol.) **99L**: 47.

Pauley, G. B., Krassner, S. M., and Chapman, F. A. 1971. Bacterial clearance in the California sea hare *Aplysia californica. J. Invert. Pathol.* **18**: 227.

Prowse, R. H., and Tait, N. N. 1969. *In vitro* phagocytosis by amoebocytes from the haemolymph of *Helix aspersa* (Müller). I. Evidence for opsonic factor(s) in serum. *Immunology* **17**: 437.

Rabinovitch, M., and DeStefano, M. 1970. Interactions of red cells with phagocytes of waxmoth (*Galleria mellonella*, L) and mouse. *Exp. Cell. Res.* **59**: 272.

Reade, P., and Reade, E. 1972. Phagocytosis in invertebrates. II. The clearance of carbon particles by the clam, *Tridacna maxima. J. Ret. Soc.* **12**: 349.

Reynolds, B. D. 1924. Interactions of protoplasmic masses in relation to the study of heredity and environment in *Arcella polypora. Biol. Bull.* **46**: 106.

Scott, M. T. 1971. Recognition of foreignness in invertebrates. II. *In vitro* studies of cockroach phagocytic haemocytes. *Immunology* **21**: 817.

Smith, M. J. 1970. The blood cells and tunic of the ascidian *Holocynthia aurantium* (Pallas). I. Hematology, tunic morphology, and partition of cells between blood and tunic. *Biol. Bull.* **138**: 354.

Stossel, T. P. 1973. Quantitative studies of phagocytosis. Kinetic effects of cations and heat-labile opsonin. *J. Cell. Biol.* **58**: 346.

Stuart, A. E. 1968. The reticuloendothelial apparatus of the lesser octopus, *Eledone cirrosa. J. Path. Bact.* **96**: 401.

Tripp, M. R. 1961. The fate of foreign materials experimentally introduced into the snail *Australorbis glabratus. J. Parasit.* **47**: 745.

Tyson, C. J., and Jenkin, C. R. 1973. The importance of opsonic factors in the removal of bacteria from the circulation of the crayfish (*Parachaeraps bicarinatus*). *Ajebak* **51**: 609.

Valembois, P. 1974. Cellular aspects of graft rejection in earthworms and some other metazoa. In *Contemporary Topics in Immunobiology*, ed. E. L. Cooper, vol. 4, pp. 121–26. New York: Plenum Press.

Werner, R. A., and Jones, J. C. 1969. Phagocytic haemocytes in unfixed *Galleria mellonella* larvae. *J. Insect Physiol.* **15**: 425.

Wittig, G. 1966. Phagocytosis by blood cells in healthy and diseased caterpillars. II. A consideration of the method of making hemocyte counts. *J. Invert. Pathol.* **8**: 461.

Wright, R. K. 1974. Protochordate immunity. I. Primary immune response of the tunicate *Ciona intestinalis* to vertebrate erythrocytes. *J. Invert. Pathol.* **24**: 29.

Chapter 5

Quasi Immunorecognition
and Primordial Cell-Mediated Immunity

INTRODUCTION

When compared to the vertebrates, the invertebrates are still a vast and relatively unexplored subject with much to contribute to our understanding of the evolution of immune responses. Characteristics of immune competence are usually defined and have been worked out according to how vertebrates respond to antigen. For many invertebrates, only *recognition* of *not-self* seems to be the sole event peculiar to their immune responses. Until antibody is described, invertebrates will be known to possess only the first two types of immunoevolution outlined by Hildemann and Reddy (1973). Vertebrates recognize antigens and have also evolved the capacity to synthesize antibody. Although there are no reports of any invertebrate synthesizing antibodies, they do recognize foreignness, an antecedent of specific cell-mediated immunity.

Specific cellular immunity can be traced in origin to the invertebrate's primordial recognition processes. Although among multicellular invertebrates we still know nothing of the receptor cell or its recognition unit, which allows it to perceive antigen, lymphocyte-like cells among populations of invertebrate coelomocytes and hemocytes are prime candidates. It is appropriate to define broadly the first stage in the evolution of immune responsiveness. In the phylogeny of immunoevolution, we encounter first *quasi immunorecognition*, which is common to coelenterates (cnidarians), tunicates, and mammals. This event only encompasses recognition. Although recognition is specific, there is still no evidence for the intervention of antibody as the primary component effecting recognition. In addition, examples of quasi immunorecognition are demonstrable in protozoans, sponges, and numerous other invertebrates. These observations emanate from studies restricted to experimental encounters designed to show that cells distinguish between *self* and *not-self*.

TRANSPLANTATIONS OF PROTOZOAN ORGANELLES

Introduction

Protozoans, or single-cell invertebrates, can be used to study organelle transplantation. Technically successful organelle transplantation is followed by specific recog-

69

nition and incompatibilities among protozoan and several metazoan invertebrates. In advanced metazoan animals, nonspecific phenomena such as inflammation and wound healing should not be confused with specific graft rejection that results from activation of the immune system. To determine whether an invertebrate recognizes foreign transplants, it is necessary to understand recognition and rejection of cell or tissue grafts in light of vertebrate immunologic concepts.

Sarcodina

The amoebae have greatly facilitated organelle transplantation studies, nuclear transfers in particular. One can easily remove the "heart" of a cell, its nucleus, and transfer it to the enucleated cytoplasm of another cell, as was demonstrated by Goldstein (1970) (Fig. 5-1). This kind of technical feat supports the view that amoebas

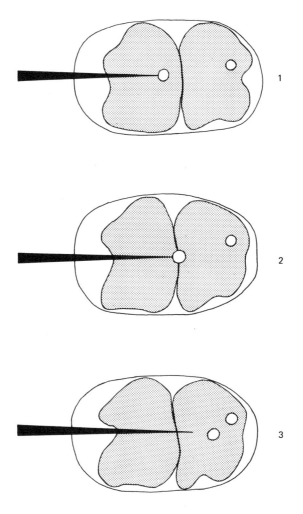

Fig. 5-1 Sequence of three steps involved in transplantation of nucleus from one amoeba to another. (*From*: Goldstein, *Transpl. Proc.* **2**: 191, 1970.)

can show specificity. When transfers are incompatible, the recipients die and clones are not produced (Table 5-1). For example, when nuclei of *Amoeba discoides* are transferred into the enucleated cytoplasm of *Amoeba proteus,* the cytoplasm may divide several times, but a viable clone rarely develops; these represent unsuccessful xeno- or hetero-transfers. Transplants of nuclei or cytoplasm of the same strain as allo- or homotransfers, are, by contrast, at least 90% successful, yielding viable mass cultures. Finally, when the nucleus is replaced in the same cytoplasm as autogeneic

Table 5-1

Type of transfer	Transfer	Expected percentage of clones	Actual percentage of clones obtained
Homotransfer	$P_{T1\ n} \longrightarrow P_{T1\ c}$	100	90
Homotransfer	$D_{T1\ n} \longrightarrow D_{T1\ c}$	100	90
Heterotransfer	$P_{T1\ n} \longrightarrow D_{T1\ c}$	< 5	< 1
Heterotransfer	$D_{T1\ n} \longrightarrow P_{T1\ c}$	< 5	< 1
Transfer into 'injected' clone	$D_{T1\ n} \longrightarrow \left(D_{T1\ c} \dashrightarrow P_{T1} \right)_c$	< 5	48
Transfer into 'injected' clone	$P_{T1\ n} \longrightarrow \left(D_{T1\ c} \dashrightarrow P_{T1} \right)_c$	100	0
'Injected' clone nuclei	$\left(D_{T1\ c} \longrightarrow P_{T1} \right)_n \dashrightarrow P_{T1\ c}$	100	0
'Injected' clone nuclei	$\left(D_{T1\ c} \longrightarrow P_{T1} \right)_n \dashrightarrow D_{T1\ c}$	< 5	0*

*30 per cent transfers divided to give more than 30 cells before death
$\longrightarrow$ Nuclear transfer. - - -$\to$ Injection of cytoplasm.
Results of transfer experiments using a clone of *A. proteus* which had received and assimilated an injection of *A. discoides* cytoplasm, compared with results obtained from homotransfer and heterotransfer experiments.
From: Hawkins, Nature, *203*: 95, 1964.

transplants, viable cells are always produced. These reactions, even in unicellular animals at the organelle level, clearly provide evidence for the presence of a universal example of *self, not-self* recognition.

When carried to technical perfection, this approach can actually make cell reassembly possible. It is sufficiently adequate so that recombinations of nucleus, cytoplasm, and cell membranes can fashion new and different cells (Jeon et al., 1970). The efficacy of such new cell clone reproduction is directly dependent upon the degree of relatedness between transferred organelles. For example, when nucleus, cytoplasm, and membranes are derived from three amoebae of the same strain, 85% viability can be achieved. However, no viable clones result when these three organelles originate from amoebae of three different strains. This represents yet another example of specific recognition at the cell organelle level.

Ciliata

Protozoans that move by cilia are somewhat more complex than those that employ pseudopodia. Tartar (1964, 1970) worked with ciliates and recognized the evolution-

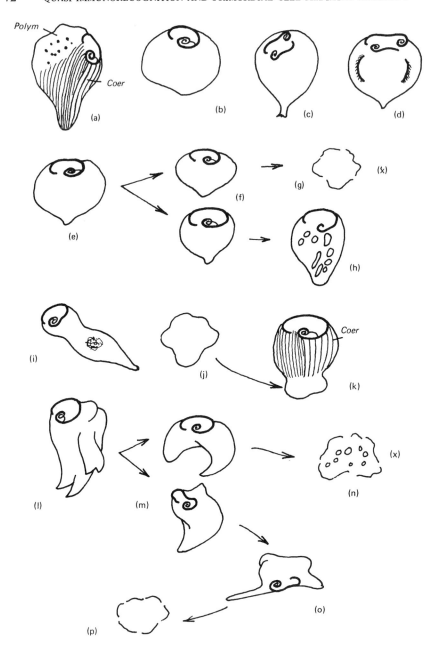

Fig. 5-2 Specificities shown in chimera of *Stentor coeruleus* and *S. polymorphus*. (a) *Polymorphus* with symbiotic chlorellae fused to twice volume of *coeruleus*. (b) Interaction of components is shown by shedding of chlorellae and fading of cerulean pigment. Some functioning is possible at first. Chimera reorganizes (c) with two sets of feeding organelles, re-reorganizes doubly, but one anlage does not develop (e). Cell divides on day 6 but one product dies (g) while other shows abnormal nucleus. This cell then becomes "snaky" (i) and loses its form (j). On day 19 (k) it was grafted to normal *coeruleus*. Product became amorphic (l) yet was able to divide (m), but both fission products eventually died. (*From*: Tartar, *Transpl.* **2**: 183, 1970.)

ary implications of protozoan incompatibilities. Such reactions are related to primordial immune phenomena and, as Tartar says, they may provide

> *evidence at the unicellular level of an anticipation of those specificities which so sharply limit the interindividual grafting of tissues in man.*

Interracial (allografts) grafts between members of the same genus, *Stentor*, from different localities reveal many affinities between animals of the same species. Although interspecific, hetero- or xenografts produce some permanent chimeras whose incompatibilities are easily measurable by the abnormal physiologic reactions that are present. For example, cytoplasm derived from *Stentor coeruleus* causes ejection of the symbiotic *Chlorella* characteristic of *Stentor polymorphus*. In a reciprocal combination, *Stentor polymorphus* cytoplasm leads to depigmentation or loss of the blue-green stentorin in *Stentor coeruleus* cytoplasm; this is followed by death of the chimera (Fig. 5-2).

AGGREGATION AND REAGGREGATION IN SPONGES

Sponges, the first metazoan diploblastic animal group, are important to understanding the phylogeny of specific cell recognition. In his classic studies on reaggregation of dissociated sponge cells, Wilson (1907) found that cells of a given species aggregate with like kind after mixing together. Galtsoff (1925) later demonstrated that specific cell sorting of *Microciona prolifera* of different cell types occurs during reformation of dissociated sponges.

The mechanisms of cell aggregation are still controversial. Humphreys (1967) believes that a large glycoprotein molecule is a component of the cell's surface coat. This glycocalix may be responsible for aggregation of dissociated sponge cells. If such cell-surface material does promote reaggregation, then the specificity existing on cell surfaces is the basis for discrete species-specific sorting and binding together of sponge cells of like type. In addition, the cell surface may have other properties that enable cells to bear antigenic determinants such as those on red blood cells or those that are transplantation antigens on other cell surfaces.

Spiegel (1954) compared recognition reactions of invertebrates to other aspects of recognition crucial to immunity. According to his hypothesis, built on an analysis of dissociated sponges, cells are held together by specific macromolecules with precise stereochemical properties. These arrangements on the cell surface make cell combinations possible by adhesion. To test that these cell macromolecules can act as antigens, we can inject them into a vertebrate such as a rabbit; this leads to antibody production. For example, three different antisera against various sponge cells are prepared in rabbits: one against *Microciona prolifera* (a large encrusting red sponge), another against *Cliona celata* (a yellow sulfur sponge), and a mixture of cells from both species. Reaggregation of dissociated cells is reversibly inhibited in the first two antiserums. Aggregates formed in normal serum containing cells of both species are of either one cell species or the other, never of both species. Thus, disaggregated xenogeneic cells do not recognize each other and therefore will not sort together. Aggregates in antiserum prepared against both species are composed of cells of both species that are distributed randomly throughout newly formed aggregates. In addition, calcium-free and high calcium media have no effect on reaggregation, a surprising observation, since calcium is involved in cell adhesions. These results are unequivocal and confirm the hypothesis that contiguous cell surfaces are held together by forces similar to those between antigens and antibodies, as proposed by Tyler (1947) and Weiss (1947).

INCOMPATIBILITY IN CNIDARIA

Introduction

We have known since the eighteenth century that animals such as hydra show incompatibilities after transplantation, much like advanced animals. Loeb (1945) introduced conflicting terminology in his accounts of tissue incompatibilities among the Cnidaria (Coelenterata). However, his important contributions to analyses of *self*, *not-self* specificity should not be minimized. Loeb's *organismal differentials* are now interpreted as antigens or gene products that determine *self* or *not-self* specificity. He states, for example, that

> in adult birds and mammals there is a very strong reaction against . . . strange orga-
> nismal differentials in general; the normal equilibrium is strictly autogenous (self); it
> depends upon the presence of the same individuality differential in all the important tissues
> and organs . . . Notable reactions (result) if small parts of tissues possessing a strange
> individuality differential are introduced into the animal body.

Introduced before much information on comparative immune responses was available, Loeb's interpretations are noteworthy.

Hydrozoa

There have been many investigations into the events accompanying grafting in cnidarians to date substantiating Loeb's predictions. *Hydra*, too, accepts autografts but rejects other types of transplants. Whereas some transplantations may not be due to recognition by the host of antigenic differences, others are unsuccessful when natural patterns are disturbed by grafting. This can occur, for example, after changing the position from the usual orthotopic one to any other heterotopic position. However, other incompatibilities arise because of genetic differences between host and donor tissues that may reflect at least underlying simple allelic differences. By direct, gross observation and the use of the electron microscope, differences after transplantation are easily viewed. Genetic control of tissue (histo-)compatibility may be more complex, as revealed by extensive genetic analyses of incompatibilities in *Hydractinia echinata*, a marine colonial encrusting hydroid. The control may be due to at least one locus with six alleles. These results were derived from precise matings over several generations, performed by Hauenschild [(1954, 1956) (recently reviewed by Du Pasquier 1974, in press)].

In addition to graft position and genetics, a third possible explanation, given by Toth (1967), ruled out the action of complementary divalent cations in studies of tissue compatibility in *Hydractinia echinata*. Fusion fails to occur if the opposing explants are of different sex, from different individuals of the same sex, or if peripheral explant contact occurs after free-growing stolons have begun to form. The findings of Ivker (1972), contrary to those of Toth, suggest that histoincompatibility in *Hydrac-*

tinia is more easily explained by invoking the current thesis of progressive phylogenetic immuno-differentiation. Tissue incompatibility develops in *Hydractinia* after any mutual contact that results in hyperplastic stolon (overgrowth) production. Overgrowth may involve surface-bound molecules produced by the ectoderm; genes ultimately control histoincompatibility and hyperplastic growth. This is consistent with studies of morphology and intermediate forms of incompatibility between related strains (i.e., parent-offspring, half-sibs).

Bibb and Campbell (1973) used several different species of the genera: *Hydra*, *Chlorohydra*, and *Pelmatohydra* in various allograft and xenograft combinations. After allografting they found by means of light and electron microscopy that "edge" cells show pseudopodial activity and attach and heal quickly; even after normal

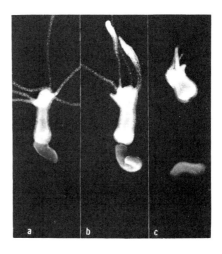

Fig. 5-3 *Hydra pseudoligactis* (apical)—*Hydra viridis* (basal) xenograft illustrating rapid separation. (a) Newly grafted animal. (b) Four hours later. (c) Separation by next day (×14). (*From*: Bibb & Campbell.) *Tissue and Cell* **5**: 199, 1973.

healing, however, xenografts eventually dissolve (Figs. 5-3 and 5-4). As a consequence of adequate xenograft healing, cell attachments develop which resemble septate desmosomes; healing is preserved for several days. Yet constrictions do develop at the graft site as a signal of incompatibility. This progresses until the incompatible

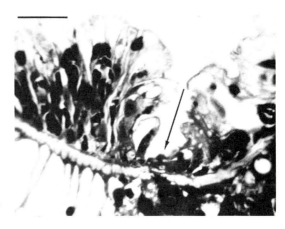

Fig. 5-4 Longitudinal section of epidermal junction of one-day-old *Hydra pseudoligactis*—*Hydra littoralis* xenograft. H. Pseudoligactis tissue at left. At site of graft (arrow), epidermis is only few microns high and cell contact is tenuous. (*From*: Bibb & Campbell.) *Tissue and Cell* **5**: 199, 1973.

tissues are finally divorced. Bibb and Campbell advance a fourth possible interpretations to account for rejection. Graft rejection is not attributed to immunological responses; rather, it may result from replacement of allospecific attachments by xenotypic cell junctions that lead to gradual tissue separations.

Anthozoa

One dramatic contribution to understanding recognition by invertebrate cells and tissues originated from studies by Theodor (1966, 1969, 1970), using species of arborescent coelenterates, the Gorgonacea. His works support the view that histo-incompatibility or quasi-immunorecognition involving allogeneic ectoderm developed early in evolution. As would be expected, autografts do succeed and survive indefinitely. Branches derived from two individuals belonging to the same species in allogeneic combinations fail to fuse. Even more striking, xenogeneic cultures of gorgonian tissue show mutual damage or histotoxicity within one to four days after contact, but allogeneic tissue disintegration is considerably slower (Fig. 5-5). The gorgonian immune reaction is not a conventional one; thus, according to Theodor's interpretations, its response represents a kind of "preimmunology." Gorgonian histotoxicity is "induced suicide" that conceivably resembles cell destructions mediated by cytotoxic or "nonimmune" reactions in cultures of vertebrate cells (Möller and Möller 1966). Thus at all phylogenetic levels, one manifestation of tissue incompatibility is the development of cytotoxicity.

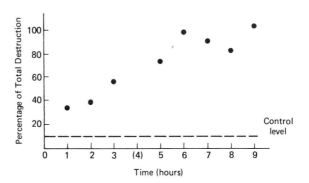

Fig. 5-5 Expression of the histopathic effect after contact (1–9 h) followed by the separation of killer and target. (*From*: Theodor, *Nature* **227**: 690, 1970.)

Despite the technical difficulties involving anesthesia, surgery, and reactions to injury, Hildemann et al. (1974) were successful in exchanging grafts in the staghorn coral *Acropora* that lives in the bays around Magnetic Island, Australia. Branches from donor staghorns can be broken 'off to make grafts and then brought into intimate contact with the coenenchyme or soft tissues of recipients. When graft donors and recipients are derived from the same colony or from the same clone, the resulting fusions (autogeneic, isogeneic) are entirely compatible for an observation period as long as 300 days. At 25°C, fusion of soft and skeletal tissues occurs in six to eight days, as it does even naturally, after accidental breakage. Such a protective response is advantageous, since it ensures an entire colony's structural integrity against occasional destructive waves.

One can test for healing of naturally occurring grafts by several experimental approaches. At the graft-host contact zone, intact polyps and pigmented zooanthellae persist. In addition, because of the primitive nerve net, the coral's characteristic nervous system, gentle probing of polyp tentacles leads to withdrawal responses perceived by and immediately transferred across the graft-recipient contact zone. This is considered to be a sensitive and unequivocal test for functional graft survival. After studying intercolonial allografts, Hildemann et al. found only moderate incompatibilities. Both morphologic and functional fusion occurs, but after several weeks, healing is always followed by destruction of soft tissues and frequent death at the graft-host contact zone. Heterografts involving transplants between several different species of *Acropora* heal rapidly, but after one week a region of cell death develops, preceded by obvious regression of soft tissues.

TRANSPLANTATION IN PLATYHELMINTHES

The transplantation experiments of Lindh (1959), using flatworms, are important to the phylogeny of recognition and transplantation reactions. Although some heterotransplants involving the same genus but different species behave as allotransplants, most heterografts are unsuccessful and result in only temporary regeneration, as between, for example *Planaria dorotocephala* and *Planaria maculata*. One generality derived from flatworm transplantation experiments is that animals that develop from three germ layers but without a coelom still show specific recognition of *self* and *not-self*.

FOREIGN GRAFTS IN SIPUNCULIDA

The sipunculids are a small group of mostly marine, worm-like creatures with certain superficial resemblances to the annelids (segmented worms). For example, in *Dendrostomum zostericolum*, a sipunculid, and many of the marine annelids the sexes are separate, but each retains its own gametes in the coelom. Transplantations of gametes can be made by injecting the eggs, sperm, or even pieces of minced tentacles from one individual into the coelom of another (Cushing et al. 1965). As in other invertebrates the coelomocytes promptly wall off all foreign material. Yet after transplanting fragments of minced auto- and allograft tentacles, each is encapsulated by host coelomocytes, surprisingly at similar rates; one would have expected different responses. With regard to eggs, the coelomocytes of neither sex recognize the antigenic differences. Whereas normal eggs are not recognized as foreign, quite the contrary occurs if the eggs are stained with eosin; they are encapsulated. In fact, any treatment such as washing, heating, and sonication, which somehow affects the egg surface, destroys its capacity to be recognized as *self* by the host, leading to encapsulation and death of the eggs. Nothing akin to antibody is demonstrable after cellular or protein antigens are injected into the coelom, nor does acceleration of the encapsulation rate or phagocytosis occur after repeat second transplants. Actually such studies merit intensive reanalysis focusing on changes that may occur in cell membranes that abrogate recognition.

INCOMPATIBILITIES IN MOLLUSCA

Pelecypoda

One of the first reports on the fate of transplanted tissues in molluscs was made by Drew and de Morgan (1910). Autogeneic gills implanted in the adductor muscle of *Pecten maximus* are eventually isolated by encapsulation. Such information is surprising and equivocal, since auto- and allotransplants behave similarly; it would seem more consistent with findings in all groups if there were a difference between auto- and allografted tissue. Cushing (1957) also found minimal cell responses to allografts. Encapsulation of autotransplants is not an example of *Pecten* recognizing *not-self*. Instead, faulty grafting techniques undoubtedly led to graft damage because of the drastic heterotopic surgery involving gills and muscles. Leukocytes (or white cells) reacted to products of autolysis. It is always desirable to graft in natural orthotopic positions to at least rule out bad techniques. Female gonads and mantle strips of grafts from *Pecten irradians* heal after forty-nine hours; however, healing does not occur if male gonads are transplanted under the mantle. Well-healed autografts retain eyes, tentacles, and contractibility for over a month. Clearly our knowledge of molluscan transplantation reactions is still hampered by lack of appropriate grafting procedures.

Des Voigne and Sparks (1969) used the oyster *Crassostrea gigas* to make small portions of mantle allografts to slits in the connective tissue near the palps. Whereas some allografts were apparently rejected by the host, others remained viable and appeared normal. The cellular response is typical. Leukocytes congregate near the wound and form a union with it and the implants so that the implant finally fuses and becomes contiguous with the host. Canzonier (1963) reports the loss of 50 % of the normal and diseased allogeneic tissue implants in *Crassostrea virginica*. Once the implants are healed, there seems to be no later indication of host rejection. The blood spaces joined with those of the host, but Canzonier observed no establishment of any cross circulation; these graft rejections are not examples of immune responses. Observation times were short without any comparison made with autograft controls. Molluscs could be more valuable to invertebrate transplantation studies if more reliable experimental procedures were employed.

Hildemann et al. (1974) began transplantation studies in the pearl oyster *Pinctada margaritifera*. Mantle tissue is accesssible and amenable to surgery. Furthermore the orange-versus-black color dimorphism of the mantle's margin in individual oysters provides a sure indication of viability; pigment should be destroyed at the time of graft destruction. The experimenters initiated the orthotopic technique, a promising approach to assessing the true condition of grafts after healing. In heterotopic positions destruction cannot be attributed to the immune system but to unknown technical factors. Apparently technical difficulties prevented unequivocal observations on the fate of some of the transplants.

Gastropoda

After transplantation, tissues that have received prior treatment suffer a more violent reaction than normal, untreated tissues. Tripp (1961) transplanted pedal tissue allografts from *Australorbis glabratus* into the cephalopedal sinus, or space between the anterior cerebral region and the foot. Fresh allogeneic tissue elicits only a transient coelomocytic infiltration, but formalin-fixed allogeneic tissue is recognized as foreign and is finally encapsulated. Xenogeneic tissues from the planorbid species *Planorbarius corneus*, transplanted to *Australorbis*, elicit a marked cellular response and, finally, graft destruction. Formalin-fixed xenogeneic tissue, however, is encapsulated within twenty-four hours by fibroblasts originating from nearby connective tissue. The cephalopedal sinus of *Hydractinia duryi normale* (strain HI-2) has also been used as a site for heterografts. Histologic studies of implants revealed more rapid and severe host reactions to xenografts than to allografts. Whereas this information strongly suggests that recipients differentiate between allografts and xenografts, there is equivocal information on the necessary controls or comparisons between autografts and allografts.

Cephalopoda

Up to the present the cephalopods have been more important to studies of leukocyte origins than to studies of their reactions against foreignness. Cushing (1962) made auto- and allotransplants of octopus skin and found no differences in the behavior of autografts or allografts. In fact, except for a few technical failures, both types of transplants survive as long as the host did in captivity. Obviously there is much to be learned in dealing with the husbandry and grafting techniques.

TRANSPLANTATION IN ARTHROPODA

Like many of the previously quoted experiments, those dealing with arthropods have often yielded conflicting reports on the outcome of transplants, especially in the case of embryonic primordia grafts such as the imaginal discs (Spinner 1969; Bhaskaran and Sivasubramanian 1969). However, certain genetically defined species are of value in learning something about the genes that control tissue recognition phenomena and immune reactions in invertebrates.

Hadorn's (1937) early studies of *Drosophila* ovarian transplants reveal the geneticist's and embryologist's viewpoint rather than that of the immunologist. Hadorn transplanted ovaries and testes into genetically normal larvae of the same age, using the transplantation methods of Ephrussi and Beadle (1936), which allow full development of normal ovaries and testes. Due to the genetic constitution of *Drosophia*, immune interference does not curtail development. Many transplants grow and elongate, the egg strings differentiate, and their apical ends contract just as they would in normal larvae. Yet development is incomplete, and the transplants never reach the size of full-grown, normal ovaries. Although eggs are formed, they degenerate before reaching their full size. According to Hadorn's interpretation, the distinct but limited development of transplanted ovaries confirms the existence within the ovaries of inherent developmental potencies unlike those of other organs such as the imaginal discs. It is the lethal genetic constitution that prevents further development in different organs at different periods of time. An alternative and more acceptable interpretation, not limited to development, assumes that gene-determined foreign antigens are present. It is the host's immune system that eventually recognizes these antigens and arrests development by graft rejection. Any given host will react differently to diverse tissue types.

Diptera

Differences between populations of *Drosophila* have been analyzed by performing interspecific or xenotransplants of larval ovaries (Kambysellis 1968, 1970). Any genetic differences should be revealed by the fate of transplantations. Although Kambysellis gave no consideration to the possibility of immune phenomena being provoked after transplantation between various groups, one of his conclusions is worth mentioning. According to Kambysellis

> the degree of gonadal development . . . is highly dependent on the genetic relationship
> of host environment and hybrid embryos or hybrid larvae can be produced between distantly isolated species.

Orthoptera

Scott (1971) attempted to determine what constitutes foreignness to an invertebrate by implanting foreign tissues into the hemocoel of the American cockroach *Periplaneta americana*; this was another approach to recognition by invertebrate cells. Nylon monofilaments are obviously foreign, and after implantation they are completely encapsulated by hemocytes from the host's body fluid, a response studied in detail by Salt (1970). Multilayered capsules composed of hemocytes isolate the particles from the blood circulation. Furthermore, interspecific or xenogeneic implants from *Nauphoeta cineria* to the blowfly *Calliphora* of the family Calliphoridae, or even implants from distantly related mice, are recognized as foreign and encapsulated twenty-four hours after implantation. Implanted allogeneic nerve cords are not encapsulated; however, allogeneic nerve cords treated with various enzymes render them more susceptible to encapsulation. For example, encapsulation occurs following treatment with collagenase and lecithinase C. Evidently recognition of antigen sites on the intact neural lamella surface is required to prevent the hemocyte reaction; here, cockroach, cells as do those of other animals, require prior treatment to provoke recognition. This work strongly supports the suggestion that specificity of recognition is at least partially determined by properties of the cell surface, particularly its antigenic composition. According to one interpretation, the destroyed receptors are those for *self*; thus hemocytes recognize the altered membrane as *not-self*.

Knowledge of certain insect hormones has been greatly increased by transplantation studies in cockroaches. Bell (1972) transplanted ovaries in eighteen cockroach species as intraspecific allografts. These grafts resulted in the initiation of yolk formation and oocyte growth rates comparable to nontransplanted controls. However, heterotransplants of roach ovaries led to sequestered host vitellogenins, but the grafts grew to terminal stages only when donor and host were closely related species. When ovaries were transplanted between species of different superfamilies or families, yolk formation did not occur. Thus, the fate of insect endocrine glands can be tested after transplantation, and the resulting fate reflects the degree of histocompatibility between donor and host, properties of the immune system.

GENETIC CONTROL OF TRANSPLANTATION IN UROCHORDATA

Genetic analysis is also possible in certain protochordates. This is not only interesting because of an additional variable that controls transplantation, but this animal group is more closely allied to the vertebrates than some of the other taxonomic groups. Freeman (1970) recently reviewed the results of Japanese workers on genetic control of transplantation specificity in *Botryllus*, a colonial ascidian. Oka and Watanabe (1960) showed that if two parental nonfusable colonies of *Botryllus primigenus* are mated, four classes of F_1 progeny develop. Each progeny class then fuses with members of its class, those of two other classes, and with both parents. Assuming that the parents are both heterozygous at a histocompatibility locus that controls colony specificity (genotypes expressed by the notation AB and CD, each letter representing one allele), then the F_1 generation possesses four classes of progeny: AC, AD, BC, and BD. Thus, colonies with at least one common allele at the colony specificity locus will fuse with each other. Matings of the F_1 progeny, producing F_2, followed by colony fusion tests, established the validity of this scheme. According to the genetic analysis of Hildemann and Reddy (1973), these results are surprising and do not agree with the immunogenetic rules of transplantation established for vertebrates. AD can fuse with BD but not with BC colonies.

Recognition events were analyzed by Tanaka (1973) in *Botryllus* and again by Tanaka and Watanabe (1973), yielding the following conclusions. They see nonfusion reaction (NFR) as allogeneic inhibition when two incompatible ascidian colonies are placed in mutual contact: ampullae to ampullae, ampullae to margin without ampullae, and cut surface of one colony to the cut surface of another. Incompatible colonies showed the nonfusion reaction. NFR is first manifested by destruction of the test (outer covering) cells around the contact area. This leads to the appearance of filaments around disintegrated test cells, followed by contraction of the ampullae. Constriction and necrosis resulted in severance of distal ampullae. Finally, the NFR is complete when the contact areas of both colonies are severed completely. The response is irreversible and progresses to completion even if one participating member is removed presumably after induction has occurred.

There is a possible interpretation from the work of Tanaka and Watanabe. Colony specific NFR resides in the test matrix and blood, causing the death of granular amoebocytes. It is noteworthy that the so-called nonimmunologic allogeneic inhibition in mammals described by Möller and Möller (1966) is interpreted as an evolutionary precursor of immune-type responses, probably related to immunologic surveillance.

According to Scott and Schuh (1963) the tunicate *Amaroecium constellatum* has remarkable powers of regeneration. If parts are separated from the body, these detached fragments regenerate all missing members, much as sponge cells do after dissociation. Such cells recognize histogenetic affinity or genetic kinship and behave according to the antigenic composition of their cell surfaces; thus, like cells will sort together. This indicates the tunicate's capacity for specific recognition.

SHORT-TERM IMMUNOLOGIC MEMORY IN ECHINODERMS

Introduction

The echinoderms are important in assessing the evolution of cell recognition mechanisms. According to some taxonomists, echinoderms are close to the vertebrates ancestrally; thus, they are excellent for sudying immune reactivities intermediate between invertebrates and vertebrates. The information on echinoderms is presented last because the approach, although less detailed, is similar to that for the earthworm. The phylum Echinodermata includes the sea cucumbers (class Holothuroidea), sea stars (class Asteroidea), brittle stars (class Ophiuroidea), sea urchins and sand dollars (class Echinoidea), sea lilies (class Crinoidea), and several extinct classes. The results from two independent earlier studies dealing with allograft recognition in echinoderms are equivocal, mainly due to faulty technique. Transplantations were performed to heterotopic sites with the animals maintained in excessively cold sea water, two parameters that create difficulty in distinguishing between graft acceptance and rejection (Ghiradella 1965; Bruslé 1967).

Cell and Tissue Transplants in Asteroidea

Despite the difficulty of the echinoderm transplantation process, Ghiradella (1965) found that the two starfishes *Patiria miniata* and *Asterias forbesi* discriminate between reciprocal allo- and xenocoelomic implants and heterogeneic pyloric caecum from two other species, *Asterias vulgaris* and *Henricia sanguinolenta*. Normal allografts, although healthy after five weeks, are surrounded by connective tissue and amoebocyte masses. Whereas amoebocytes are usually associated with damaged allograft areas, amoebocytic attack, phagocytosis, and encapsulation are apparently not associated with the elimination of xenotransplants. Xenografts are eliminated by the hosts one week after transplantation. *Henricia* caecum is extruded through the dermal branchiae by both hosts; *Patiria* disposes of *Asterias* caecum by transferring it from the host ray to the cardiac stomach where it is digested or extruded through the mouth.

Self-Recognition in Asteroidea-Echinoidea

To understand cell recognition, Reinisch and Bang (1971) injected *Arbacia* (sea urchin) coelomocytes, about half of which are deeply pigmented, into *Asterias* (sea star); circulating amoebocyte numbers in the hosts dropped abruptly. Amoebocytes from *Arbacia* adhered to and were phagocytosed by host amoebocytes, which clumped consistently within the papulae, out-pushings of the body wall. The reverse, i.e., injection of *Asterias* cells into *Asterias*, does not elicit cell clumping, nor is it followed by a drop in circulating amoebocytes. Recognition by *Asterias* of intact foreign cells evokes a defense mechanism distinct from its reaction to allogeneic cells. In fact, this echinoderm response closely resembles the type of *self, not-self* cell recognition without memory that is demonstrable in vertebrates, except that in allogeneic combinations, observations could have been longer to be sure of signs of possible incompatibilities.

Tests for Short-Term Memory

Because of the echinoderm body structure (rigid exoskeleton), enormous technical difficulties must be surmounted before successful grafting can be achieved. Yet Hildemann and Dix (1972) made substantial progress toward revealing specific recognition as well as an immunologic memory component in echinoderms. To define the events in allograft destruction, they chose the sea cucumber *Cucumaria tricolor* and the horned sea star *Protoreaster nodosus*, which inhabits the Great Barrier Reef.

The coloration is strikingly different; thus pigment cell destruction is the easiest external criterion of a transplanted graft's condition. Intact pigment cells indicate viability, but dissolved cells reflect graft destruction.

In *Cucumaria*, three distinct cell layers are evident in permanently surviving auto-grafts. These are the epidermis, an outer muscle layer, and a deep muscle layer. *Protoreaster* integumentary autografts show similar normal morphology characterized by an outer epithelium with secretory cells and muscle fiber bundles. Three layers are distinguishable; epidermis, thick dermis with loose connective tissue, and an under-lying muscle layer into which crypts extend. Macrophages and small lymphocytes make up the remainder of the cellular components (Fig. 5-6).

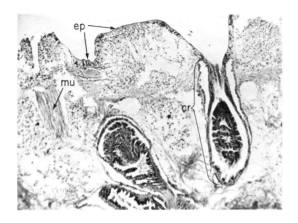

Fig. 5-6 *Protoreaster* integumentary autograft in cross section at 4 months after grafting showing normal morphology. Outer epithelium (oep), sensory secretory (?) crypts (cr), and muscle fiber bundles (mu) are intact. Three-cell layers are distinguishable: epidermis, thick dermis with loose connective tissue, and an underlying muscle layer into which crypts extend. ×*165*. (*From*: Hildemann & Dix, *Transpl.,* **15**: 624, 1972.)

Chronic, slow allograft destruction responses occur in both species as in other invertebrates. Progressive pigment cell destruction heralds gross rejection. Micro-scopic events, studied more intensively in the sea cucumber than in the sea star, show the following characteristics. The epidermis becomes edematous initially; this is ac-companied by vacuolation and loss of cytoplasm in some areas. Macrophages are abundant at 173 days, but may have appeared earlier. At later rejection stages the most important feature is the presence of varying leukocyte types, especially macro-phages and lymphocytes in association with *Cucumaria* grafts. By contrast, at terminal stages of rejection, *Protoreaster* grafts show less infiltration by macrophages and more eosinophils into the dermis and loose connective tissue. First-set allograft destruction occurs four to six months at 21°C (Fig. 5-7).

To test for immunologic memory, second-set grafts were performed in a few cases when first-set transplants were still only rejected by approximately 50–75%. All showed pronounced accelerated rejection (positive memory). As further evidence of

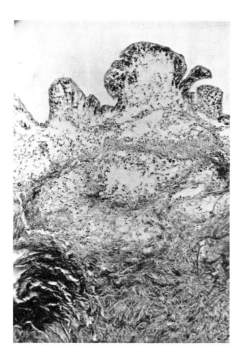

Fig. 5-7 *Protoreaster* integumentary allograft at zero survival end point based on progressive disappearance of red donor pigmentation in tan pigmented recipient area at 160 days after grafting. Both epidermis and dermis appear atrophic and vacuolated with an absence of crypts at this stage. Diffuse small lymphocyte or hemocyte infiltration is seen throughout dermis and loose connective tissue. Numerous eosinophils are observed in epidermis, but macrophages are not abundant. (*From*: Hildemann & Dix, *Transpl.,* **15**: 624, 1972.)

this second-set response, several characteristics were obvious. Early inflammatory discoloration and hyperplasia produced invasive resorption of grafts, a type of response that occurs readily, perhaps due to short-term memory. Alternatively, it may be a continuation of the inductive phase, since there was no evidence of complete graft destruction. After second-set graft destruction, the first-set response continues unaffected. If this is indeed an example of short-term memory, one must predict that long-term memory also exists. This would be demonstrable by showing accelerated rejection of second transplants performed after first-set transplant destruction.

SUMMARY

The ability to recognize the difference between *self* and *not-self* is an attribute not restricted to multicellular metazoans. Indeed, this characteristic can be traced to the simplest protozoans. Transplantations of cell organelles in protozoans produce incompatibility reactions that are to immunity what primitive irritability is to the vertebrate nervous system. *Quasi immunorecognition* is the capacity for *not-self* recognition of allogeneic tissue followed by incompatibility reactions. Unicellular protozoans also show quasi immunorecognition, a universal characteristic that evolved earlier than primordial cell-mediated immunity. Memory could conceivably be demonstrable, but careful techniques are required for confronting hosts with second transplants of organelles, cells, and tissue grafts. Furthermore, well-defined criteria for assessing graft viability and animal husbandry are prime requisites for future consideration. Alternatively, specific immunologic memory may not have evolved at these levels of phylogeny.

BIBLIOGRAPHY

Bell, W. J. 1972. Yolk formation by transplanted cockroach oocytes. J. Exptl. Zool. **181**: 41.

Bhaskaran, G., and Sivasubramanian, P. 1969. Metamorphosis of imaginal disks of the housefly: evagination of transplanted disks. J. Exptl. Zool. **171**: 385.

Bibb, C., and Campbell, R. D. 1973. Cell affinity determining heterospecific graft intolerance in Hydra. Tissue and Cell **5**: 199.

Bruslé, J. 1967. Homogreffes et heterogreffes du tegument et des gonades chez *Asterina gibbosa* et *Asterina pancerii* (Echinodermes, Asterides). Cahiers de Biologie Marine **8**: 417.

Canzonier, W. J. 1963. Histological observations on the response of oysters to tissue implants. Proc. Nat. Shellf. Assoc. **54**: 1.

Cushing, J., 1957. Tissue transplantation in *Pecten irradians*. Biol. Bull. **113**: 327.

————. Blood groups in marine animals and immune mechanisms of lower vertebrates and invertebrates (comparative immunology). Proc. Conf. on Immuno-Reproduction: La Jolla, Calif. Sept. 1962. Issued by the Population Council, New York, New York.

Cushing, J. E., Boraker, D. and Keough, E. 1965. Reactions of sipunculid worms to intracoelomic injections of homologous eggs. Fed. Proc. **24**: 504.

Des Voigne, D. M., and Sparks, A. K. 1969. The reaction of the Pacific oyster, *Crassostrea gigas*, to homologous tissue implants. J. Invert. Pathol. **14**: 293.

Drew, G. H., and De Morgan, W. 1910. The origin and formation of fibrous tissue produced as a reaction to injury in *Pectin maximus*, as a type of lamellibranchiata. Quart. J. Micros. Sci. **55**: 595.

Du Pasquier, L. 1974. The genetic control of histo-compatibility reactions: phylogenetic aspects. Arch. de Biol. (in press).

Ephrussi, B., and Beadle, G. W. 1936. A technique for transplantation for *Drosophila*. Am. Nat. **70**: 218.

Freeman, G. 1970. Transplantation specificity in echinoderms and lower chordates. Transpl. Proc. **2**: 236.

Galtsoff, P. S. 1925. Regeneration after dissociation (an experimental study on sponges). I. Behavior of dissociated cells of *Microciona prolifera* under normal and altered conditions. J. Exp. Zool. **42**: 183.

Ghiradella, H. T. 1965. The reaction of two starfishes, *Patiria miniata* and *Asterias forbesi*, to foreign tissue in the coelom. Biol. Bull. **128**: 77.

Goldstein, L. 1970. Nucleo-cytoplasmic incompatibilities in free-living amoeba. Trans. Proc. **2**: 191.

Hadorn, E. 1937. Transplantation of gonads from lethal to normal larvae in *Drosophila melanogaster*. Proc. Soc. Exp. Biol. Med. **36**: 632.

Hauenschild, C. 1954. Genetische und entwicklungs-physiologische untersuchungen über intersexualität und gewebeverträglichkeit bei *Hydractinia echinata* Flemm (Hydroz. Baugainvill.) Roux Arch. Entwick lungs-mechanik **147**: 1.

————. 1956. Ueber die vererbung einer gewebertiäg lichkeits-eigenschaft bei dem hydroidpolypen *Hydractinia echinata*. Z. Naturforsch **2**: 132.

Hildemann, W. H., and Reddy, A. L. 1973. Phylogeny of immune responsiveness: marine invertebrates. Fed. Proc. **32**: 2188.

Hildemann, W. H., Dix, T. G., and Collins, J. D. 1974. "Tissue Transplantation in Diverse Marine Invertebrates, in *Contemporary Topics in Immunobiology*, vol. 4, ed. E. L. Cooper. New York: Plenum Press.

Humphreys, T. 1967. "The Cell Surfaces and Specific Cell Aggregation," in *The Specificity of Cell Surfaces*, pp. 199–210, eds. B. D. Davis and L. Warren. Englewood Cliffs, N. J.: Prentice-Hall, Inc.

Ivker, F. 1972. A hierarchy of histo-incompatibility in *Hydractinia echinata*. Biol. Bull. **143**: 162.

Jeon, K. W., Lorch, I. J., and Danielli, J. F. 1970. Reassembly of living cells from dissociated components. Science **167**: 1626.

Kambysellis, M. P. 1968. Interspecific transplantation as a tool for indicating phylogenetic relationships. Proc. Nat. Acad. Sci. **59**: 1166.

———. 1970. Compatibility in insect tissue transplantations. 1. Ovarian transplantations and hybrid formation between *Drosophila* species endemic to Hawaii. J. Exptl. Zool. **175**: 169.

Lindh, N. O. 1959. Heteroplastic transplantation of transversal body sections in flatworms. Arkiv für Zoologi, Serie 2, Band 12, nr. 14, 183.

Loeb, L. 1945. *The Biological Basis of Individuality*. Springfield, Illinois: C. C. Thomas Pub.

Möller G., and Möller, E. 1966. Interaction between allogeneic cells in tissue transplantation. *Ann. N. Y. Acad. Sci.*, **129**: 735.

Oka, H., and Watanabe, H. 1960. Problems of colony specificity in compound ascidians. *Bull Biol.* **10**: 153.

Reinisch, C. L., and Bang, F. B. 1971. Cell recognition: Reaction of the sea star (*Asterias vulgaris*) to the injection of amoebocytes of sea urchin (*Arbacia punctulata*). Cell. Immun. **2**: 496.

Salt, G. 1970. *The Cellular Defense Reactions of Insects*. Cambridge, England: The University Press.

Scott, F. M., and Schuh, J. E. 1963. Intraspecific reaggregation in *Amaroecium constellatum* labelled with tritiated thymidine. *Acta Emb. Morph. Exp.* **6**: 39.

Scott, M. T. 1971. Recognition of foreignness in invertebrates. Transplantation studies using the American cockroach, *Periplaneta americana. Transplantation* **11**: 78.

Spiegel, M. 1954. The role of specific surface antigens in cell adhesion. I. The reaggregation of sponge cells. *Biol. Bull.* **106**: 130.

Spinner, W. 1969. Transplantationsversuche zur blastemgliederung, regenerations and differen zierungsleistung der beinanlagen von *Culex pipiens* (L.). *Wilhelm Roux Archiv.* **163**: 259.

Tanaka, K. 1973. Allogeneic inhibition in a compound ascidian, *Botryllus primigenus* Oka. II. Cellular and humoral responses in "nonfusion" reaction. *Cell. Immunol.* **7**: 427.

Tanaka, K., and Watanabe, H. 1973. Allogeneic inhibition in a compound ascidian, *Botryllus primigenus* Oka. I. Processes and features of "nonfusion" reaction. *Cell Immunol.* **7**: 410.

Tartar, V. 1964. "Experimental Techniques with Ciliates," in *Methods in Cell Physiology*, 1, p. 109, ed. D. M. Prescott. New York: Academic Press.

———. 1970. Transplantation in protozoa. *Transplantation Proc.* **2**: 183.

Theodor, J. 1966. Contribution á l'étude des gorgones (V) Les greffes chez les gorgones: etude d'un systéme de reconnaissant de tissu. *Bull. Inst. Oceanogr. Monaco* **66**: 3.

———. 1969. Histotoxicité *in vivo* et *in vitro* entre tissue xénogénique et entre tissue allogéniques chez un invertébré. *C. R. Acad. Sci. Paris* **268**: 2534.

———. 1970. Distinction between *self* and *not-self* in lower invertebrates. *Nature* **227**: 690.

Toth, S. E. 1967. Tissue compatibility in regenerating explants from the colonial marine hydroid *Hydractinia echinata* (Flem). *J. Cell. Physiol.* **69**: 125.

Tripp, M. R. 1961. The fate of foreign materials experimentally introduced into the snail *Australorbis glabratus. J. Parasitol.* **47**: 745.

Tyler, A. 1947. An autoantibody concept of cell structure growth and differentiation. Symp. Soc. Study Develop. *Growth* **6**: 7.

Weiss, P. 1947. The problem of specificity in growth and development. *Yale J. Biol. Med.* **19**: 235.

Wilson, H. V. 1907. On some phenomena of coalescence and regeneration in sponges. *J. Exp. Zool.* **5**: 245.

Chapter 6

Primordial Cell-Mediated Immunity

INTRODUCTION

The second stage of immunoevolution is termed *primordial cell-mediated immunity*. Unlike the most primitive stage, immunorecognition, there is memory and specificity. Since memory (either positive or negative) is characteristic, a population of leukocytes exists capable of reproducing upon a second encounter with closely related tissue antigens. At this level of phylogeny, the number of antigenic determinants that are recognized specifically by leukocytes are more restricted in comparison to those encountered by leukocytes of animals at the most advanced level of immunoevolution (i.e., integrated cell and humoral immunity) where antibody synthesis occurs. Coelomocytes are cells of coelomate invertebrates that react to antigen, reproduce after antigen challenge, but do not synthesize antibody. Absence of antibody in itself makes the continued analysis of this form of immunity even more challenging. According to Acton et al. (1972):

> the exact relationship of all aspects of invertebrate immunity to that of the vertebrates will, of course, require much additional study. However it is now clear that these primitive animals not only have cellular capabilities to ward off intrusion by infectious agents, but also have been shown to possess a whole system of components which interact to provide a type of immune response analogous to the vertebrates. While all the criteria established to determine vertebrate immunity cannot be met by the invertebrate species, only the purist would argue that these animals do not possess immune capabilities.

Studies of primordial cell-mediated immunity had roots in early tissue transplantation experiments (Joest 1897; Korschelt 1896–1898; Korschelt 1927a, b; Leypoldt 1911; Rabes 1902; Korschelt 1929). However, in the nineteenth century, investigators were not concerned with graft rejection as an immunologic phenomenon, since thinking then was relatively nonimmunologic with regard to graft rejection in primitive animals. However, at that time earthworms were considered excellent for studying tissue transplantation. Now, because we have a greater understanding of cellular immunity, primitive animal reactions to autografts, allografts, or xenografts aid in a continued characterization of immune responses.

FIRST-SET ALLOGRAFT REJECTION IN *LUMBRICUS* AND *EISENIA*

Cell-mediated immunity in invertebrates may, indeed, be the evolutionary precursor of vertebrate cellular immunity as revealed by the results from earthworm studies. Three laboratories (Cooper 1965a, b, 1969, Duprat 1964, Izoard 1964, Valembois 1963, 1968, 1970) have demonstrated independently, by using several criteria, the earthworm's capacity to reject allografts and xenografts. Two of the most important characteristics that link earthworm graft rejection to the vertebrate response are *specificity* and *anamnesis*. Other invertebrates of similar structural complexity probably possess the same degree of cellular immune capability as the earthworm, but studies have not been pursued rigorously; for this reason the earthworm is discussed in greater detail. Earthworms are highly motile; therefore, they are anesthetized before grafting. Grafts, usually three segments of body wall, are cut and exchanged between host and donor. Postoperative care with sutures or adhesives are unnecessary, since the grafts adhere while the worms are anesthetized. Autografts are grossly healed after twenty-four hours, microscopically healed after forty-eight hours, and survive permanently. Allografts, after healing, exhibit varying degrees of incompatibility and are eventually rejected; the same is true for xenografts.

Lumbricus

Allografts from different geographical locales heal normally but much later and show varying signs of incompatibility as measured by pigment cell destruction. However, if allografts are exchanged within populations there is little or no incompatibility, suggesting a kind of inbreeding. Perhaps, within populations, the number of recognizable alloantigenic differences are less than the differences that exist between populations. It is unknown if this results from the fact that the earthworm mode of reproduction is sexual even though it is hermaphroditic. Absence of alloantigenic differences was recognizable by the lack of intrapopulation allograft rejections in earthworms derived from Oregon. Similarly, only 10% of intrapopulation Canadian allografts were destroyed.

Eisenia

Allograft destruction is possible in another earthworm, *Eisenia foetida*, a member, like *Lumbricus*, of the family Lumbricidae. Although *Eisenia* shows greater variability in external physical appearance, displaying phenotypic "red" and "stripe" worms, (according to Dr. G. E. Gates of Bangor, Maine, a noted earthworm systematist), they are still the same species. All allografts exchanged between pairs of *Eisenia* always heal, but eventually a larger percentage are completely destroyed than in *Lumbricus*: actually 23%. According to Duprat (1970), first-set allografts exchanged between *Eisenia foetida* from the same geographical location, like autografts, heal promptly and may remain intact grossly. Presumably, genetic homogeneity results from the inbreeding of worms from the same locale. Normally, both first- and second-set transplants between worms from different regions that are genetically heterogeneous are always rejected.

Xenograft Rejection

Introduction

One different approach to an analysis of the earthworm's capacity for recognition and sequestration of transplantation antigens took into account the fact that 100%

rejection was never observed when allografts were exchanged, suggesting

a) the absence of recognition of strong alloantigenic differences;
b) the absence of the existence of strong alloantigenic differences; or
c) either one and two combined.

If we assume that the immune system is capable of adequate recognition, then absence of complete rejections is probably due to the second alternative. Thus, if there are no antigens to recognize, even the most efficient immune system is incapable of responding. To rule out the existence of strong alloantigenic differences, and to support our contention of a vigorous immune system, we exchanged xenografts between *Eisenia* and *Lumbricus* and, in so doing, confronted each genus with diverse xenoantigenic differences. Xenografts can be exchanged easily despite the difference in size, which is counteracted by transplanting a two-segment *Lumbricus* graft and a three-segment *Eisenia* graft.

Healing of Autografts

Earthworm autografts heal rapidly and are always accepted permanently even if the normal graft polarity is intentionally rotated (Fig. 6-1). Grafts rotated so that the antero-posterior axis is now perpendicular to the worm's long axis still heal normally. When grafts are healed they can be touched with sharp instruments and in response

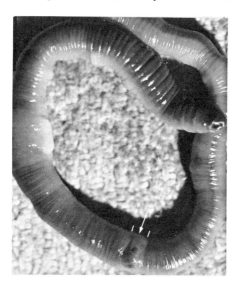

Fig. 6-1 This is a *Lumbricus* bearing a perfectly healed autograft indicated by the arrow. Graft polarity has been rotated so that the graft is healed perpendicular to the antero-posterior axis. This is at 75 days post-grafting, *×1.8*. (*After* Cooper, *Transpl.,* **6**: 322, 1968a.)

they often show immediate contraction. Similarly, strong pressure with other instruments never provokes dislodging of firmly healed autografts or xenografts. At twenty days an autograft is indistinguishable from surrounding host tissue. Heat-killed or alcohol-treated autografts never heal. If frog skin is transplanted to the worms, it remains totally unrecognized; the host's graft bed remains empty and its edges merely heal together leaving the isolated frog skin unaffected. Thus, there must be some recognizable antigens; otherwise, a graft would never be recognized.

First-Set Rejection of Xenografts Within the Family Lumbricidae

There are other ways of showing specificity of recognition. When an *Eisenia* autograft and *Lumbricus* xenograft are transplanted into the same graft bed of an *Eisenia* host, both grafts heal together and to the surrounding host tissue, but later the xenograft is always destroyed and the autograft remains. The position of the grafts in the bed does not affect the response. Earthworm coelomocytes are leukocytes that distinguish sharply between autografts and xenografts. It is easy to imagine coelomocytes confronted with *self* and *not-self*, "choosing" between the two and ultimately destroying the xenograft. Such a confrontation has no effect on the rejection time, since a single *Lumbricus* graft to *Eisenia* yields an equivalent survival time. Diverse intrafamilial specificities are likewise easily demonstrable. *Lumbricus* hosts respond differently to *Eisenia* xenografts, yielding a mean survival time of twenty-six days. However, an *Allolobophora* graft on a *Lumbricus* host leads to a survival time of approximately forty days. When *Eisenia* is host and *Allolobophora* is donor, the rejection time is thirty-five days, similar to that when *Lumbricus* is used as donor.

First-set *Eisenia* xenografts on *Lumbricus* hosts heal initially but eventually show signs of incompatibility and rejection at varying times (Fig. 6-2). At 15°C, four groups based on such times can be distinguished. For example an acute response occurs in eleven days or less; a rapid chronic response from twelve to nineteen days; intermediate chronic responses from twenty to forty-nine days; and those in the prolonged chronic class from fifty to more than 100 days. The highest number of rejections fall into the period from twelve to fifty days (Fig. 6-3). Obviously the condition of the host and the transplanted antigens affect the outcome of the response so that four groups are recognizable.

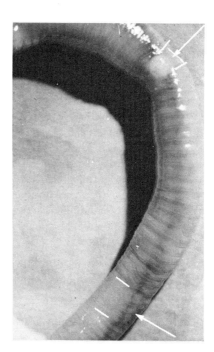

Fig. 6-2 A *Lumbricus* well-healed autograft (bottom arrow) and a rejected xenograft (top arrow). The xenograft shows blanching, swelling, and edema at 20 days post-grafting, ×2.5. (*After* Cooper, *Transpl.,* **6**: 322, 1968a).

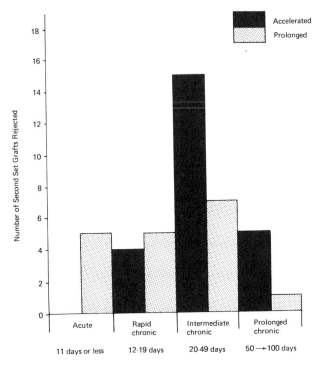

Fig. 6-3 The relationship between rate of rejection of first-set xenografts and rejection of second-set grafts. When first-set grafts are rejected in an acute or rapid-chronic fashion, second-set grafts show prolonged survival (negative responders). First-set grafts, rejected in an intermediate, chronic, prolonged fashion, are always followed by second-set grafts rejected at an accelerated rate (positive responders). (*After* Cooper, *Transpl.*, **6**: 322, 1968a).

First-Set Rejection of Interfamilial Xenografts (Eudrilidae-Lumbricidae)

Longer survival times of intrafamilial transplants suggests a greater sharing of cellular and tissue antigens, whereas the converse—faster rejection of tissues—reflects more distantly related individuals. Grafts from *Eudrilus* to *Lumbricus* yield a survival time of thirteen days and *Eudrilus* on to *Eisenia*, seventeen days. Both survive for a significantly shorter time than those involving intrafamilial combinations. Xenografts are always destroyed; thus, the absence of rejections in allogeneic combinations does not reflect a defective immune recognition mechanism, but may represent an absence of recognizable antigens. Such information defines the existence of an immune system capable of recognizing and reacting to antigen.

POSITIVE AND NEGATIVE MEMORY DURING XENOGRAFT REJECTION

It is a fascinating fact that any invertebrate can reject a graft. However, it is still necessary to define certain events that transpire before, during, and after rejection.

For example, are the two essential parameters, *specificity* and *anamnesis*, demonstrable as characteristics of earthworm transplant rejection? Specificity is inherent in the differential recognition and reaction to auto-, allo-, and xenografts and memory is the capacity to react faster to a second encounter with an antigen.

When grafted immediately after first-set rejection, second-sets are destroyed in a biphasic manner at 15°C. Most second-set transplant destructions occur faster than the first-set; however, a significant number are destroyed at longer times. Apparently there exists a relationship between first-set xenograft rejection class and positive and negative memory responses. Worms showing acute rejection of first-set grafts always react to repeat grafts by prolonged graft survival. The greatest number of positive responders results from those second-sets transplanted to worms that had first-sets destroyed during the intermediate chronic period of twenty to forty-nine days.

The interval between first-set rejection and second-set grafting can be correlated with the type of memory response to a second graft (Fig. 6-4). For example, short intervals tend to produce more positive responders than longer intervals. Short intervals of five days or less give significantly more accelerated reactions (positive responders). Furthermore, onset of rejection of a first-graft seems to affect the time of

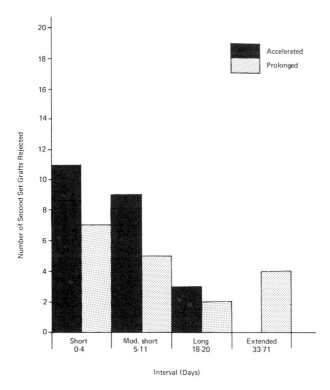

Fig. 6-4 Relationship of first-set graft rejection class to number, interval, and type of second-set rejection. Shorter intervals produced both positive and negative responders in similar proportions; extended intervals yielded only negative and no positive responders. (*After* Cooper, *Transpl.*, **6** : 322, 1968a).

second-set rejection (Fig. 6-5). Onsets of rejection that are moderately short (e.g., six to twelve days) result in slightly more accelerated rejections (positive responders) than

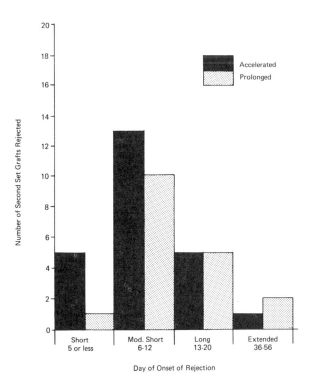

Fig. 6-5 Relationship between onset of second-set graft rejection and rejection type. Shorter onset times generally produced positive responders but extended onsets were followed by negative responders. (*After* Cooper, *Transpl.,* **6** : 322, 1968a).

prolonged survivers (negative responders). The character of the response is likewise affected by the time required for the appearance of the first response and the time that the second antigen is presented.

Interrupting the Inductive Phase

Rapid destruction of second-set xenografts is evidence that graft rejection mechanisms in earthworms are characterized by a memory component reminiscent of vertebrate anamnesis. In fact, prolonged survival, interpreted as negative memory, also recalls certain vertebrate-like responses. To manipulate the immune system such that responses were either all positive or all negative was the aim of one experiment (Cooper 1969a). It was determined that short intervals between first-set rejection and second-set grafting tend to produce positive responders. In addition, a maximal coelomocyte response occurs immediately after first-set grafting and during the first five days post-transplantation. This information and the assumption that coelomocytes are important in earthworm immune responses suggested that memory was short-lived. Control *Lumbricus* hosts transplanted with two *Eisenia* grafts at 15°C are destroyed at approximately thirty-three days.

Lumbricus hosts transplanted with a single *Eisenia* graft, followed five days later by a second-set graft from the same donor as the first, rapidly destroy the first- and second-set grafts, a strikingly unexpected result. This heightened reactivity to both grafts at about eighteen and fifteen days respectively can be interpreted in the following way. The induction phase of the immune response to the first graft is already in progress when the second graft is performed. Thus, the second serves as a booster for an already ongoing reaction. A second challenge with the same antigen that induced the first response during the latent period augments the response to both antigens. When *Lumbricus* hosts are grafted with a single *Eisenia* transplant and, five days later a second *Eisenia* transplant is made simultaneously with a third graft from a completely independent donor, *Allelobophora* (family Lumbricidae), the *Eisenia* grafts are destroyed at the same time. The rejection time of *Allelobophora*, however, is independent of the two *Eisenia* transplants and is equivalent to that of a single *Allelobophora* on a *Lumbricus* host. Once again, the inductive phase is interrupted, suggesting evidence for memory and specificity. As a further interpretation, if the coelomocytes of *Lumbricus* could not distinguish specifically between any of these grafts, then the host would have confused the *Eisenia* rejection times with the time induced by a donor graft from *Allelobophora*. Thus, the second-set response is probably regulated by antigen challenge time and temperature.

A HISTOLOGIC DESCRIPTION OF GRAFT REJECTION

The First Two Weeks

The earthworm's immune system is highly differentiated so that it can destroy foreign tissue antigens. The gross response is quantifiable, and there is strong evidence for active coelomocyte participation in the graft destruction process. After twenty-four hours, both autografts and xenografts are well healed by scar tissue that is identical histologically. Scar tissue associated with grafts is tissue that grows from the severed ends of muscle and the connective tissue between the muscle; its growth connects with tissue similar to that in the graft. In Figs. 6-6 and 6-7 epithelial cells are rediffer-

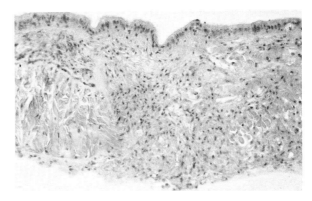

Fig. 6-6 A *Lumbricus* autograft at 11 days post-grafting, showing host tissue (at left) and graft (at right). The epithelium covering the scar tissue shows differentiation into cell types similar to those seen on host and graft sides, ×320. (*After* Cooper, *Transpl.,* **6**: 322, 1968a).

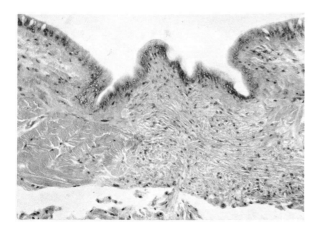

Fig. 6-7 An *Eisenia* xenograft 12 days post-grafting. Note the scar tissue between the host (at left) and the graft (at right). Many circular and longitudinal muscle bundles and epithelium show essentially no difference on either side. At biopsy this xenograft was well healed with no signs of rejection, ×*256*. (*After* Cooper, *Transpl.,* **6**: 322, 1968a).

entiated and are apparent as young mucus-secreting cells. At twenty-four hours, coelomocytes congregate at both autograft and xenograft sites, suggesting general nonspecific responses to injury and healing. This response occurs primarily at the graft-host contact zone in association with scar tissue; however, the central portion of grafts is not without profuse coelomocyte activity. The coelomic cavity is bathed by the coelomic fluid wherein numerous coelomocytes are suspended. There they serve as second-line sentinels after the epithelium of the body wall is broken (Fig. 6-8). The origin of coelomocytes is disputed, but one favored region is the loose aggregation of acidophilic-staining tissue found in the dorsal gut identified as *lymph gland* by nineteenth century German workers.

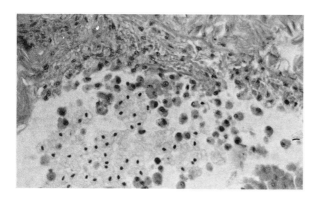

Fig. 6-8 An *Eisenia* xenograft on a *Lumbricus* host 8 days post-grafting. Note the intense coelomocyte reaction at the base of the graft, ×*400*. (*After* Cooper, *Transpl.,* **6**: 322, 1968a).

Revascularization of Transplants

The presence of blood vessels as early as day 1 reveals circulation to grafts. Blood vessels usually begin growth as extensions from thin sheets of the host peritoneal tissue where they are contained; later they are found in the surrounding scar tissue (Fig. 6-9). Growth of host vascular twigs may occur directly into transplants, or it may proceed by inosculation of host vessels with those in the graft. Transplants show sensitivity that suggests at least partial reestablishment of branches of integumentary nerves during the first few days after the transplants are healed.

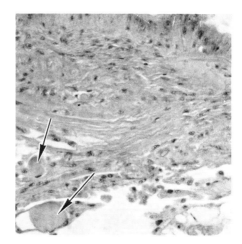

Fig. 6-9 A well healed *Eisenia* xenograft on a *Lumbricus* host 8 days post-grafting. Graft tissue is at the left. Arrows indicate a cross-section through two blood vessels at the base of the graft, ×410. (*After* Cooper, *Transpl.,* **6**: 322, 1968a).

ADOPTIVE TRANSFER OF GRAFT REJECTION BY COELOMOCYTES

Because coelomocytes aggregate at the site of xenografts, they must play a significant role in mediating immunity. There may be two explanations: namely, that coelomocytes are involved in recognition or that coelomocytes actually effect rejection. As a test, *Lumbricus* hosts were xenografted with *Eisenia*, and the coelomocytes from such hosts were tested for their capacity to transfer memory. To confirm memory, coelomocytes were harvested from host *Lumbricus* (A_1) at five days posttransplantation and injected into ungrafted *Lumbricus* (A_2). Then hosts were transplanted with the same xenografts derived from *Eisenia* donors as those used to induce immunity in A_1. Because *Lumbricus* shows only negligible allograft responses, no early allo-incompatibility toward coelomocytes was anticipated prior to their action against the *Eisenia* graft on *Lumbricus* A_2. The predicted result occurred, and at 15°C the *Lumbricus A* hosts showed accelerated rejection of their test transplant due to adoptive transfer by primed coelomocytes. At least one major aspect of the graft rejection response is cell mediated, since transfer with coelomic fluid alone, free of coelomocytes, is ineffective. Furthermore, coelomocytes from unprimed *Lumbricus* and those from *Lumbricus* primed with saline do not transfer the response, strongly suggesting the primary role of coelomocytes. Experiments designed to test for specificity, the duration of memory, and the effects of temperature on adoptive transfer responses remain to be determined.

REGULATION OF PRIMITIVE MEMORY BY TEMPERATURE

Both positive and negative memory responses develop when earthworm hosts are challenged after first-set grafts are destroyed. To study the role of antigen challenge time and temperature on the regulation of immune responsiveness, the ambient temperature is raised to 20°C and second-set transplants are performed after destruction of first-set grafts. In addition, coelomocytes are harvested and quantitated by removing them from the area just beneath the graft surface. Using these techniques, coelomocyte specificity can be deduced and gross aspects of graft survival can be quantitated and correlated at the same time with coelomocyte activity.

At 20°C, the mean survival time of first-set xenografts is approximately seventeen days, clearly different from previous results at 15°C (Fig. 6-10). Coelomocytes more than double their numbers at forty-eight hours after receiving second-set xenografts that only survive to 6 days. Thus a typical memory response occurs at the cellular level and is correlated grossly with accelerated rejection of repeat second-set xenografts. This higher temperature of 20°C does not lead to widespread first-set graft sur-

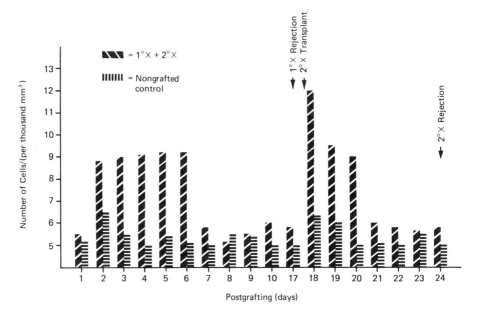

Fig. 6-10 Coelomocyte counts from *Lumbricus* hosts which received a second-set *Eisenia* xenograft after rejecting a first-set. Note the background values for coelomocytes from ungrafted worms. At day 2, after grafting, coelomocytes rise rapidly and return to normal long before gross rejection of the graft at day 17. The second anamnestic coelomocyte response is faster than the first. Gross rejection of the second graft is, similarly, faster. (*After* Hostetter and Cooper, *Cont. Topics in Immunobiol.,* **4**: 91, 1974).

vival times; instead survival times are narrowed significantly, and second-set grafts are rejected uniformly faster than both accelerated (positive) and prolonged (negative) memory rejections at 15°C. Finally, and of obvious significance, coelomocytes respond differently to autografts, nonspecific wounds, and both first- and second-set xenografts, revealing the necessity, in earthworms as in other animals, for both non-specific and immunologic reactions (Fig. 6-11).

A comparison of coelomocyte numbers from *Lumbricus* with no grafts, or first autografts only, with coelomocytes responding to second-set xenografts reveals a specific heightened cellular response to second xenografts. The first rise in coelomocytes is a general and nonspecific response, since autografts or simple injury provoke similar reactions.

There is an interdependency among the induction phase, the primary response, and the secondary reactions that influence anamnesis. Coelomocytes respond to first

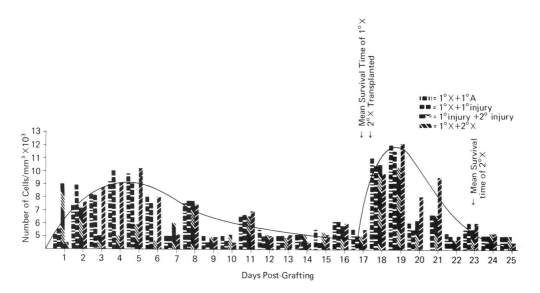

Fig. 6-11 Coelomocyte counts from another group similar to Fig. 6-10. Note the additional number of controls incorporated into the experiment to add further support to specific anamnesis and to rule out non-specific responses. (*After* Hostetter and Cooper, *Cont. Topics in Immunobiol.,* **4**: 91, 1974).

xenografts by increasing in number and then declining gradually during primary reactions. Presumably during this time primary xenografts stimulate the production of specific memory cells, this accounting for the abrupt increase in coelomocytes after a second-set challenge. This differs from the slow coelomocyte build-up after a first-set challenge. Quantitation of coelomocyte responses provides further confirmation for the existence of immunologic memory in earthworms.

A Summary of Primordial Cell-mediated Immunity

The earthworm coelomic cavity with the coelomocytes contained therein can be likened to vertebrate immune organs such as bone marrow. In the coelomic cavity, as in this organ, there are several varieties of immunocompetent cells. Earthworm coelomocytes respond just as vertebrate immunocytes do, by sequestering potential pathogens. Effecting tissue graft rejection is one example of how coelomocytes function. Coelomocytes may utilize the same or similar mechanisms for dealing with allografts and xenografts as those observed during cellular reactions against bacteria and parasites (Figs. 6-12, 6-13). Upon contact with a foreign antigen, coelomocytes become immobilized, and it is conceivable that they release humoral factors analogous to opsonins, lysins, agglutinins, and substances similar to mammalian migration inhibitory factor (MIF). The presence of antigen or the release of humoral agents may cause additional coelomocyte differentiation by stimulating sites of coelomo-cytopoiesis, leading to cell accumulations around foreign antigens. Once degraded, the stimulus for coelomocyte activation is removed. Coelomocytes produced in excess

CELLULAR RESPONSE TO AUTOGRAFTS

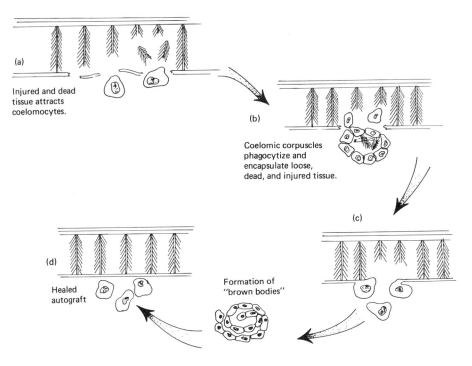

Fig. 6-12 Coelomocyte response to autografts. Phagocytosis clears dead and injured tissue from graft or injury sites. Injured tissue attracts coelomocytes which ultimately form brown bodies. Autografts are self-tissue, therefore no foreign response is evoked and the graft heals without coelomocyte damage. (*After* Hostetter and Cooper, *Cont. Topics in Immunobiol.,* **4**: 91, 1974).

because of antigen stimulation become attached to surrounding organs, and the total coelomocyte population returns to normal. This aids in rapid coelomocyte accumulations at antigen sites; because of greater coelomocyte numbers, a more rapid destruction of foreign antigens ensues.

Earthworms are excellent invertebrates to use in the search for the phylogenetic origins of cell-mediated immunity. Their immune responses are easily measurable after immunization with foreign xenogeneic tissue antigens from other earthworms. Although earthworms show no humoral immunity to certain bacterial antigens (Cooper et al. 1969), the coelomocyte may possess interesting surface properties that would be useful in studying origins of receptors (Fig. 6-14). We would then be able to speculate less on how coelomocytes recognize foreign antigens introduced normally or experimentally into the coelom. Also, this would suggest how coelomocytes may function as the earthworm's policing system against other natural threats such as tumors and neoplastic changes (Cooper 1968c; Cooper and Baculi 1968b; Cooper 1969c). Finally, a new model would emerge for analyzing mechanisms of antigen recognition and the manner by which antigen-stimulated coelomocytes reproduce.

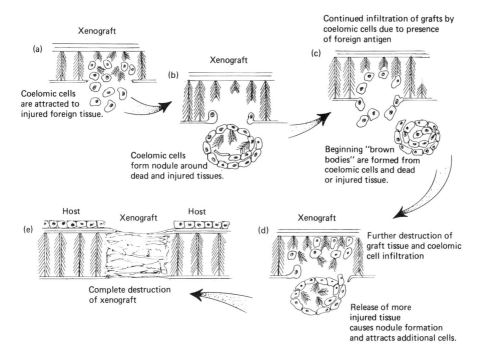

Fig. 6-13 Coelomocyte response to xenografts. Essentially the same first general non-specific reactions occur when coelomocytes recognize a foreign, *not-self* xenograft. However, the response is much more intense. Brown bodies are formed, but at least some of the coelomocytes continue to effect xenograft destruction leaving no transplant and only collagenous scar tissue. Coelomocytes then migrate elsewhere, carrying memory to effect a second-response after second-set transplantation. (*After* Hostetter and Cooper, *Cont. Topics in Immunobiol.,* **4**: 91, 1974).

Fig. 6-14 Hypothetical Model of Coelomocyte Recognition of Self vs. Not-Self Exemplified by Responses to Transplants (Primordial *T* Cell Response). Three representative coelomocyte types bearing receptors for allograft and xenograft antigens are at the left side. Coelomocytes have no recptors for *self* antigens, thus they are unable to recognize autografts. With regard to allografts, only few allo-antigens are present and correspondingly few specific coelomocyte receptors. Rejection is slow. Xenografts elicit strong recognition responses and ultimately rejection of all grafts due to many xenogeneic antigens. Such specificity, accompanied by memory, represents a primordial *T* cell response. Certain coelomocytes probably divide leaving daughter cells carrying memory information.

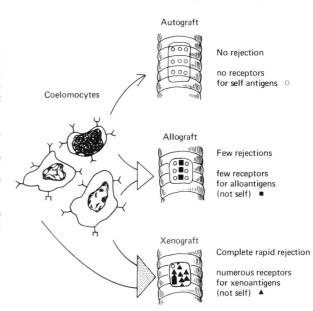

Hypothetical Model of Coelomocyte Recognition of Self — Not-Self Antigens Primordial T Cell Response

BIBLIOGRAPHY

Acton, R. T., Evans, E. E., Weinheimer, P. F., Cooper, E. L., Campbell, R. D., Prowse, R. H., Bizott, M., Stewart, J. E., Fuller, G. M., et al. 1972. Invertebrate immune defense mechanisms. MSS Information, New York.

Cooper, E. L. 1965a. Rejection of body wall xenografts exchanged between *Lumbricus terrestris* and *Eisenia foetida*. Am. Zool **5**: 665.

———. 1965b. Method of tissue grafting in the earthworm *Lumbricus terrestris*. Am. Zool. **5**: 254.

———. 1968a. Transplantation immunity in annelids. I. Rejection of xenografts exchanged between *Lumbricus terrestris* and *Eisenia foetida*. *Transplantation* **6**: 322.

Cooper, E. L., and Baculi, B. S. 1968b. Degenerative changes in the annelid, *Lumbricus terrestris*. *J. Geront.* **23**: 375.

Cooper, E. L. 1968c. Multinucleate giant cells, granulomata and "myoblastomas" in annelid worms. *J. Invert. Pathol.* **11**: 123.

———. 1969a. Specific tissue graft rejection in earthworms. *Science* **166**: 1414.

———. 1969b. Chronic allograft rejection in *Lumbricus terrestris*. *J. Exptl. Zool.* **171**: 69.

———. 1969c. Neoplasia and transplantation immunity in annelids. *J. Nat. Can. Inst.* **31**: 655.

Cooper, E. L., and Rubilotta, L. M. 1969. Allograft rejection in *Eisenia foetida*. *Transplantation* **8**: 220.

Cooper, E. L. 1970. Transplantation immunity in helminths and annelids. *Transpl. Proc.* **2**: 216.

———. 1971. Phylogeny of transplantation immunity. Graft rejection in earthworms. *Transpl. Proc.* **3**: 214.

———. 1973. Evolution of cellular immunity. In *Symposium on Non-Specific Factors Influencing Host Resistence*, eds. W. Braun and J. Ungar, p. 11. Basel: S. Karger.

———. 1973. Earthworm coelomocytes: Role in understanding the evolution of cellular immunity. I. Formation of monolayers and cytotoxicity. In *Proc. III international colloquium on invertebrate tissue culture*, eds. J. Rehácek, D. Blaskovic, W. F. Hink, p. 381. Bratislava: Publishing House of the Slovak Academy of Sciences.

———. 1974b. Phylogeny of leucocytes: Earthworm coelomocytes *in vitro* and *in vivo*. In *Proc. 8th leukocyte culture conference*, p. 155. University of Uppsala: Academic Press.

Du Pasquier, L., and Duprat, P. 1968. Aspects humoreaux et cellulaires d'une immunité naturelle non spécifique chez l'oligachéte *Eisenia foetida* sur (Lombricidae). C. R. Acad. Sci. Paris **266**: 538.

Duprat, P. 1964. Mise en evidence de reaction immunitaire dans les homogreffes de paroi du corps chez le Lombricien *Eisenia foetida*. C. R. Acad. Sci. Paris **259**: 4177.

———. 1967. Etude de la prise et du maintien d'un greffon de paroi du corps chez le lombricien *Eisenia foetida* typica. Ann. Inst. Past. **113**: 867.

Duprat-Chateaureynaud, P. 1970. Specificity of the allograft rejection in *Eisenia foetida*. In *Symposium on phylogeny of transplantation reactions*, eds. W. H. Hildemann and E. L. Cooper. *Trans. Proc.* **2**: 222.

———. 1971. Etude des reactions de défense de nature humorale chez le Lombricien *Eisenia foetida*. C. R. Acad. Sci. Paris **273**: 1647.

Duprat-Chateaureynaud, P., and Izoard, F. 1972. Etude *in vitro* de l'histocompatibilité chez les Lombriciens. C. R. Acad. Sci. Paris **275**: 2795.

Duprat, P., and Lassalle, A. M. 1967. Etude du liquide coelomique du Lombricien *Eisenia foetida* Sav. dans quelques cas experimentaux. C. R. Acad. Sci. Paris **264**: 386.

Hostetter, R. K., and Cooper, E. L. 1972. Coelomocytes as effector cells in earthworm immunity. *Immunol. Comm.* **1**: 155.

———. 1973. Cellular anamnesis in earthworms. *Cell. Immunol.* **9**: 384.

———. 1974. Earthworm cellular immunity. In *Contemporary Topics in Immunobiology*, **4**, 91, ed. E. L. Cooper. New York: Plenum Press.

Izoard, F. 1964. Evolution de greffes heteroplastiques de paroi du corps realisees, chez les Lombriciens, entre animaux de meme genre mais d'espéces differentes. Recherches sur le genre *Lumbricus*. C. R. Acad. Sci. Paris **258**: 5972.

Joest, E. 1897. Transplantationsversuche an Lumbriciden. Morphologie und physiologie der transplantationen. Archiv für Entwicklungsmechanik der Organismen **5**: 419.

Korschelt, E. 1896–8. Über regenerations und transplantations veguche an Lumbriciden. Verh. Deutsch. Zoolog. Gesellsch **6–8**: 79.

———. 1927a. Kapitel 7 Transplantations versuche an anneliden. Regeneration und Transplantation, Verlag von Gebrüder Borntraeger, Berlin 304.

———. 1927b. Regeneration und Transplantation. Verlag von Gebrüder Borntraeger, Berlin, 332.

———. 1929. Zur frage der morphogenetischen induktion nach transplantation. Archiv. f. Entwicklungsmechanik **117**: 1.

Leypoldt, H. 1911. Transplantationsversuche an Lumbriciden. Zur Beeinflussung der Regeneration eines kleinen Pfropfstückes durch einen grösseren Komponenten. Archiv. f. Entwicklungsmechanik **31**: 1.

Rabes, O., 1902. Transplantationsversuche an Lumbriciden. Archiv f. Entwicklungsmechanik. **13**: 239.

Valembois, P., 1963. Étude anatomique de l'évolution de greffons hétéroplastiques de paroi du corps chez quelques Lombriciens. C. R. Acad. Sci. Paris **257**: 3227.

———. 1968. Libération de phosphatase acide dans les cellules musculaires d'un greffon de paroi du corps chez un Lombricien. J. Microscopic. **7**: 61a.

———. 1970. Etude d'une heterogreffe de paroi du corps chez les Lombriciens. Aspects cytologiques, physiologiques et immunologiques de l'evolution du greffon (*Allolobophora caliginosa* Duges) et de la reaction du porte-greffe *Eisenia foetida* Sav. Study of heterografts of body wall in earthworms. Thesis for Doctor of Natural Science, No. 281 Bordeaux.

Chapter 7

The Machinery of the Immune System

Cells, Tissues, and Organs of the Immune System

The lymphoid organs are central to the immune system in generating cells that effect *integrated cellular and humoral immunity*. These organs are the thymus, the spleen, the lymph nodes, and various aggregations in mammals. In addition, these same organs and the bursa of Fabricius occur in birds. Among the fishes, amphibians, and reptiles, the thymus and spleen are present, but there are several additional lymphomyeloid organs. These are well defined, particularly in the anuran amphibians, and include the larval lymph gland, jugular, procoracoid, and prepericardial bodies of adults. Bone marrow, although primarily myeloid, is significant in the development of immune competence in all groups where it is present; it is absent in fishes, apodan, and larval anuran amphibians. Obviously, bone marrow function must be effected by other structure(s).

Lymphoid organs generate lymphocytes. Even in microdrops, lymph node cell suspensions are a heterogeneous population with several recognizable cell types. Small lymphocytes (68–71 %) are cells 5–8 μ in diameter with a relatively large nucleus rich in densely aggregated chromatin granules and a thin cytoplasmic rim. Medium lymphocytes are 8–10 μ in diameter with a more abundant cytoplasm than the small type and less compact chromatin arrangement in the nucleus (2–3 %). Immature plasma cells are 12–15 μ in diameter with an eccentric nucleus that contains diffusely dispersed chromatin granules and one or two nucleoli; the cytoplasm is basophilic with a clear area along one side of the nucleus (5–11 %). Mature plasma cells range from 8–14 μ in diameter with an eccentric nucleus; it possesses the characteristic cart-wheel arrangement of the chromatin and one or two small nucleoli. The cytoplasm is markedly basophilic and relatively more abundant than the immature types. Mature plasma cells also possess the characteristic clear area adjacent to the nucleus in the area of the cytocentrum. Often, mature plasma cells show two nuclei (5–9 %).

Stem or blast cells are large cells, 15–20 μ in diameter with intensely basophilic cytoplasm and a voluminous nucleus; a stem cell contains relatively scanty chromatin and multiple large nucleoli. It closely resembles the stem cell that gives rise to myeloid types in the marrow or, by other terminologies, lymphoblast, plasmablast or transitional cell (1–5 %). Reticulum cells are also large, 15–25 μ in diameter with an irregular outline, an oval shaped nucleus that contains scanty chromatin and abundant non-basophilic cytoplasm that sometimes has a foamy appearance (1–3 %). Finally,

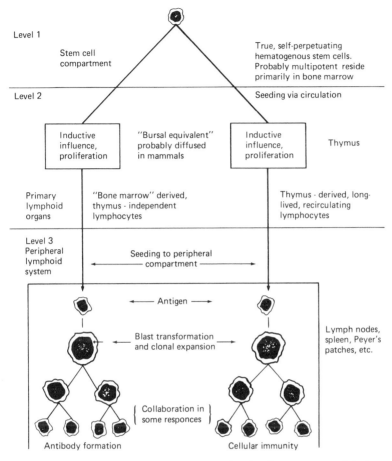

Level 1

Stem cell
compartment

True, self-perpetuating
hematogenous stem cells.
Probably multipotent reside
primarily in bone marrow

Level 2   Seeding via circulation

Inductive   "Bursal equivalent"   Inductive
influence,   probably diffused   influence,   Thymus
proliferation   in mammals   proliferation

Primary   "Bone marrow" derived,   Thymus - derived, long-
lymphoid   thymus - independent   lived, recirculating
organs   lymphocytes   lymphocytes

Level 3
Peripheral   Seeding to peripheral
lymphoid   ←————— compartment ——————→
system

←—— Antigen ——→

Blast transformation
and clonal expansion   Lymph nodes,
                                           spleen, Peyer's
                                           patches, etc.

            { Collaboration in }
            { some responces   }

Antibody formation   Cellular immunity

Fig. 7-1 A schematic overview of the three main functional compartments of the lymphoid system. (*From*: Nossal & Ada, 1971, *Antigens, Lymphoid Cells and the Immune Response.*)

granulocytes (3–9%) are cells with a kidney-shaped or lobulated nucleus and a cytoplasm crowded with distinct acidophilic granules.

Bone marrow gives rise to stem cells that can differentiate into erythrocytes, granulocytes, thrombocytes (involved in clotting), monocytes, plasma cells, and lymphocytes. Before their appearance in adult marrow, they originated from the yolk sac in the embryo or fetus. Stem cells, destined to participate chiefly in cellular immune reactions, are thought to pass through the thymus, where they receive the necessary "education" for becoming thymus-derived T cells. Stem cells that will differentiate into antibody-secreting B cells must receive further information by passing through the equivalent of the avian bursa of Fabricius. Thus, the immune system— of birds, mammals, and probably that of fishes, amphibians, and reptiles—is distributed throughout the body and is ubiquitous; however, it is basically a two-compartment system as outlined in Fig. 7-1. Such a precise bipartite system in fishes, amphibians, and reptiles requires clarification. Presumably there are strong resemblances, and, predictably, there should be divergence. With regard to phylogeny in general and invertebrates in particular, the T-type cell may emerge as the earliest lymphocyte giving evolutionary preeminence to cellular immune reactions.

The ways by which immunocompetent cells are identified are as important as their function. Both cell types (T and B cells) participate in two distinct kinds of immune reactions. First, tissue antigens such as foreign tissue grafts elicit T cell reactions or cell-mediated responses. It is not clear if antigen recognition occurs by means of cell surface antibody as receptors for detecting *self* vs. *not-self*. Second, soluble large protein antigens stimulate the humoral response. This occurs by activation of B cells or antibody-secreting cells.

Most organs of the immune system originated embryologically from either endoderm (thymus, bursa of Fabricius) or mesoderm (spleen); none are derived from ectoderm. Regardless of origin, the epithelium provides the first line of defense, and if this defense is broken, the underlying lymphocytes then react. Fichtelius (1970) suggests that immunity evolved with the invertebrate's ability to react to *not-self*, or antigens, on either their external or internal epithelial surfaces. According to this view, the coelom separates the outer body wall from that of the gastrointestinal tract, leaving the potential immunologically competent coelomocytes capable of reacting immediately to antigenic insult. Perhaps these lymphocytes, closely associated with the epithelium, particularly in the vertebrates, receive signals and from there, execute the instructions in other sites. This lymphoepithelial relationship is important to the study of the development of immunity.

Fänge (1966) considers the anterior kidney (or pronephros, an epithelial derivative common to all vertebrate excretory systems) to be an evolutionary precursor of certain lymphoid structures. Figure 7-2 exhibits the relationship between excretory tissues and those of the immune system. In addition to the excretory system, the digestive system, which is derived from endoderm, contributed to the differentiation of immunocompetent cells and tissues. In most animals, though, digestion and immunity evolved to become separate structural and functional systems. Vertebrates possess both the Von Kuppfer, or phagocytic, cells of the liver and the macrophages of the lymphomyeloid organs.

Cell, tissue, and organ components of representative immune systems are emphasized. Good and his group, pioneers in studies of the phylogenesis of immunity (Good et al. 1966), emphasized some of the anatomic features of the immune systems in the entire animal kingdom. In the invertebrates, a presentation of tissues and organs is, of course, limited because these are largely undetermined. Similarly, as there are

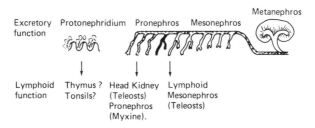

Fig. 7-2 Possible evolution of lymphoid structures from parts of the chordate excretory system. (*From*: Fange, 1966, *Phylogeny of Immunity*.)

many features of primitive vertebrates that have not been fully examined, there is an enormous need in phylogeny for further investigation into the sources of lymphoid cell precursors. With the exception of Chapter 11, all the other chapters of this book deal with some aspect of cell-mediated and humoral immunity.

REPRESENTATIVE EXAMPLES FROM THE ANIMAL KINGDOM

The Invertebrates: The Octopus

It is perhaps worthwhile at this point to present an example of an invertebrate organ that bears a morphological similarity to the immune organs of vertebrates. The absence of functional studies, long overdue, forces a histological description only. Surely there are similar organs in invertebrates that require description (Cooper, 1974). Leukocyte-forming organs have been described in tunicates, scorpions, and earthworms, but octopus "white bodies" have received more attention. Cowden (1972) renewed interest in these organs and offered concrete evidence for a discrete source of leukocytes (chiefly lymphocytes). The white body of cephalopod molluscs, located behind the eyes of *Octopus vulgaris*, is bilateral in the orbital pits of the cranial cartilages. The general structure of octopus white bodies bears a striking resemblance to descriptions of vertebrate lymphoid organs. The outer surface is covered with connective tissue. Encased within it is the medulla, composed of stem cells. These form strings separated by sinusoids where mature cells enter the circulation. Internally it is supported by a loose connective tissue network. This network is predominant on

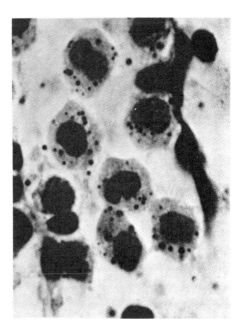

Fig. 7-3 "Mature" leukocytes as seen in touch preparations from *Octopus* white body; note presence of multiple basophilic cytoplasmic inclusions. (Azure A. Eosin B. *×1,025*.) (*From*: Cowden, *J. Invert. Pathol.*, **19**: 113, 1972.)

the outer surface, and, like the leukopoietic cell cords, it also traverses close to blood vessels.

Primary leukoblasts, the most primitive cells found in the cords, contain large vesicular nuclei, abundant cytoplasm rich in RNA, and yellowish brown inclusion droplets. Secondary and tertiary leukoblasts divide regularly, even *in vitro*, and possess deeply staining nucleoli. Mature leukocytes have nuclei of irregular shape similar to those of vertebrate monocytes, and imprints or sections reveal basophilic cytoplasmic inclusions (Fig. 7-3). Mature leukocytes are found chiefly in the sinusoids between the leukopoietic cell cords (Fig. 7-4). The octopus white body is intriguing; it awaits vigorous experimental analysis to elucidate its role in cellular and humoral immunity. The octopus may then be as important for comparative immunology as it is for comparative neurophysiology.

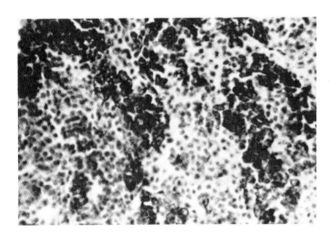

Fig. 7-4 A section near the center of the "white body" showing both strings of leukoblasts and extensive sinusoids containing "mature" leukocytes. (DNase, pH 4.0, azure B. ×*250*.) (*From*: Cowden, *J. Invert. Pathol.*, **19**: 113, 1972.)

Class Agnatha (Jawless Vertebrates); Order—Cyclostomata
(*the Most Primitive Vertebrates*)

The cyclostome (agnathan jawless) fishes are considered by most systematists to be the most primitive living vertebrates. These fishes have a single nostril, multiple hearts, and rudimentary eyes, but no stomach, jaws, or paired fins. Hemopoietic or blood-forming tissue in the California hagfish *Eptatretus stoutii* is reminiscent of the spleen, and is found in the *lamina propria* (epithelium and underlying connective tissue) along the entire length of the gut wall. This collection of cells consists of erythrocyte-like precursors, but there is no apparent evidence of plasma cells. Another focus of hemopoiesis, particularly for lymphoid cell activity, is found in the protovertebral arch, but here, too, plasma cells are absent. Even repeated stimulation with various antigens leads to no plasma cell development. Whether a primitive thymus appears just beneath the epithelium of the pharyngeal gutter between the second and fifth pharyngeal pouches, or is present in hagfishes at all, still remains a matter of controversy. Recently Riviere et al (1975) concluded that the hagfish thymus may be a part of an anterior pharyngeal muscle complex. Hagfish regularly destroy allografts and synthesize antibody to several antigens. Thus, despite the apparent absence of a typical vertebrate thymus, functional T cells are found some-place, as evidenced by graft rejection; B cell activity is evident by antibody synthesis. As will be detailed later, the hagfish is an immunologically competent animal, capable of both cellular and humoral responses when husbanded correctly.

There is actual morphological evidence for a possible evolution of lymphoid structures from the excretory system. According to Holmgren (1950) a hematopoietic organ in the hagfish *Myxine* is located in the derivative of the pronephros or anterior kidney. According to Fänge (1966) the cells possess at least all the appearances of lymphoid cells. What is lacking still is a thorough study using certain functional markers as a further definition of their lymphoid character.

Ammocoetes are larval or juvenile lampreys that live as mud-burrowing filter feeders; lampreys represent another group of cyclostomes. Their bodies contain several primitive hemopoietic centers similar to those of the hagfish. One focus is in the typhlosole, a spiral invagination of the midgut wall, roughly the location of the spleen; another focus is in the thymic area of the gill region.

Class Chondrichthyes (Cartilaginous Fishes)
    Subclass Elasmobranchii (sharks and related forms)

The primitive elasmobranchs exhibit a much more vigorous immune response than the agnatha; this naturally accompanies a more complicated morphology of their immune cells, tissues, and organs. The primitive ray (order Batoidea), *Rhino-batos productus*, is born with a fully developed discrete thymus. It is an encapsulated lymphoid organ located dorsal to the gill region, between the second and fifth gill bars. It consists of an outer *cortex* and an inner *medulla*. The spleen, at birth, is also an encapsulated organ composed of red and white pulp. Foci of lymphoid tissue, as white pulp, appear after a few weeks and surround the blood vessels. Additional accumulations of lymphoid cells are apparent in the gut, the renal parenchyma, and even the gonads. Rays can reject allografts and they produce serum antibodies; thus, manifestations of the two-compartment immune system are present, and at least for the thymus, the presumed source of T cells is structurally identifiable.

Both the horned shark *Heterodontus francisci* and the guitar fish *Rhinobatos productus* develop destructive, delayed necrotizing lesions after adjuvant stimulation. In addition to having all of the ray's immunologic characteristics, the horned shark has a family of lymphoid cells in the peripheral circulation. Lymphoid accumulations also occur in the anterior region of holocephalan fishes. The spleen of the newborn guitar fish contains large amounts of reticular, erythropoietic, and myelopoietic tissue. Lymphoid cells develop around small blood vessels, giving rise to white pulp. Although an epithelial rectal gland is found in these fishes in the same region as the avian bursa of Fabricius, it apparently lacks lymphoid cells, and it may be involved in the regulation of salt metabolism much like the nasal glands of birds.

Typical sharks (order Selachii) show advanced immune capabilities concomitant with more complex lymphoid differentiation. In the nurse and leopard sharks, a discrete lymphoid thymus is separated into cortex and medulla with bodies reminiscent of Hassall's corpuscles. The shark thymus corresponds to the histological appearance of the mammalian thymus divisible into cortex and medulla. Hassall's corpuscles, best known in mammals, are spherical epithelial structures found in the medulla and are closely associated with blood vessels; thymic corpuscles, or Hassall's corpuscles, are of disputed function. Conceivably, too, these bodies may be similar to the typical myoid cells of the amphibian and reptilian thymus as revealed in electron micrographs. The spleen is divided into red and white pulp. In addition, abundant lymphoid tissues occur in the gonads and gastrointestinal tract. Sharks are the first vertebrates in which plasma cells identical to those of mammals and birds are identifiable.

Subclass, Holocephalii (*Like Sharks Except for Presence of Operculum and Jaws Fused to Skull*)

The chimaeroids (Holocephalii) differ from ordinary Elasmobranchii in that they show similarities to extinct ptychodontids. According to Fänge's review (1966), the chimaeroids are unlike other elasmobranchs. They lack lymphoid tissue in their excretory systems; however they do possess a thymus and prominent lymph gland-like hemopoietic structures in the cranial region. There is a whitish gland-like organ found in the orbit of *Chimaera monstrosa* (from the depths near Espegrand, Norway). The organ has no distinct connective tissue capsule and it is penetrated by blood vessels. It contains three cell types: 1) small cells that cluster in groups, 2) large cells with prominent nucleoli, 3) cells containing numerous basophilic cytoplasmic inclusions. These three types resemble small lymphocytes, blast cells, and monocytes. In a later work, Fänge and Sundell (1969) conclude that lymphocytopoiesis takes place in the spleen, the cranial lymphomyeloid tissue, the thymus, and possibly in other less well defined lymphomyeloid structures. Although the animals are rare, a further investigation of this structure, emphasizing functional characteristics, is necessary.

Class Osteichthyes (*Advanced Bony Fishes*)
Subclass Actinopterygii (*ray-finned fishes*)
Superorder Chondrostei (*primitive ray-finned fishes*)

The paddlefish, *Polyodon spathula*, possesses a highly developed hematopoietic system. It is capable of antibody formation with primary and secondary responses and it can readily reject allografts. The paddlefish's thymus, too, is well developed; it is organized into lobes and lobules. Structures that may represent primitive Hassall's corpuscles are obvious. The presence of small and medium thymic lymphocytes (thymocytes), as well as large, blast-like cells, is circumstantial evidence that such cells are immunologically competent. Among the lymphocytes, large cells are the least differentiated. Although small lymphocytes were once considered to be fully differentiated and effete, they can dedifferentiate and divide by mitosis in the presence of antigens or mitogens. Blast cells can then divide further and differentiate in directions that produce immune reactivities.

The spleen is divided into a red and white pulp. A bone marrow precursor is situated over the base of the heart in association with the atrium and ventricle. Various stages in plasma cell and lymphocyte differentiation are also found in this tissue. Plasma cells proliferate heavily in *Polyodon*, and this correlates with intense antibody production to a wide variety of antigens. Furthermore, repeated antigenic stimulation results in the active participation of eosinophils, one of the three types of vertebrate granular leukocytes. This seems peculiar, since eosinophils increase during parasitic infections in mammals. Evidently the same cell structurally may often function differently at two levels of phylogeny.

Superorder Holostei (ray-finned fishes from the Mesozoic)

In the bowfin, *Amia calva*, the thymus is divided into cortex and medulla, but it appears to be less complex than in the previously described fishes; this remains to be confirmed. The spleen is similar in morphology to that of the chondrosteans, and plasma cells are typical, with the basophilic cytoplasm and nuclear chromatin condensed toward the periphery.

Superorder Teleostei (Cenozoic and recent times)

The teleosts are endowed with a thymus, spleen, and subsidiary discrete lymphocyte aggregations accumulated in an interesting organ, the *pronephros* or *head*

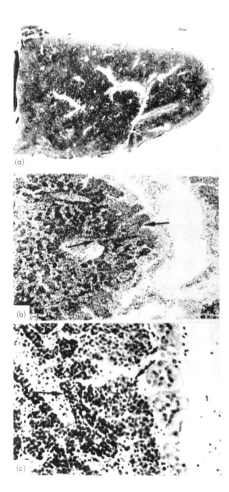

Fig. 7-5 Sections of one pronephros of adult *Lepomis*. (a) section at low magnification showing the predominant lympho-reticular composition of the pronephros and the large vascular channels. (b) cord-like arrangement of lympho-reticular tissue, arrows pointing right in this section and section (c) point to the lymphoid component while the arrows to the left point to the reticular component. Note the renal cuboidal epithelium to the right of the reticular tissue. Note sinusoidal character of the lympho-reticular tissue in (b) and (c). (Magnifications (a) ×35; (b) ×105; (c) ×250.) (From Smith et al., *J. Immunol.*, **99**: 876, 1967.)

kidney. Plasma cells that secrete antibody are present, and there are lymphoid cells capable of eliciting cellular immune responses. In *L. macrochirus,* the bluegill, the spleen and the pronephros are active sites of antibody synthesis. The pronephros contains more antibody-releasing cells than the spleen, which seems to be a consequence of its more prominent lymphoreticular morphology. The cellular architecture of the pronephros is markedly similar to that of mammalian lymph nodes. This implies its phylogenetic involvement in the filtration of tissue fluids and in antibody formation. The teleost pronephros may, in fact, represent a prototype of the mammalian lymph node (Fig. 7-5).

Class Amphibia [Tetrapods (Largely Terrestrial), Anamniote Development]
  Subclass Lissamphibia (modern, smooth skinned)
    Order Apoda (worm-like, burrowing types)

Graft rejection is one of the first experimental studies of any kind to be performed on the *apodans* or *legless amphibians.* Garcia-Herrera and Cooper (1968) found that at least three organs, the liver, spleen, and thymus, are involved in the production of leukocytes. Liver hemopoiesis especially involves the production of granulocytes. The spleen shows typical lymphoid and myeloid cells. The thymus is composed of a parenchyma consisting of lymphocytes and reticular cells; reticular cells and their thinly drawn-out processes provide support for lymphocytes. Acidophil bodies are present in the typical medulla and are reminiscent of mammalian Hassall's corpuscles.

Order Urodela (Salamanders and Newts with Many Degenerate Characteristics)

The thymus in the metamorphosed axolotl lies under the skin in front of the muscles that move the gill arches. With regard to development in some salamanders such as *Amblystoma,* only the first five visceral pouches that are derived from endoderm develop buds. As illustrated in Fig. 7-6, the first two buds degenerate. Note,

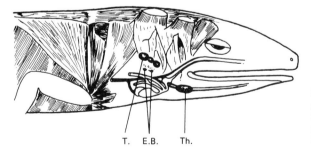

T.   E.B.   Th.

Fig. 7-6 Diagram of the head of an adult *Ambystoma* showing position of the thymus. *e.b.,* epithelial bodies; *t.,* thymus; *th.,* thyroid glands and associate blood vessels. (*From:* Noble, 1931, *The Biology of the Amphibia.*)

too, that the epithelial bodies are considered to be components of the lymphomyeloid system. Usually, three thymi are situated on each side of the body. The thymus in the salamander lies immediately under the skin in the posterior margin of the parotid glands. It is irregular in shape and is divided by connective tissue into separate, or even groups of lobules. In *Triturus,* the thymus lies directly under the skin near the posterior ends of the hyoids and has a compact, uniform shape.

Order Anura (Frogs and Toads)

Anuran amphibians are in a unique position in evolution, for they have structural and functional similarities to fishes, reptiles, birds, and mammals; with regard to organs of the immune system the anuran larva most closely resembles those of fish. Evolutionary precursors of the entire array of lymphoid and myeloid organs in mammals are first apparent in anuran amphibians. These are the thymus, spleen, and extralymphoid organs suggestive of mammalian hemal nodes; bone marrow appears after anurans metamorphose into adults. As they have been subjects of a great deal of investigation, the discussion here is quite detailed and representative of most vertebrates.

The frog spleen is a reddish, bean-shaped body lying dorsal to the anterior end of the cloaca and attached to the supporting mesentery. It receives blood from a branch of the anterior mesenteric artery and releases it through the splenic vein. Both vessels enter the spleen at a common point called the *hilus*, which lies at the concave end opposite the rounded convex surface. The spleen is surrounded by a fibrous membrane, the outside of which is coated by the peritoneum. The internal structure is composed of splenic white pulp, which in turn is made up of several cell types repre-

Table 7-1

Terminology of lympho-myeloid and lympho-epithelial organs in certain anuran amphibia

Older names employed	Proposed new term for organ	Stage in development where best observed
Dorsal or subthymic tonsils (paired)		Larvae: *Rana fusca*
Corpus lymphaticum		Tadpole and adult *Rana esculenta*
Dorsal cavity body		42 day old larvae *Rana temporaria*
Lymph gland	LM1	Larvae
Dorsal gill remnant		Larvae: *Bufo, Rana;* Adults: *Bufo*
Glandula interposita or inclusa		Larvae, adults: *Rana esculenta, tigrina, ribunda, mugiens, occidentalis*
Ventral cavity bodies		Larvae
Ventral tonsils (paired)	LM2	Larvae: *Rana fusca*
Anterior gill remnant		
Lymphatic ganglion		
Jugular body		
Kiemenreste	LM3	Adults
Pseudothyroid		
Ventral gill remnant		
Corpus lymphaticum		
Median or pre-epiglottic tonsils (unpaired)		Larvae: *Rana fusca*
Middle gill remnant	LM4	Larvae: *Bufo, Rana*; Adults: *Bufo*
Epithelial bodies	LM5	Adults
Corpus prepericardiale		
Prepericardial body	LM6	Adults
Corpus procoracoidale		
Procoracoid body	LM7	Adults
Glandula interpositas or inclusa		

From: Cooper, *Morph.,* **122**: 381, 1967.

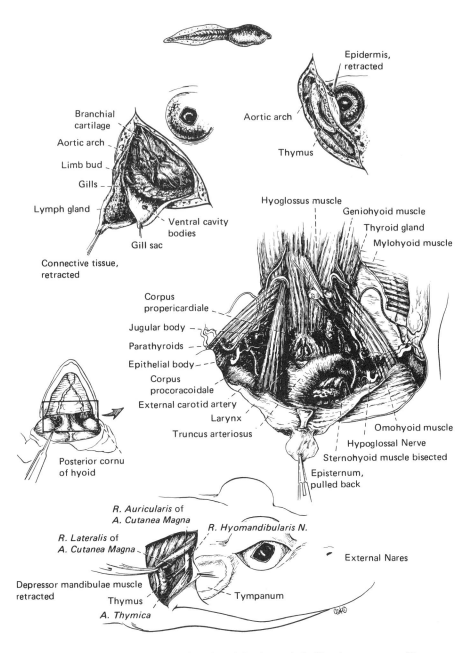

Fig. 7-7 This figure shows the location of the thymus in bullfrog larvae at stage 25. Note the relationship of the thymus to other branchial structures, ear and eye. The thymus in the adult frog is located in close proximity to the muscles of the head and pectoral girdle and the tympanic membrane. The branchial region reveals two types of lympho-myeloid organs found in bullfrog larvae at stage 25. Note the large pear-shaped lymph gland located close to the developing anterior limb. Also enclosed within the gill basket in the ventral region are several smaller nodules (ventral cavity bodies). In the same region can be seen the gills and aortic arches. In this section the lymphomyeloid organs are located in the neck and lower jaw region of an adult bullfrog. One pair (prepericardial bodies) lies anterior and lateral to the larynx. A second pair (procoracoid bodies) is located just anterior to the truncus arteriosus. Lateral to the sternohyoid muscle near the insertion of the geniohyoid and posterior end of the hyoid apparatus are the large jugular bodies. The fourth pair (epithelial bodies) is lateral to the previous organ near the parathyroid glands. (*From*: Cooper, 1967, *Ontogeny of Immunity*.)

senting different periods in lymphocyte development. As the spleen is a site for the deposition of worn-out cells captured by phagocytosis, erythrocytes are found in various stages of degeneration. Large numbers of melanocytes or black pigment cells are present, a condition typical of amphibian internal organs. The distinction between red and white pulp is apparent, but well-defined germinal centers in the white pulp, equivalent to those of mammalian spleen, are lacking. Removal of the spleen in adult *Rana pipiens* does not lead to a prolonged survival of allografts; in other words, grafts are rejected normally, suggesting the absence of splenic T cells. However, splenectomy inhibits antibody synthesis, implicating the spleen as a major producer of antibody-secreting or B cells.

The thymus of adult frogs is a three-lobed structure, perhaps formed by a fusion of the three embryonic endodermal buds from which it is derived. Its position, just posterior to the eye, remains essentially unchanged, even after metamorphosis. However, the lymphomyeloid organs comprising LM 1-7 (Table 7-1) are associated with the branchial cavity and gills as larval structures. At metamorphosis these organs disappear or contribute to the formation of adult structures situated in the ventral neck region. The anterior head organs of a typical anuran, the bullfrog, is represented during larval and adult stages of development in Fig. 7-7.

Normal development of lymphoid organs in amphibians is typified by the condition in *Xenopus laevis*, the clawed toad. The thymus, the first of all the lymphoid organs to develop, arises from a thickening in the dorsal portion of the visceral pouches; these later become epithelial. All amphibian development, like that of any vertebrate, is described by stages defined by some obvious physical condition, for example, limb development; different authors use arbitrary numbers. Manning and Horton (1969) described the thymic analagen at stage 42 as still contiguous with the pharyngeal epithelium of the second branchial pouch. As can be seen in Fig. 7-8, small lymphocytes are conspicuous in the thymus at stage 49, and the cortex and medulla appear at stage 51. At stages 45–46 the spleen anlaga is a well-defined condensation of cells in the dorsal mesogastrium. Differentiation into red and white pulp occurs at stages 47–48. The anlaga, or developmental precursor of the ventral cavity bodies, can be distinguished at stage 49. Furthermore, there are signs of blood cell formation in the liver and mesonephros. As Fig. 7-9 indicates, by stage 50 the spleen and ventral cavity bodies have greatly increased in size and exhibit pronounced lymphoid differentiation.

A feature of special interest in the clawed toad and other amphibians and even in fishes, in contrast to mammals, is the presence of antibody-forming cells in the thymus. In mammals, antibody production by the thymus must be a consequence of injecting antigen directly into the organ. However, active antibody secretion by the thymus seems to be a characteristic of fishes and amphibians, not birds or mammals (see Chap. 14). The thymus in young *Xenopus* at one point in its life history is the only functioning lymphoid organ. For example, when lymphocytes in the *Xenopus* thymus and no other place are fully mature, they invade foreign tissue grafts. Organs with phagocytic cells, such as lymph nodes, are not present. Turner found that carbon injections sequestered only by the spleen and liver seem to represent a more primitive system than that of either *Rana* or *Bufo* (Fig. 7-10), where carbon-trapping lymphomyeloid organs are present (Turner 1969).

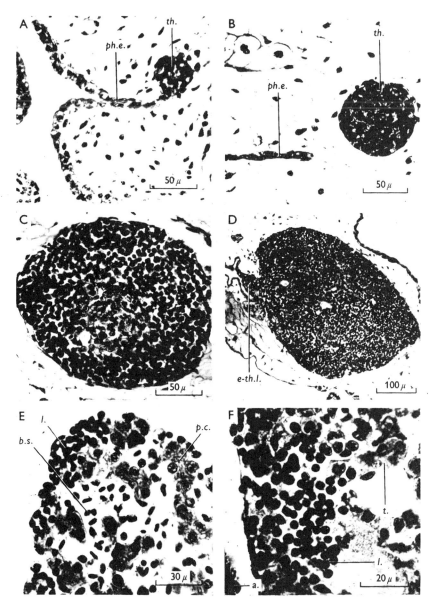

Fig. 7-8 (a) Pharynx of a stage-42 larva in the region of the left second branchial pouch; the thymus bud is still in continuity with the pharyngeal epithelium. (b) Thymus of a stage-48 larva; the thymus is now detached. *ph.e.*, Pharyngeal epithelium; *th.*, thymus. (c) Thymus of a stage-49 larva showing cortico-medullary differentiation. (d) Thymus of a stage-54 larva showing the fully differentiated cortex and medulla. This section also shows an extra-thymic accumulation of lymphocytes in the area of the pharyngeal epithelium. *e-th.l.*, Extra-thymic accumulation of lymphocytes. (e) Liver of a stage-51 larva; groups of lymphocytes can be seen at the periphery. *b.s.*, Liver sinuses with blood cells. *l.*, lymphocytes. *p.e.* cells of the liver parenchyma. (f) Mesonephros of a stage-59 larva showing lymphocytes in the medial wall. a., Wall of the dorsal aorta, *l.*, lymphocytes, *t.*, cells of the kidney tubule. (*From:* Manning & Horton, *J. E. E. M.,* **22**: 265, 1969.)

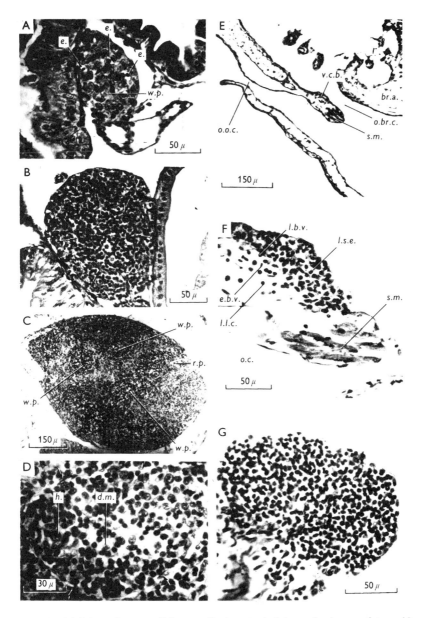

Fig. 7-9 (a) Spleen of a stage-48 larva. *e.*, Erythrocytes in future red pulp; *w.p.*, future white pulp. (b) Spleen of a stage-50 larva showing the white pulp with many small lymphocytes. The white pulp is delimited by the boundary layer. Arrows to boundary layer *ce.* (c) Spleen of a stage-59 larva showing the distribution of red pulp and white pulp; *r.p.*, red pulp; *w.p.*, white pulp. (d) One of the white pulp areas shown in (c) seen at a higher magnification. Some lymphocytes predominate within the white pulp and also extend beyond boundary layer into the red pulp. Arrows to boundary layer cells. *d.m.*, Degenerate macrolymphocyte, *h.*, nucleus of a haemocytoblast. (e) Pharynx of a stage-49 larva in the region of the right opercular opening showing the *anlage* of the second right ventral cavity body, *br.a.* Cartilage of the tri-branchial arch; *o.br. c.*, opening of the second branchial chamber into the opercular cavity; *o.o.c.*, opening of the opercular chamber; *s.m.*, third subarcualis muscle; *v.c.b.*, *anlage* of second right ventral cavity body. (f) Second ventral cavity body of a stage-50 larva; lymphocytes are now present in the organ. *c.b.v.*, Erythrocyte in blood vessel; *i.b.v.*, lymphocyte in blood vessel; *l.l.c.*, lymphocyte in lymphatic channel; *l.s.e.*, subepithelial accumulation of lymphocytes; *o.c.*, opercular chamber; *s.sm.*, third subarcualis muscle. (g) First ventral cavity body of a stage-56 larva; the organ now contains many lymphocytes and has reached its maximum development. (*From*: Manning & Horton, *J. E. E. M.*, **22**: 265, 1969.)

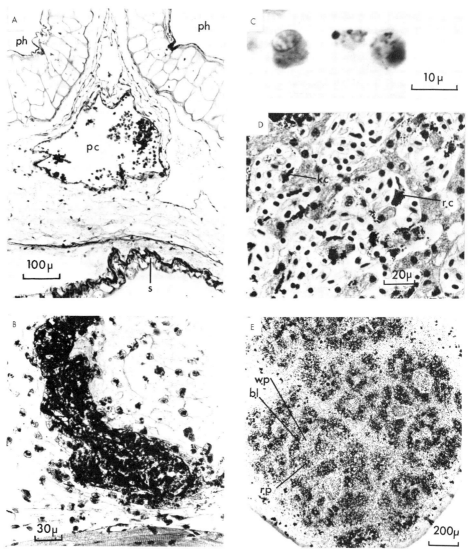

Fig. 7-10 (a) Photomicrograph of a stage-59 tadpole 24 hours after intraperitoneal injection of carbon, taken through the region of the pericardium just anterior to the heart (*p.c.*, pericardial cavity; *p.h.*, pharynx; *s.*, skin). Note the large population of macrophages in the pericardial cavity; some of these cells contain densely packed carbon granules. (b) Stage 57 tadpole, 24 hours after injection of carbon through the interhyoideus muscle (bottom of figure) into the connective tissue of the region just anterior to that depicted in (a). The carbon mass is enclosed in "pocket" of connective tissue, and a large number of macrophages, some containing carbon, can be seen surrounding it. (c) Pericardial macrophages of a stage-48 tadpole, 24 hours after intraperitoneal carbon injection. The cell on the left shows a typical excentric elliptical necleus; some carbon is seen in the cytoplasm of the other cells. (d) Adult liver after uptake of carbon injected via the dorsal lymph sac. Note that some carbon (shown as long, flattened, black aggregations) is in Kupffer cells, *k, c,* but that some of it is in rounder cells, *r.c.,* of less certain origin. (e) Spleen of adult 24 hours after injection of carbon into the dorsal lymph sac, showing selective localization of particules. A ring of heavily aggregated carbon can be seen surrounding each white pulp island, *w.p.*; the clear areas which can be seen within the dense rings are the red pulp sinuses, *r.p.* The white pulp and the boundary layer, *b.l.,* are almost or completely clear. (*From*: Turner, *J. Anat.,* **108**: 13, 1971).

Class Reptilia (Amniotes with no Avian or Mammalian Characteristics)
Thymic Development

With regard to lymphoid organ development, the thymus of reptiles is unique. The reptilian thymus, like that of fish, amphibians, and birds, originates from the germ layer endoderm that produces thymic primordia, which are dorsal outgrowths of the pharyngeal walls. By contrast, the mammalian thymus differentiates from ventral outgrowths. Even among the reptiles, the thymus can differ in origin. The thymus of lizards, snakes, and turtles each develops from different pairs of the five pharyngeal pouches.

One other interesting feature of the amphibian and reptilian thymus is the presence of the so-called myoid cells. With ordinary light microscopy, myoid cells appear to be many times the diameter of thymocytes. Since the nineteenth century, myoid cells have been referred to by a variety of names. Some investigators stressed their superficial resemblence to mammalian Hassall's corpuscles. Hassall's corpuscles, found in the medulla of the mammalian thymus, consist of concentrically arranged epithelial reticular cells that are acidophilic, i.e., sensitive to the red stain eosin. Myoid cells are also found in the medulla as distinct cell types. It is with the use of electron microscopy that myoid cell morphology has been elucidated more clearly. In reptiles, myoid cells are actually muscle cells. They may be round or highly elongated with a centrally placed nucleus. The myofibrils are arranged circumferentially around the nucleus and these are composed of thick and thin myofilaments like those of skeletal muscle. It is assumed that the muscle elements represent differentiations from embryonic mesenchyme, which also contribute to thymic differentiation.

Of significance to clinical immunology is the possible relationship of myoid cells and the autoimmune disease, myasthenia gravis. *Autoimmunity* is a state of immunity against *self* components resulting, often, in the development of a disease. Ordinarily individuals do not react against *self* components. In some patients with myasthenia gravis, serum gamma globulins containing antibodies react against the antigens of mammalian skeletal and cardiac muscle, as well as reptilian thymic myoid cells. One can envision how important amphibians and reptiles could be for studying the evolutionary development of a disease.

Subclass Anapsida (Without Temporal Opening)
Order Chelonia (the turtles)

Borysenko and Cooper (1972) found that the thymus and spleen of the snapping turtle, *Chelydra serpentina*, are similar to those of other ectothermic vertebrates. Certain gut-associated lymphoid aggregates suggest the presence of reptilian equivalents of tonsils and Peyer's patches reminiscent of mammalian GALT (gut-associated lymphoid tissues). Those found in the cloaca may be ancestral to the avian bursa of Fabricius. Lymphoid aggregates located in the axillary and inguinal regions are apparent for the first time in the ectothermic vertebrate lung and kidney (Figs. 7-11—7-15). In another turtle, *Pseudemys scripta*, lymphoid nodules and diffuse lymphocytic infiltration are common in the urinary bladder just beneath the epithelium. In addition to lymphocytes, plasma cells are present, but germinal centers are absent. The snapping turtle is not deficient in lymphoid tissue, although there is a conspicuous

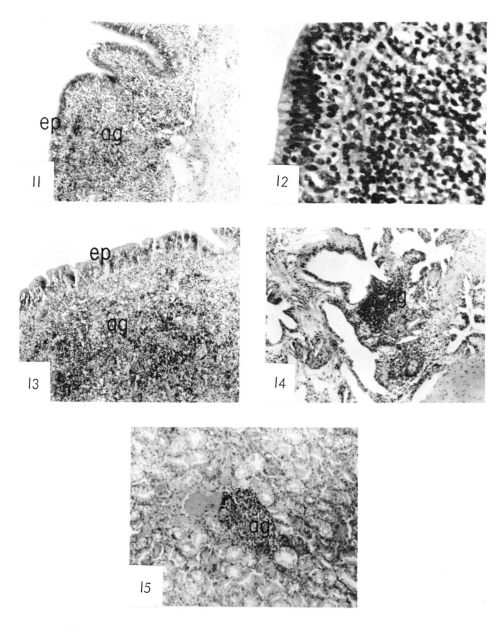

Fig. 7-11 A lymphoid cell aggregate, *ag*, in the ileum. Note that the lymphocye accumulation is extensive, filling the connective tissue space (lamina propria) beneath the epithelium, *ep*. (×75).

Fig. 7-12 Higher magnification of part of Fig. 7-11. (×300).

Fig. 7-13 A lymphoid cell aggregate, *ag*, in the cloaca. Here the cellular accumulations are extensive, although only the area of the lamina propria directly beneath the epithelium, *ep*, is shown. (×75).

Fig. 7-14 A small lymphoid cell aggregate, *ag*, in the lung. (×75).

Fig. 7-15 A small lymphoid cell aggregate, *ag*, in the kidney. (×75). (*From*: Borysenko & Cooper, *J. Morphol.*, **138**: 487, 1972.)

absence of typical germinal centers, which are characteristic of mammalian organs. Still these lymphoid aggregations are of particular interest, since they may represent ancestors of true lymph nodes in analogous locations in mammals.

Subclass Lipidosauria
   Order Squamata (Lizards and Snakes)

The structure of the spleen in the garden lizard, *Calotes versicolor*, may be unique. A definite demarcation into red and white pulp is absent, a slight departure from earlier examples. The normal spleen consists of an outer thin capsule and an inner splenic pulp. Splenic pulp is darkly stained and extends continuously throughout the spleen, but it also contains several scattered, lightly stained areas. Dense accumulations of lymphocytes comprise the darkly stained area, composed further of fixed macrophages and narrow blood spaces filled with erythrocytes. This portion of the spleen is comparable to the white pulp of mammals and constitutes the lizard's white pulp. One important distinction, though, is its lack of organization into discrete follicles. The light areas contain reticular cells that enclose arterioles. According to Kanakambika and Muthukkaruppan (1972), the typical red pulp as found in mammals is absent.

The gecko, *Gehyra variegata*, is interesting because of the discovery by Johnston (1973) of lymphoid tissue in the axillae closely associated with the lymphatic and blood systems. Within the perivascular space, a part of the lymphatic system, perivascular lymphoid tissue occurs in both axillary sinuses. This lymphoid tissue invests the veins draining the body wall as they cross the axillary sinus to join the lateral vein (Fig. 7-16). As in all lymphoid tissues gecko lymphocytes are provided with an internal support composed of reticular cells and fibers (Fig. 7-17).

The axillary sinus, because of its location, may be continuous with the lateral lymphatics; it is lined with endothelium. All lymphatics and blood vessels are lined by simple squamous, flattened epithelial cells, through which mobile leukocytes can squeeze by diapedesis. Lymph is carried in the lateral lymphatics, flows into the sinus, and bathes the vein and the perivascular lymphoid tissue before continuing to

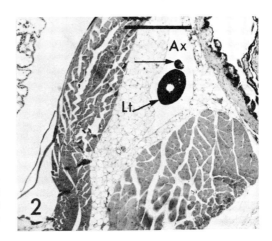

Fig. 7-16 A small vein (*arrow*) from the body wall is here sectioned transversely as it crosses the axillary sinus, *ax*, to join the lateral vein which is invested by lymphoid tissue, *lt*. (*From*: Johnston, *J. Morphol.*, **139**: 431, 1973).

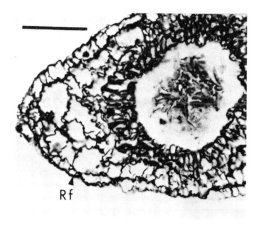

Rf

Fig. 7-17 The appearance of the reticular fiber network within the perivascular lymphoid tissue following impregantion with silver. Erythrocytes are seen in the lumen of the laterial vein. (Scale, 0.05 mm.) (From: Johnston, J. Morphol, **139**: 437, 1973).

the lymphatico-venous junction. Such an arrangement represents a fundamental difference in structure and function between the gecko's organs and analogous amphibian organs; these are blood filtering, and all blood cells, erythrocytes, and leukocytes must pass through such organs. Of even more importance to immunity is how mature lymphocytes can enter either of the systems. The difference lies in the fact that the lymph on the lymphatic end should consist only of lymphocytes, with no myeloid leukocytes or granulocytes, or erythrocytes. Thus, in regard to lymph filtration the gecko lymph nodule is closer to that of mammals.

The axillary position of the gecko node-like structure, interesting as it is, calls to mind such locations of primary nodes in mammals; primary nodes lack germinal centers. The basic architecture of the gecko node, i.e., lymphoid tissue, supported by a reticular framework surrounding a blood vessel and all enclosed within a lymphatic, confirms its striking similarity to that of the monotreme mammal, the echidna (see Mammalia). In the snake *Elaphe*, lymphoid tissue occurs in the wall of the cardinal lymphatic, giving it superficial resemblance to nodes in the domestic fowl (Kotani 1959; Biggs 1957). Modern analyses of reptilian lymphoid organs raises the issue of the possible evolution of avian and mammalian lymph nodes from a common extant reptilian ancestor.

Class Aves (Winged Archeosaur Descendents with Feathers and Temperature Control)
  Subclass Neornithes (Modern Birds)
    Superorder Neognathae (Birds Other than Ostrich-like Birds)

The immune system of birds is no more complex than that of amphibians or reptiles, if we compare only the number of lymphoid organs present in each group. Yet, since the T and B concept was derived from studies of the avian immune system, the immediate impression is that birds are more complex; this is not the case. Earlier descriptions of the avian immune system stressed the morphology of the thymus, bursa of Fabricius, and spleen. Birds do possess bone marrow, ubiquitous subcutaneously located patches of lymphoid aggregations, and others found in association with the gut. According to Kampmeier (1969) the lymph nodes of birds, unlike mammalian nodes, apparently offer little resistance to lymph flow. Avian nodes are elongate and occur as an enlargement of a lymphatic. The afferent and efferent vessels are at opposite ends of the structure. There is a central lymphatic sinus bordered by dense lymphoid tissue containing germinal centers; loose lymphoid tissue occurs at the periphery.

Recently a lymphoid aggregation was described by Mueller, et al. (1971) in association with the eye. This organ, the gland of Harder, is dorsal and anterior to the optic nerve, medial to the eyeball and overlapped by an eye muscle. It is flattened against the eyeball and positioned more medially at its ventral end than at its dorsal end. A thin duct is attached anteriorly and runs ventrally toward the anterior wall of the orbit (Fig. 7-18). In a fourteen-week-old chicken the gland measures approximately $15 \times 15 \times 1$ mm; it grows in size with age. Histologically, the Harderian gland shows a progressive increase with age in methyl green pyronin-staining cells, lymphocytes, and plasma cells. This stain is specific for the cytoplasmic endoplasmic reticulum of antibody synthesizing cells. In fact, within the gland, germinal centers reminiscent of those found in the spleen and caecal tonsil increase in size up to approximately

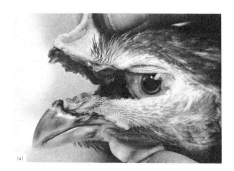

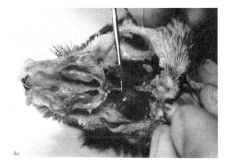

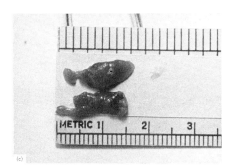

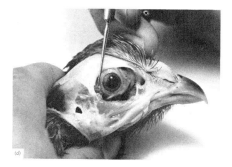

Fig. 7-18 Gross photographs of 10-week old NHR chickens showing (a) the location of an incision through the nasal bone to expose the gland of Harder, (b) the pointer beneath the gland of Harder and above the eyeball, (c) the excised Harderian glands, and (d) the pointer at the anterior edge of the lacrimal gland. (*From*: Mueller, et al., *Cell. Immunol.*, **2**: 140, 1971).

fourteen weeks of age. The normal pattern of pyronin-positive cell development is dependent on the presence of the bursa of Fabricius. Birds that have been chemically bursectomized, by dipping an egg on the third day of incubation in a testosterone proprionate alcohol solution, show pronounced depletion of pyronin-positive cells in the Harderian gland. Another organ, the lacrimal gland, is located posterior to and slightly dorsal to the posterior lateral eye fold, and is more firmly attached to the orbital wall than the eyeball. It is small, measuring approximately $3 \times 2 \times 1$ mm in eight-week-old chickens. The histology is basically similar to the gland of Harder.

The thymus in birds is best exemplified by Fig. 7-19. Here the characteristic multilobulated condition of the avian thymus is obvious. These lobulations can be traced to early developmental stages (Fig. 7-20). This is best evident during lympho-blastic transformation coincident with mesenchymal condensation and formation of the dense connective tissue capsule. The whole organ is in the neck region in close contact with the jugular veins on either side, reminiscent of the position of the jugular body in the neck of adult anuran frogs. The thymus of normal two-month-old antigen-stimulated chicks shows a fairly uniform group of thymocytes; when compared with lymphocytes from the bursa of Fabricius, they are considerably smaller (Fig. 7-21). Thymic lymphocytes show a thin rim of cytoplasm that surrounds a nucleus with densely clumped chromatin material.

The bursa of Fabricius is a lymphoid organ attached to the dorsal surface of the proctodaeum of birds. As is well known, it plays a vital role in the development of antibody potential during the earliest period of a bird's life. In the mallard duck, when dissected the bursa appears grossly as shown in Fig. 7-22 at approximately three weeks post hatching. A cross section reveals that it is surrounded by a serosa and muscle layers, but the most striking feature is the large number of lymphoid

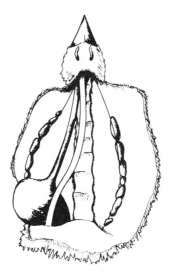

Fig. 7-19 A sketch of the open neck region of the chick showing the position of the thymus lobes lining the jugular veins on either side of the neck. (*After*: Aspinall et al., *J. Immunol.*, **90**: 872, 1963).

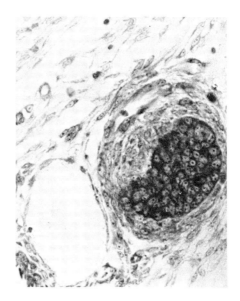

Fig. 7-20 The association of the developing thyms, *t*, the condensation of the capsular mesenchyme, *m*, the jugular vein, *j*, is illustrated. Note the deeply basophilic lymphoblastic cell (*arrow*) present in the central portion of the thymus and the absence of similar cells or lymphocytes in the surrounding connective tissues; vascularity is limited to the periphery of the thymic capsular connective tissue. The indentation of the thymic tissue represents the first evidence of lobular formation. $7\frac{1}{2}$ day chick embryo. (Formol-sublimate-acetic fixation. Giemsa stain. ×*180*.) (*From*: Ackerman & Knouff, *Anat. Rec.*, **149**: 191, 1964).

follicles (Fig. 7-23). At the end of sixteen days of development in the chick, developing follicles of the bursa show endodermal cells from which it, like the thymus, is derived. Furthermore, there is a full array of cells: blast types and even differentiated lymphocytes of various sizes (Fig. 7-24). At two months of age the chicken bursa of Fabricius is composed of numerous discrete lymphoid follicles. Each follicle is further subdivided into a cortex and medulla separated by a thin layer of epithelial cells and

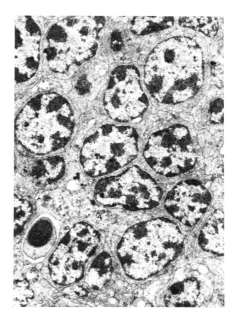

Fig. 7-21 Thymus of a normal 2-month-old antigen-stimulated chicken. This population of thymic lymphocytes does not range in size as widely as those of the bursa of Fabricius. Most of these cells contain a relatively thin rim of cytoplam surrounding a nucleus with densely clumped chromatin material. Large blastoid-appearing cells, found in the bursa of this same bird were not found in the thymus. (×*5,280*). (*From*: Clawson et al., *Lab. Invest.*, **16**: 407, 1967).

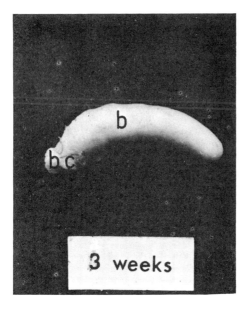

Fig. 7-22 Bursa from a mallard 3 weeks old. (*b*, bursa; *b.c.*, bursal canal). (*From*: Ward & Middleton, *Canad. J. Zool.*, **49**: 11, 1971).

a well-delineated basement membrane. Lymphocytes from both the cortex and medulla of the bursa vary in size from 4 to 8μ (Fig. 7-25). Small or large bursal cells have proportionate amounts of cytoplasm. Chromatin in the smaller cells is more clumped than it is in the large cells. The cytoplasm of small lymphocytes shows predictably fewer organelles in comparison with the larger cells; these larger cells

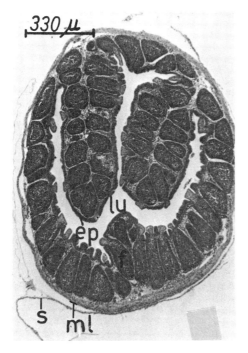

Fig. 7-23 Photomicrograph of the cross section of a mallard bursa illustrating serosa (*s*), muscle layers (*m.l.*), lymphoid follicles (*f*), lumen (*lu*) and epithelial layer (*ep*). H and E (haematoxylin and eosin). (*From*: Ward & Middleton, *Canad. J. Zool.*, **49**: 11, 1971).

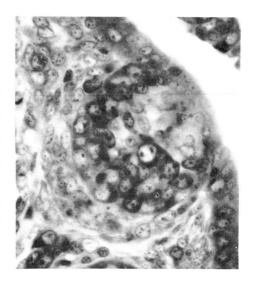

Fig. 7-24 A lympho-epithelial nodule showing the surface endodermal epithelium, *s*. the epithelial-nodular junction (*arrow*), and basement membrane, *x*, separating the medullary and cortical portions of the developing follicle. Various cells comprising the follicle may be recognized: undifferentiated basal epithelial cells, *u*, lymphoblasts, *b*, large lymphocytes, *p*, medium lymphocytes, *l*, reticular-epithelial cells, *e*, modified epithelial cells of the epithelial tuft of the nodule, *t*, mesenchymal cells, *m*, and an erythrocyte, *r*, in a capillary in the cortex. A primitive lymphocytic cell, *j*, is located in the cortex in contact with the basement membrane. 16-day-old chick embryo. Bursa fixed in Zenker's formol, embedded in paraffin, and stained with Giemsa. Light micrograph. (×*1,030*). (*From*: Ackerman, *J. Cell. Biol.*, **13**: 127, 1962).

are reasonably well equipped with the Golgi apparatus, mitochondria, and endoplasmic reticulum.

Although there is less emphasis in description on the avian bone marrow, undoubtedly it is a locale for the genesis of most blood cells. The spleen, also, surely plays a vital role in hemopoiesis, and in the immune system generally. In the spleen, for example, stem cells (the hemocytoblasts) are found in the germinal centers (Fig. 7-26). It is perhaps at the phylogenetic level of the birds that true, distinct germinal centers begin to appear in the spleen. Germinal centers are well-delineated areas in the center of white pulp where lymphocytes differentiate from stem cells. The precise arrangement of lymphocytes in this region and the contiguous red pulp functionally characterize the spleen, especially in its interactions with the thymus.

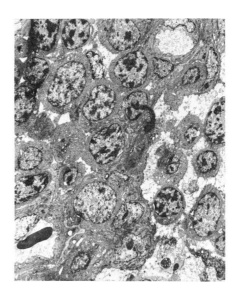

Fig. 7-25 Normal chicken bursa of Fabricus. The basement membrane which surrounds each bursal lymphoid follicle can be seen here (arrows) extending between two perifollicular capillaries, *c*, and separating the follicle (*lower right*) from the perifollicular cuff of lymphocytes (*upper left*). Both the follicle proper and the cuff contain a variety of sizes of lymphocytes ranging from 4 to 8 μ in diameter. No ultrastructural distinction could be made between the lymphocytes in these two locations. (×*2,000*). (*From*: Clawson et al., *Lab. Invest.*, **16**: 407, 1967.)

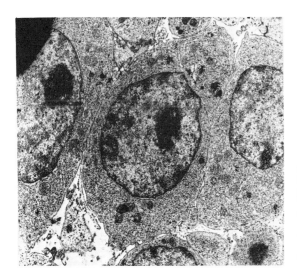

Fig. 7-26 Hemocytoblasts of the splenic germinal center of the chicken. These large cells contain an abundant polyribosome population predominately in a clustered configuration. Transitional appearing cells were seen within the germinal centers which suggested that the hemocytoblasts were derived from the bursal form of lymphocyte but not from the thymic form. (×7,560). (*From*: Clawson et al., *Lab. Inves.*, **16**: 407, 1967).

Class Mammalia (Animals with Hair or Fur, Which Suckle Their Young; Advanced Brain)
  Subclass Prototheria (Egg-laying Mammals)
    Order Monotremata (Duckbill and Spiny Anteater of Australia)

Although the lymphoid apparatus is complex throughout the class Mammalia, in general the eutherian, or placental mammals, possess a greater variety of lymphoid organs in more diverse locations than those identified in either the prototherian (monotreme) or metatherian (marsupial) mammals. Mammals, like other vertebrates, show lymphocyte accumulations, either diffuse or as discrete organs, closely associated with epithelial surfaces and near orifices. Recall the predictions, based on studies of the advanced invertebrates and primitive vertebrates, that in phylogeny, the epithelium provides the first line of defense against threatening pathogens. If successful in breaking the epithelial coat, bacteria or other harmful pathogens are met by leukocytes, particularly neutrophils and lymphocytes. Thus, destruction of the epithelial wall activates a sentinel of leukocytes ready to sequester, quickly and nonspecifically, foreign material or antigens by phagocytosis. Furthermore this triggers a chain of specific events that ultimately leads to immune responses characterized by specificity and memory.

The mammalian lymphoid system consists of oropharyngeal aggregations or tonsils, GI tract aggregations (as Peyer's patches), and appendix (GALT). At present there is no known precise equivalent of the avian bursa of Fabricius among mammals, even in the monotremes, the most likely mammalian group, because of their superficial developmental and anatomic analogies. Monotreme mammals lay eggs, but the hatched young suckle like other mammals. There is a thymus, a spleen, and extradigestive tract lymph nodes that are structurally discrete and located in rather consistent groups.

A prototherian mammal of much interest is the Australian echidna, *Tachyglossus aculeatus*. The thymus of this animal is divided into numerous highly vacularized lobules that are in turn subdivided into cortical and medullary regions. The medulla contains numerous Hassall's corpuscles, and in essence it is hardly different from that of placental mammals. However, one distinct feature should be stressed, namely the pattern of labelling after the injection of ^{125}I-labelled flagella antigen. At twenty-four hours, antigen is selectively taken up by Hassall's corpuscles in the medulla. Hassall's corpuscles consist of whorls of acidophilic-staining epithelial-reticular cells. The significance of this finding awaits further analysis, as does an elucidation of the function of Hassall's corpuscles. As a reminder, the thymus of amphibians and reptiles contains myoid cells with a significant number of characters similar to those of muscle cells.

The echidna spleen is typical of advanced vertebrate spleens. Both red and white pulp are readily distinguishable. The red pulp is characterized mainly by the presence of erythrocytes and phagocytic cells, readily demonstrable twenty-four hours after the intravenous injection of carbon. Germinal centers distinguish the white pulp. It is interesting that erythrocytes appear scattered specifically within white pulp follicles between the marginal zones and the germinal centers. From the comparative viewpoint, it should be emphasized that the white pulp of the echidna and the eutherian mammals, as well as that of the marine toad *Bufo marinus*, contains no carbon after injections.

The echidna appendix shows a striking similarity to the rabbit appendix and the avian bursa of Fabricius, as there are clear separations of follicles into cortical and medullary zones (Fig. 7-27). We are cautioned, for according to Diener and Ealey (1965),

> there is no reason, however, to suggest any homology between the echidna appendix and the bursa of Fabricius in birds. The anatomical situation is quite different, and paleontological opinion is that birds were derived from the same archaic group, the Diadectomorpha, as modern reptiles and are far removed from the line of monotreme evolution.

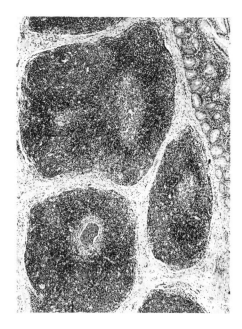

Fig. 7-27 Appendix of echidna showing lymphoid follicles each divided into cortical and medullary zone. Note the crypt in the center of one of the follicles filled with polymorpho nuclear cells (*arrow*). (Haematoxylin and eosin, xc.41). (*From*: Diener & Ealey, *Nature*, **208**: 950, 1965).

The interesting organ of the echidna's immune system is the lymph nodule. By means of a lymphogram, injections of an x-ray detectable, radio-opaque dye, the patterns of the thoracic duct and clusters of lymph nodules of the echidna become obvious (Fig. 7-28). A comparison of the echidna's lymph nodules with those of a

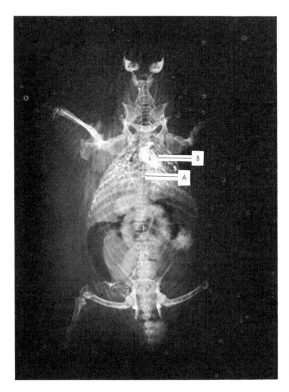

Fig. 7-28 Lymphogram of an echidna. *a,* thoracic duct; *b,* clusters of lymph nodules. (*From*: Diener et al., *Immunol.,* **13**: 339, 1967).

placental mammal, the rat, shows that they are fundamentally different (Fig. 7-29). Whereas a single rat node is composed of many nodules and lies in the path of a lymphatic vessel with afferent and efferent channels, several echidna nodules lie within the lumen of a lymphatic vessel suspended by a vascular bundle. A large circular sinus represents the interspace between the lymphatic vascular wall and the lymph nodule (Fig. 7-30).

There are other obvious differences. Echidna nodules are composed primarily of small lymphocytes, located in the periphery, that are vascularized by postcapillary venules; there are no primary lymphoid follicles in the periphery of the nodule. In eutherian or placental mammals, primary nodules such as these are composed of densely packed lymphocytes arranged in the outer portion of the node and referred to as the *cortex*. The *medulla*, the inner area of a eutherian mammalian node, is absent in the echidna. Labelling echidna nodes after antigen stimulation with ^{3}H thymidine reveals the presence of highly active germinal centers, usually one per nodule. Antigen is localized first around the entire nodule, but later it appears in the germinal center. Occassionally germinal centers are located eccentrically; then the

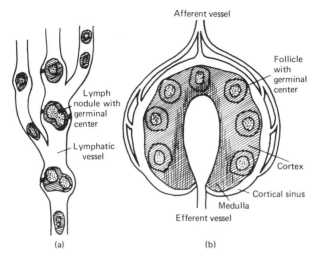

Fig. 7-29 Schematic diagram of (a) lymph nodules of the echidna within lymphatic vessels, and (b) lymph node of the rat. (*From*: Diener et al., *Immunology*, **13**: 339, 1967.)

labelled antigen forms a typical germinal center cap, characteristic of secondary follicles of rat lymph nodes. Labelled antigen also occurs in the appendix and Peyer's patches of the ileum.

With regard to the evolutionary significance of diffuse single or primary follicles in monotreme mammals, it is interesting to correlate morphology with function. Follicles are involved in antibody synthesis, and the multifollicular lymph node of

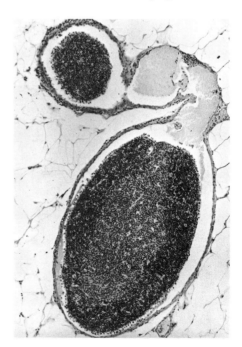

Fig. 7-30 Lymph nodules of an echidna: The "circular sinus" is defined by the interspace between the periphery of the nodule and the wall of the lymphatic vessel. (H & E, ×*50*). (*From*: Diener et al., *Immunology,* **13**: 339, 1967).

eutherian mammals may be more efficient in encountering the same antigen a second time to produce both primary and secondary responses. In other words, in eutherian nodes, germinal centers characteristic of secondary follicles seem to stand ready for encounter with antigens. Such complexity of follicular arrangement into a single node is absent in monotremes; this difference may account for the atypical secondary or memory response of monotremes. It is assumed that the monotreme lymph node represents a primitive stage in the phylogeny of placental mammalian lymph nodes. It recalls the fish, amphibian, reptile, and even avian lymph node situation.

> Subclass Theria (*Mammals Bearing Live Young*)
> Infraclass Metatheria
> Order Marsupialia (*Pouched Mammals*)

We are all aware that marsupial mammals are born relatively immature, and development is completed in a pouch. In North America, particularly the southern part of the USA, the opossum is the typical marsupial; in Australia and New Zealand the kangaroo and its near kin are common marsupials. To complete our presentation of the machinery involved in the immune system throughout the phylogenetic scale, we turn now to a well-studied marsupial, the opossum *Didelphys virginiana* Kerr.

The most elegant and by far the most complete study of the cells and organs of the opossum immune system to be published recently was done by Block (1964).

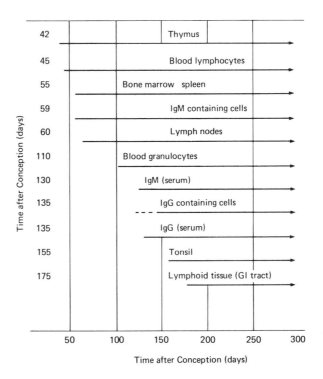

Fig. 7-31 Timetable of development of lymphoid tissue and immunoglobulins in the bovine fetus. (*From*: Schultz, *The Cornell Veterinarian*, **63**: 507, 1973).

To provide a complete picture of the development of the liver, thymus, spleen, bone marrow, and lymph node, Table 7-2 has been reproduced almost in its entirety; it more than adequately summarizes development from day 1 through to days 65 to 100. It will be interesting to compare the various developmental events and ultimate maturation with the conditions reviewed for other vertebrates in this chapter. See for example the timetable of development in the bovine fetus compiled by Schultz (Fig. 7-31).

The opossum is unusual at birth. It closely resembles a ten-day-old rat or mouse embryo, an eight-week-old human embryo, and a twelve-day-old guinea pig embryo. At this time it weighs 0.1 gm. It is evident that, despite the technical difficulties encountered, breeding the opossum is particularly advantageous, since in the marsupial it is possible to analyze crucial developmental events in a mammalian vertebrate without tampering with the uterus. Not only has the opossum's anatomy been elucidated, but sophisticated immunology studies have been done on these and other marsupials from Australia and New Zealand.

For those interested in other lymphoid organs, Zimmerman (1943) has provided an excellent review of tonsil development in the opossum. He found that the earliest appearance of lymphoid tissue in the mesenchyme surrounding the tonsilar sinus begins at about the same time as it does in other areas, approximately 3 weeks after birth. Lymphoid accumulations become more prevalent at approximately forty days old. The first primary nodules appear at sixty days, near the weaning period, and secondary nodules, with germinal centers, are present in weaned opossums. This is similar to the time observed by Block (1964) for peripheral lymph node development.

Infraclass Eutheria (Higher Mammals with Placentas)

Any of the commonly studied laboratory mammals are representative and contain all of the varying kinds and distributions of lymphoid tissues. It is perhaps significant for phylogenetic perspective that from the anuran amphibians, particularly the *Rana* species, we have viewed for the first time nodes composed of lymphoid cells and phagocytic cells, but arranged so as to filter blood. In many placental mammals, hemal nodes occur. It is believed that such hemal nodes represent discrete organized remnants of these phylogenetically earlier organs that are first recognizable in the amphibians. In fact, Turner's (1971) observations of the hemal nodes of rats show that the arrangement of the cell components is strikingly reminiscent of the lymph gland in *Rana* larvae that supercede, but may not necessarily contribute to, the development and differentiation of adult lymphomyeloid organs. For example, cords of lymphocytes are separated by blood-filled sinusoids lined by macrophages. Stellate reticular cells comprise the framework or *stroma*.

All eutherian or placental mammals possess commonly known lymphoid organs located strategically for antigen trapping. Again, as in phylogeny, lymphocytes are found almost constantly in association with epithelial surfaces. The degree of lymphocyte aggregation determines the presence or absence of a defined lymphoid organ. In general, the gastrointestinal tract is best equipped with lymphocytes in varying quantities or aggregations; however, other lymphocytes are found in association with the nasal mucosa and the bronchi of the lungs. The oropharyngeal region is ringed by tonsils. It is only now that tonsils have been shown to play a vital role in immunity.

Table 7-2

Normal development of the blood-forming tissues and blood of the newborn opossum.

	Liver	Thymus	Spleen	Marrow	Lymph node
1 day	50% hematopoietic; maturation to basophil erythroblasts; fewer cells in granulocytic than erythroblastic lineage but more maturation; megakaryocytoblasts without platelet formation	Pure epithelial sheet; large lymphocytes bordering capillaries between lobules.	Avascular but mesenchyme more dense than in embryo as a whole; rare transitional form between mesenchymal cell and large lymphocyte.	Endochondral bones solidly cartilagenous; diaphyseal cartilage cells more swollen than in rest of bone; membranous bone irregular bone spicules.	
2 days	Increased concentration of hematopoietic tissue; maturation to polychromatophil erythroblast; fine granulation in megakaryocyte cytoplasm.	Large and a few medium lymphocytes in center; periphery mostly stroma with many transitions between stroma and large lymphocytes; many mitoses and degenerating cells.	Increased mitoses, more closely packed mesenchymal cells, more prominent sinusoids; rare large lymphocyte.	No change except increase in size.	
3 days	Erythroblast maturation to eosinophil stage; granulocytopoiesis in capsule and portal connective tissue, neutrophil precursors more frequent than eosinophil or basophil; coarse megakaryocytic granulation.	Rapid growth in size; medium lymphocytes in center, large lymphocytes and transitional forms at periphery; further increases in mitoses and karyorrhexis.	More transitional stages between mesenchymal cells and large lymphocytes; still no hematopoiesis; small amount of nuclear debris.	Mesenchyme of membranous bones more vascular and edematous; spicules lined by osteoblast and osteoclasts.	
4 days	Greater increase in erythroblasts than in granulocytes; platelet formation in some megakaryocytes.	Marked increase in size; primarily medium lymphocytes; smaller lymphocyte-poor edge.	Rare small foci of basophil erythroblasts and rare single megakaryocytes; more prominent sinusoids.	Periosteum formed at diaphysis, diaphyseal cartilage cells more swollen.	1 of 7 animals first evidence of node near thymus.

134

5 days	Hematopoiesis more focalized; increased ratio of granulo- to erythropoiesis; eosinophil precursors appear.	Decrease in ratio of large to medium lymphocytes, small lymphocytes at center; very thin lymphocyte-poor growing edge, numerous mitoses and karyorrhexis; primitive Hassall's corpuscles.	Many discrete islands of erythroblasts, myelocytes; less maturation than in liver; arterioles only near hilum.	Diaphysis of endochondral bones in cranial half contain 1° marrow; primary marrow in membranous bone.	Only in mediastinum; consist of mesenchymal network crossing sinusoid with histioid wandering cells and transitions between latter and mesenchymal cells; intrasinusoidal erythroblasts.
6 and 7 days	Eosinophils and precursors as numerous as neutrophils and precursors.	Small lymphocytes predominate in center, medium at periphery; thin lymphocyte-poor growing edge persists, more mitoses and karyorrhexis than any other area; Hassall's corpuscles have swollen epithelial cells and nuclear debris.	Marked increase in number, size and maturation of hematopoietic foci; eosinophils as numerous as neutrophils; less maturation but same distribution of cell lineages as liver; arterial capillaries distributed through red pulp.	Mature eosinophil and neutrophil granulocytes in extravascular mesenchyme in endochondral bones.	Only cranial to diaphragm; small and medium lymphocytes and myelocytes among mesenchymal cells, basophil erythroblasts in sinusoids.
8 and 9 days	Beginning decrease in concentration of hematopoietic cells and increase in ratio of mature to immature hematopoietic cells.	Center occupied by small lymphocytes, decrease in karyorrhexis and mitoses but still more than in any other area.	Increase in number and size of hematopoietic foci and of mitoses.	Increase in percentage of endochondral bone occupied by marrow.	Found caudal to diaphragm; myeloid cells still as numerous as medium and small lymphocytes.
10 to 12 days	Continued decrease in concentration of hematopoietic cells especially neutrophil precursors; most of mitoses in erythroblasts; nuclear debris in Kupffer cells.	Thymus except for Hassall's corpuscles filled with small lymphocytes; very small lymphocyte-poor growing edge.	More rapid increase in erythroblasts than in granulocyte precursors; granulocytopoiesis near connective tissue, trabeculae, arterioles and capsule, eosinophils more numerous than neutrophils; perivascular mesenchymal cells separate arterioles from myeloid tissue of red pulp.	Increased number of eosinophil granulocytes separated from cortex by myxoid mesenchyme; a few intravascular large lymphocytes and basophil erythroblasts.	Recognizable cortex with dense diffuse lymphatic tissues; medulla with medullary cords with scattered small and medium lymphocytes; myelocytes, erythroblasts and megakaryocytes in sinusoids.

Table 7-2 Continued.

	Liver	Thymus	Spleen	Marrow	Lymph node
13 to 16 days	Decrease in number and increase in focalization of hematopoietic cells.	First appearance of medullary lymphatic tissue with fewer lymphocytes than cortex; small lymphocytes fill cortex to capsule; eosinophil droplets in Hassall's corpuscles; decrease in mitoses and karyorrhexis.	Rapid growth of spleen due more to increase in erythroblasts than granulocyte precursors or megakaryocytes; more mitoses than any other organ.	Increase in amount of marrow in endochondral bone.	Decrease in myeloid metaplasia; loss of anterior-posterior gradient of maturation.
17 to 22 days	Decrease in hematopoiesis; erythroblasts in lobules, granulocyte precursors in portal tissue; no change in ratio of immature to mature cells; a few eosinophil precursors persist in lobules, eosinophil lineage outnumbers neutrophil lineage.	Increase in ratio of medullary to cortical tissue; persistence of epithelial lined cysts and formation of eosinophil material in Hassall's corpuscles.	Solidly filled with erythroblasts, lesser increase in granulocytopoiesis and megakaryocytes; first appearance of medium lymphocytes and transitional forms between latter and reticular cells in periarteriolar mesenchyme.	Sinusoids filled with large lymphocytes and erythroblasts; higher ratio of immature to mature cells in sinusoids than in granulocytic tissue outside sinusoids.	Increase in number and size; increased number of small lymphocytes in cortex; decrease in myelocytes and megakaryocytes, to lesser extent in erythroblasts.
23 to 32 days	Decrease in amount of hematopoietic tissue; eosinophil lineage no more numerous than neutrophil lineage.	Resembled fully developed thymus.	Decrease in myeloid tissue, especially granulocytopoiesis; white pulp found in all animals, lymphocytes outnumbered by mesenchymal cells.	Endochondral bones filled with marrow except at epiphyses; ratio of intravascular to extravascular hematopoiesis increased.	Clear separation of cortex and medulla; large lymphocytes found in cortex, small lymphocytes in medullary sinusoids and in walls of medullary veins.
33 to 45 days	Only occasional hematopoietic foci, no change in ratio of immature to mature cells, cessation of subcapsular granulocytopoiesis.		Decrease in myeloid tissue; increase in amount of white pulp with increase in ratio of lymphocytes to mesenchymal cells.	Increase in ratio of immature to mature granulocytes and of intrasinusoidal erythroblasts and megakaryocytes to extravascular granulocytes and precursors; occasional myelocytes in membraneous bone marrow.	Increase in size due to increased number of lymphocytes.

45 to 65 days	One small island of hematopoiesis (usually erythroblasts or megakaryocyte) per 3–4 lobules.	Increased ratio of white to red pulp; decrease in myeloid hematopoiesis in red pulp; white pulp consists of inner densely lymphocytic core and outer less lymphocyte rich rim.	More intrasinusoidal erythropoiesis and megakaryocytopoiesis than extravascular granulocytopoiesis; increase in ratio of mature to immature erythroblasts, and of immature to mature granulocytes.	Diffuse increase in lymphocytes; cortex forms complete crescent separating subcapsular sinus from medulla, islands of large lymphocytes in cortex; increase in large lymphocytes and proplasma cells in medullary cords, rare plasma cells; very slight myeloid metaplasia; nuclear debris in cortex and medulla.
65 to 100 days	One or two foci of erythroblasts and rare megakaryocyte in each section; no iron by Prussian blue stain.	Differentiation of lymphatic nodules with reactionary and germinal centers.	Similar to marrow of mature animal.	Persistent rapid increase in size due to increase in number of lymphocytes; decrease in area occupied by medullary sinusoids; nodules with reaction and germinal centers in cortex; increase in plasma and proplasma cells.

From: Block, Ergebnisse der Anatomie u. Entwicklungsgeschichte 37 : 237, 1964.

Lingual tonsils are associated with the tongue, usually the posterior end. The tonsils that guard the entrance to the digestive and respiratory systems are referred to as the *palatine tonsils*. The pharynx is equipped with pharyngeal tonsils or *adenoids*. Tonsils first appeared in the anuran amphibians.

The esophagus, stomach, and intestines contain aggregations that are defined into discrete nodules. In the ileal portion of the small intestine, these nodules are aggregated into definite organs known as *Peyer's patches*. Continuing further, the all important appendix is a constant feature of the large intestine. Peyer's patches and the appendix constitute the major components of the gut-associated lymphoid tissue or GALT, which is often considered, because of its location and function, to be a mammalian counterpart of the avian bursa of Fabricius. The urinary system of mammals does not have great quantities of lymphocytes, though they are phylogenetically part of analogous filtration organs related to primitive urinary systems.

That lymph nodes filter lymph is true, but, as with other systems, mammals have more highly developed organ systems that tend to be restricted functionally. The need to filter remains in both immune and urinary systems, but filtrations for immunity are attributed to lymphoid organs that must sequester certain potentially antigenic pathogens. The urinary system filters, but not necessarily those elements capable of antigenicity, unless perhaps these can combine with *self* proteins to become antigenic, leading to autoimmune phenomena. Other systems (e.g., the nervous system) are relatively devoid of lymphocytes or other adjunct immune cells such as phagocytes.

Because the rabbit appendix is often likened to the avian bursa of Fabricius, the rabbit provides a good representative placental mammal for description from the viewpoint of ontogeny and phylogeny. Furthermore, if the two functional divisions of the immune system are to be made structurally relevant to mammals and all other vertebrates, we probably should ultimately recognize an organ source of the B cell, since the T cell is derived universally from the thymus. In the rabbit the thymus, common to all vertebrates, develops first. Following thymic development, lymphoid differentiation occurs in the spleen and aggregations in association with gut and peripheral lymph nodes. That the thymus is the first lymphoid organ to develop phylogenetically was recognized in cartilaginous fishes in the pioneer work of Beard (1900). With regard to ontogeny, Auerbach's (1961) elegant experiments on the contributions of both endodermal epithelium and mesenchyme to the development of the mouse thymus are important. According to the findings of Archer et al. (1964), the rabbit thymus is still an epithelial organ at day 18, part of the total gestation period of thirty-two days. Differentiation is rapid, so that by day 20 the thymus is a fully formed lymphoid organ; then it compares favorably with the typical thymus of other vertebrates.

The mammalian thymus is representative of that of most vertebrates; its overall anatomy and location are dependent upon the species, making it quite variable. In the African black rhinoceros, *Diceros bicornis*, the thymus is bilobed and weighs approximately 85 gms. According to Cave (1964), when fully dissected it

> *has an appearance not unlike that of a vascular tree bearing minor glandular lobules for leaves, so that Galen's term θύμος for this organ is demonstrated to be not inapt.*

Completely dissected, the thymus strongly resembles the thyme plant, *Thymus vulgaris* (Fig. 7-32). According to Cave, Galen may have had prior knowledge of a nonhuman (probably ungulate) mammalian thymus.

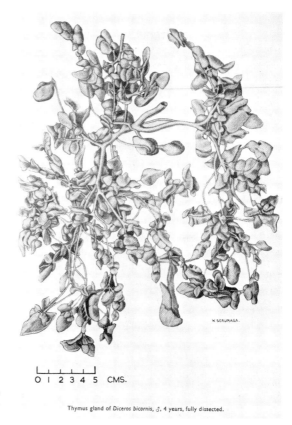

O I 2 3 4 5 CMS.

Fig. 7-32 Thymus gland of *Diceros bicornis*, 4 years, fully dissected. (*From*: Cave, *Proc. Zool., Soc. Lond.*, **142**: 73, 1964.)

Thymus gland of *Diceros bicornis*, ♂, 4 years, fully dissected.

The thymus is surrounded by a capsule of collagen, which penetrates the parenchyma as numerous stout collagenous trabeculae; this adds further subdivisions. Each thymus lobe is divided into numerous subsidiary lobules separated from each other by thick fibrous penetrations. Blood vessels usually accompany the trabeculae. It is intensely vascular due to abundant, relatively large thymic blood vessels, an arrangement necessary for routing lymphocytes into the blood stream. The thymus is divided by virtue of lymphocyte density into a cortex and medulla. The medulla, or outermost portion, contains dense accumulations of lymphocytes that are thinner

Fig. 7-33 Transverse section of rat thymus. This is a microphotograph of 5-μ thick sections of rat thymus with fixation in Bouin-Hollande and staining in Dominici. The connective tissue line which crosses the thymus in center (*arrow*) separates right and left lobes. Similar, though shorter, lines across the parenchyma are the trabecule which outline the lobules. Within the lobules, the dark cortex surrounds the pale medulla. (Elastic arteries may be seen below and mediastinal lymph nodes at each side.) (Magnification about ×7.8.) (*From*: Sainte-Marie & Leblond, *Blood*, **23**: 275, 1964.)

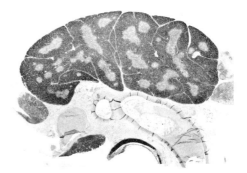

in arrangement in the medulla where the epithelial cells are more obvious (Fig. 7-33). The medulla contains Hassall's corpuscle, concentrically arranged epithelial cells whose function is controversial. Because of their associations with the epithelial-reticular stroma, they may have an endocrine function. The hormone thymosin is thought to be derived from the medullary region of the thymus. The best evidence was gained from studies of the restorative potential of thymus fragments placed in cell-tight millipore filter chambers and inserted into immune-deficient mice. Shortly thereafter, lymphocytes die, the epithelial reticular stroma remains, and immune function is restored, implicating restoration by humoral product(s) from the remaining epithelial stroma.

It is not until eight to ten days later, at day 28, that the spleen shows lymphoid follicles for the first time. At 36 days, four days after birth, splenic lymphocytes are aggregated around small penicillary arteries. At this same time, lymphoid tissue develops in the gut, primarily in the ileum and the appendicular portion of the caecum. This early development precedes final differentiation of Peyer's patches and the appendix. Peripheral lymph nodes show early development of primary follicles also in four-day-old rabbits. At ten days, the spleen is clearly divisible into red and white pulp and lymphoid follicles are obvious in the appendix and ileum. The adult state is reached at approximately nine weeks, a time when a remarkable degree of interdependence is demonstrable between lymphoid organs.

In addition to its vital role in the vertebrate immune response, the spleen, at least in mammals, is of interest because of its involvement in blood circulation. With regard to splenic circulation, there is controversy over the presence or absence of venous sinuses. In fact, mammalian spleens can be classified either as *sinusal* or *nonsinusal*. According to Hayes (1970), the armadillo spleen is invested by a capsule composed predominantly of smooth muscle; it is therefore capable of altering its size changing its blood content. The capsule penetrates the interior as trabeculae but these carry no blood vessels (Fig. 7-34). The white pulp shows typical follicles and the red pulp is permeated by anastomosing venous sinuses. In mammals more primitive than man, the arterioles continue to subdivide into several small branches that lie close together like a brush or penicillus. By still further subdivisions, structures eventually appear called *sheathed arterioles* or *ellipsoids*, with markedly thickened walls. This Schweigger-Seidel sheath is composed of a mass of concentrically arranged cells and fibers that are peripherally continuous with the reticulum of the red pulp. The reticular cells that make up the sheath exhibit various sized vacuoles and inclusion bodies, suggesting a phagocytic function. By means of light and electron microscopy, it has been found that venous sinuses lie in proximity to the peripheral cells of the ellipsoid sheaths (Figs. 7-35, 7-36). In fact, within the walls of venous sinuses, patent openings are apparent between the lining cells, and if these exist functionally, a better means of communication can occur between blood and cellular elements, particularly for phagocytosis; this facilitates a way to capture antigen.

Rabbits can be thymectomized and appendectomized on the first day of life. At nine weeks the spleen and lymph nodes can be examined. It is clear that early removal of the thymus and appendix (the latter to show the resemblance of the rabbit appendix to the avian bursa of Fabricius) leads to marked depletion of lymphocytes. Actually, lymph nodes or spleen, even at this late date, show much similarity to nodes with no lymphocytes that are derived from neonatal rabbits that have only been thymectomiz-

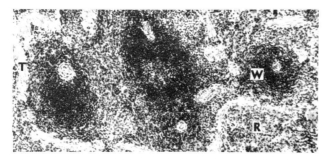

Fig. 7-34 Armadillo spleen. Photomicrograph demonstrating relationship of white pulp, *w.p.*, to the surrounding red pulp, *r.p.* The majority of the trabeculae, *t*, are of the non-vascular type. (Hematoxylin and eosin, ×*70*.)

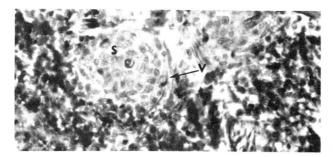

Fig. 7-35 Armadillo spleen. Photomicrograph of a cross-section of an ellipsoid sheath, *e.s.* The reticular cells are organized about the lumen of the capillary. The endothelial cells lining the capillary lumen appear swollen and tend to bulge into the lumen. A portion of a venous sinus, *v*, is evident at the periphery of the ellipsoid sheath. (Masson's Trichrome stain, ×*315*.)

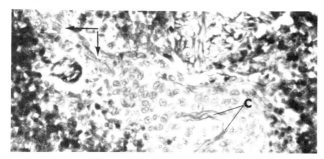

Fig. 7-36 Armadillo spleen. Photomicrograph demonstrating branching of the sheathed capillary, *s.c.* The arrows indicate a segment of the terminal capillary within the red pulp. (Masson's Trichrome stain, ×*315*.) (*From*: Hayes, *J. Morphol.*, **132**: 207, 1970.)

ed. In other words, the two operations (thymectomy and appendectomy), performed during the neonatal period, interfere with the apparent recovery of peripheral lymphoid tissue. At the end of nine weeks, a spleen from a rabbit with no thymus or appendix looks like a ten-day-old spleen and lymph node from rabbits neonatally thymectomized (only). At nine weeks such rabbits are fully recovered, suggesting that appendix-derived lymphocytes can make good any loss in lymph node lymphocytes caused by thymectomy.

SUMMARY

This chapter documented examples of an intriguing collection of lymphoid organs that occur throughout the animal kingdom. It should be stressed that the presentation consists of interesting cases, especially those drawn from poikilothermic vertebrates, that are generally neglected in the usual discourses on immunology. In instances not involving fishes, amphibians, reptiles, or birds, other animals such as certain invertebrates or prototherian and metatherian mammals were selected for discussion; hopefully, these choices will arouse an urge to study the immunology of exotic animals. In examples such as the octopus, the echidna, and the opossum, there is still room for much critical study. The animal kingdom is replete with other intriguing species; because of lack of space the presentation here is certainly not complete. With such abundance of subjects, we should never tire in our quest for new problems in immunology.

BIBLIOGRAPHY

Archer, O. K., Sutherland, D. E. R., and Good, R. A. 1964. The developmental biology of lymphoid tissue in the rabbit. Consideration of the role of thymus and appendix. Lab. Invest. **13**: 259.

Auerbach, R. 1961. Experimental analysis of the origin of cell types in the development of the mouse thymus. Develop. Biol. **3**: 336.

Beard, J. 1900. The source of leucocytes and the true function of the thymus. Anat. Anz. **18**: 561.

Biggs, P. M. 1957. The association of lymphoid tissue with the lymph vessels in the domestic chicken (*Gallus domesticus*). Acta Anat. **29**: 36.

Block, M. 1964. The blood-forming tissues and blood of the new born opossum (*Didelphys virginiana*). I. Normal development through about the one hundredth day of life. Ergebnisse der Anatomie u. Entwickslungsgeschichte **37**: 237.

Borysenko, M., and Cooper, E. L. 1972. Lymphoid tissue in the snapping turtle, *Chelydra serpentina*. J. Morph. **138**: 487.

Cave, A. J. E. 1964. The thymus gland in three genera of Rhinoceros. Proc. Zool. Soc. Lond. **142**: 73.

Cooper, E. L. [ed.], 1974. *Invertebrate Immunology in Contemporary Topics in Immunobiology*, Vol. 4. New York: Plenum Press, 299 pp.

Cowden, R. R. 1972. Some cytological and cytochemical observations on the leucopoietic organs, the "white bodies" of *Octopus vulgaris*. J. Invert. Pathol. **19**: 113.

Diener, E. and Ealey, E. H. M. 1965. Immune system in a monotreme: Studies on the Australian Echidna (*Tachyglossus aculeatus*). Nature **208**: 950.

Fänge, R., 1966. Comparative aspects of excretory and lymphoid tissue. In *Phylogeny of Immunity*, eds. R. Smith, P. Miescher, and R. Good, p. 142. Gainesville: University of Florida Press.

Fänge, R. and Sundell, G. 1969. Lymphomyeloid tissues, blood cells and plasma proteins in *Chimaera monstrosa* (Pisces, Holocephali). Acta Zoologica **50**: 155.

Fichtelius, K. E. 1970. Cellular aspects of the phylogeny of immunity. Lymphology **3**: 52.

Garcia-Herrera, F., and Cooper, E. L. 1968. Organos linfoides del anfibio apoda, *Typhlonectes compressicauda*. Acta Medica **4**: 157.

Good, R. A., Finstad, F., Pollara, B., and Gabrielsen, A. E. 1966. Morphologic studies on the evolution of the lymphoid tissues among the lower vertebrates. In *Phylogeny of Immunity* eds. R. Smith, P. Miescher, and R. Good, p. 149. Gainesville: University of Florida Press.

Hayes, T. G., 1970. Structure of the ellipsoid sheath in the spleen of the armadillo (*Dasypus novemcinctus*). A light and electron microscopic study. J. Morph. **132**: 207.

Holmgren, N. 1950. On the pronephros and the blood in *Myxine glutinosa*. Acta Zool. **31**: 234.

Johnston, M. R. L. 1973. Perivascular lymphoid tissue associated with the axillary lymph sinus and the lateral vein of *Gehyra variegata* (Reptilia: Gekkonidae). J. Morph. **139**: 431.

Kampmeier, D. F. 1969. *Evolution and Comparative Morphology of the Lymphatic System.* Springfield, Illinois: Charles C. Thomas.

Kanakambika, P. and Muthukkaruppan, V. R. 1972. The immune response to sheep erythrocytes in the lizard, *Calotes versicolor*. J. Immunol. **109**: 415.

Kotani, M. 1959. Lymphgefässe, lymphatische, apparate und extravaskuläre saftbohnen der schlange (*Elaphe quadrivirgata Boie*). Acta Scholae Med. Univ. Kioto, Japan **36**: 121.

Manning, M. J., and Horton, J. D. 1969. Histogenesis of lymphoid organs in larvae of the South African clawed toad, *Xenopus laevis* (Daudin). J. Embryol., Exp. Morph. **22**: 265.

Mueller, A. P., Sato, K., and Glick, B. 1971. The chicken lacrimal gland, gland of Harder, caecal tonsil, and accessory spleens as sources of antibody-producing cells. Cell. *Immun.* **2**: 140.

Riviere, H. B., Cooper, E. L., Reddy, A. L. and Hildemann W. H. 1975. In search of the hagfish thymus. Am Zool **15**: 39.

Turner, D. R. 1971. The reticulo-endothelial components of the haemal node. A light and electron microscopic study. J. Anat. **108**: 13.

Zimmerman, A. A. 1943. The origin, development and adult structure of the palatine and pharyngeal tonsils in the oppssum (*Didelphys virginiana*, Kerr). Supplement to the Transactions of the American Academy of Ophthalmology and Otolaryngology.

Chapter 8

Development of Transplantation Immunity

INTRODUCTION

The immune system, like all other systems, develops and matures in a regular, sequential manner. The ability to distinguish between *self* and *not-self*, revealed by the destruction of foreign cells or tissue transplants, develops ontogenetically in all vertebrate animals. If an animal is challenged with an antigen at a period when it is immunologically incompetent, it will not develop immunity to the antigen, but instead, develops tolerance. Tolerance is the inability of an animal to respond to a given antigen if it has encountered it during the period when it is developing immune competence. At birth or hatching, the immune response usually has matured completely. Hence, antigens are no longer accepted as *self*, as they are prior to birth, but are destroyed.

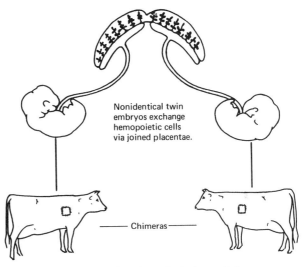

Late rejection of skin grafts
exchanged between chimeric cattle twins

Nonidentical twin
embryos exchange
hemopoietic cells
via joined placentae.

———— Chimeras ————

Exchanged skin grafts survive for long periods,
but some are eventually rejected.

Fig. 8-1 (*From*: Anfinsen et al., 1973, *Current Research in Oncology*)

144

The concept of tolerance grew out of Owen's (1945) observations on the fate of blood cells in dizygotic (nonidentical) fraternal cattle twins. As they share placental circulation *in utero*, their blood cells invariably develop as natural blood cell chimeras (Fig. 8-1). Because of a free exchange of erythrocytes, grafts exchanged between these now tolerant twins are accepted. Burnet subsequently predicted that if mammalian animals are given foreign cells during their *in utero* developmental period, a time when the fetus is unable to distinguish between *self* and *not-self*, when challenged later with a graft from the tolerizing cell donor, the animals would accept the foreign material as *self* (Burnet and Fenner 1949). Subsequently a team of investigators headed by Medawar (Billingham et al 1953), verified this prediction in the laboratory.

Since these discoveries, there have been a substantial number of basic experiments concerning tolerance to cellular antigens. Like many other approaches in cellular immunology, these have been restricted to mammals. Yet, despite this restriction, some are novel in that less common mammals have been employed. Opossum adults (marsupials) readily show first- and second-set skin allograft rejection. By contrast, pouch young less than twelve days old do not reject such grafts (La Plante et al 1969, Fig. 8-2). To test for induced tolerance, young opposums can be regrafted with skin from the same donor. Less than half reject their second grafts in a first-set response, but the remainder maintain a viable second graft for over ninety days. Grafts from different donors are rejected within twenty days on these same animals, leaving the initial graft unchanged. In marmosets, small South American primates, the incidence of hematopoietic chimerism is high because fraternal twinning is the rule and a syn-

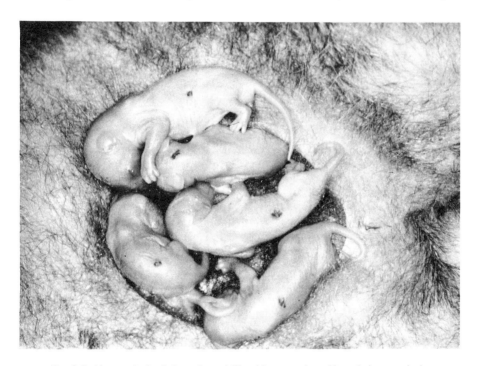

Fig. 8-2 Litter grafted at 3 days of pouch life with maternal ear skin and photographed at 40 days of pouch life. Initial grafts measured 1 × 2 mm in size. (*From*: LaPlante et al., *Transplantation*, **7**: 67, 1969.)

chorion allows fetal parabiosis. As in cattle, the mechanism producing hematopoietic chimerism also induces specific tolerance for histocompatibility antigens (Porter and Gengozian 1969).

The erythrocyte mosaicism first described in cattle occurs naturally and is influenced by the genetic background of the animal. To overcome these limitations in other mammals, techniques have been developed in mice with distinctive genotypes. One such technique developed by Mintz (1962) consists of fusing blastomeres from two (or more) genetically dissimilar cleavage stage embryos to form a single embryo. After the genetic composite reaches the morula or blastocyst stage *in vitro*, it is allowed to complete its prenatal life by transferring it to the uterus of a foster mother. From these experiments Mintz has obtained at least thirty-eight different genotypic combinations tolerant to erythropoietic cells.

SELF-RECOGNITION PRIOR TO IMMUNOLOGICAL MATURATION

The amphibian larval pituitary gland is ideal for an analysis of the embryonic development of *self*-recognition. It is easily extirpated *in toto*, produces its own unique antigens, and the health of its component cells can be conveniently and accurately determined by the frog's pigmentation. Normal cells secrete a hormone which causes the melanophores to expand, giving the frog its characteristic coloring. Damaged or unhealthy cells do not secrete this hormone, so the melanophores do not expand, and the animal becomes permanently blanched or albino. Triplett (1962) removed the pituitary gland from amphibian larvae of the tree frog *Hyla regilla* before it had reached the initial stages of differentiation and produced its own organ-specific proteins. When the explanted pituitary was regrafted to the original metamorphosed owners as dermal implants, most of the albino frogs promptly darkened. Subsequently, most of the frogs rejected their own pituitaries and again became albinos. The behavior of the now "foreign" autografted glands reveals that the frog is capable of an immune response against its own tissues provided it has never been in contact with the adult antigens of that tissue.

On the other hand, if one-half of a pituitary is cultivated in an allogeneic host and returned to the original donor, it is not destroyed. The graft area becomes darkened in response to the transplanted fragment, and the grafts are accepted and remain healthy. Moreover, all transplants of tail-tip autografts from hypophysectomized larvae are accepted. Thus, the reason for the rejection of the whole pituitary can not be metamorphic changes in antigenic specificity. These results suggest that the immunologic system has no memory of *self* that is genetically transmitted. Furthermore, it appears that the ability to recognize a graft as *self* depends on embryonic contact between graft tissue and host reticuloendothelial system.

TOLERANCE IN ANURAN AMPHIBIAN LARVAE

Partial Tolerance in Pattern Mutants of the Leopard Frog, Rana pipiens

The dorsal spotting patterns of the common leopard frog *Rana pipiens* are Mendelian variants (Moore 1942). At least three mutant patterns of the normal leopard-like spots are easily identified (Fig. 8-3). The burnsi frog is a Mendelian dominant with large dorsal spots. The kandiyohi frog has melanotic blotches in the interspaces

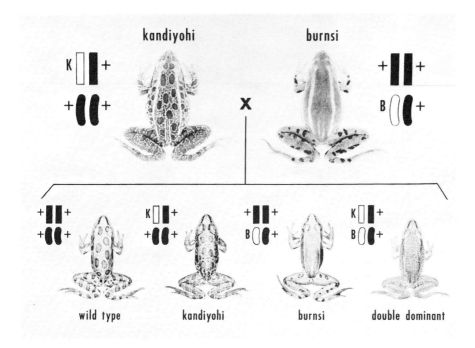

Fig. 8-3 Four patterns recovered in a ratio 1 : 1 : 1 : 1 from a cross of a heterozygous kandiyohi and a heterozygous burnsi frog. The dominant mutant genes, kandiyohi (K) and burnsi (B), assort independently. (*From*: Volpe, *J. Exp. Zool.*, **157** : 179, 1964.)

between the normal dorsal spots (Volpe 1964). Both of these mutant genes are non-allelic; thus, each expresses its distinct effect when all are combined within the same genotype. A third mutant has both the burnsi's large dorsal spots and the kandiyohi's mottlings and is therefore a double dominant. The resulting melanocyte pattern is advantageous for studying partial tolerance to neural crest transplants performed during the embryonic stage.

To induce partial tolerance in embryonic frogs, the right trunk neural fold of one embryo can be transplanted to the midventral region of a second embryo (Fig. 8-4). Allotransplantation of the neural crest to the abdominal region can not only reveal whether propigment cells of mutants develop autonomously or by interaction with different genotypes, but at the same time, this information shows degrees of tolerance or its opposite, recognition of foreign allografts. Both points are important to developmental immunology. Although there is usually no subsequent adverse host reaction to a neural crest allograft during the early and middle periods of larval development, host antagonism to the graft is demonstrable late in larval life.

In addition to pigment cell destruction in neural crest allografts, there is an infiltration by host lymphocytes, confirming a cellular immune response (Fig. 8-5). Initially, one would be hesitant to accept this later immunological response by hosts, since it was not observed in classical transplantation studies using amphibian pattern mutants. However, these early transplantation experiments were done before information was available on all aspects of the development of immunity, including such variables as

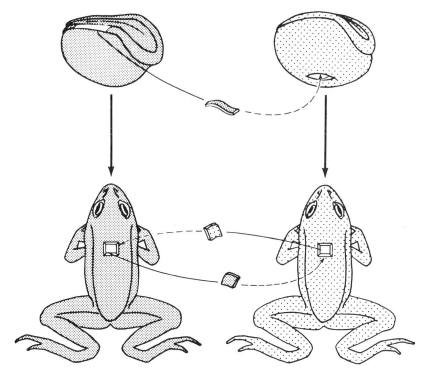

Fig. 8-4 Two-part scheme of operations. Right trunk neural fold of one embryo transplanted to the mid-ventral region of a second embryo in the early neurula stage. Subsequently, when both donor and host embryos transformed into juvenile frogs, pieces of dorsal skin were reciprocally exchanged. (*From*: Volpe, *J. Exp. Zool.*, **157**: 179, 1964.)

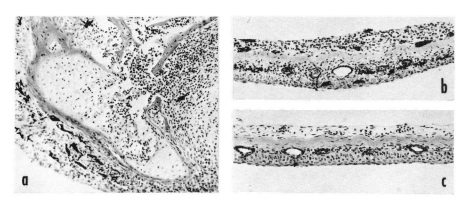

Fig. 8-5 Incipient stage of degeneration of the differentiated tissues of the neural crest homograft at larval stage XIX. A strong lymphocytic reaction is evident on the surface in the graft cartilage (a). Closely packed lymphocytes, identifiable by their round, darkly stained nuclei, have invaded the interior of the cartilage, where degeneration has already begun. The skin overlying the graft (b) is contrasted with a normal piece of skin (c) taken from a region lateral to the graft area. In the latter may be seen the stratified epithelium of the epidermis, through which multicellullar simple alveolar glands open; the thin dermal stratum spongiosum; the deeper stratum compactum, composed of parallel bundles of collagenous fibers; and the subcutis (tela subjunctiva), a region of loose fibroelastic tissue. In the skin overlying the graft (b), both the stratum spongiesum and the subcutis are packed with lymphocytes. (*From*. Volpe, *J. Exp. Zool.*, **157**: 179, 1964.)

age and dosage. The experiments were usually terminated before incompatibilities appeared, since the concern was for testing the *self*-differentiative potencies of transplanted embryonic primordia.

Effect of Dosage on Tolerance of Embryonic Allotransplants in the Leopard Frog, Rana pipiens

Many biologists have studied the effects of tissue antigen dosage on subsequent tolerance to transplants. The greater the dosage, the more likely the host is to develop tolerance and therefore to accept the transplant. According to Volpe and Gebhardt (1965), the anuran embryo becomes tolerant to the sensitizing properties of an embryonic allograft only if the dose of the antigenic stimulus is large enough and not, as many have assumed, because of its early introduction and protracted residence in the host before the immunological response faculty has matured.

Pigment pattern mutants of the common spotted leopard frog have been used to study such dosage effects. When different quantities of neural fold tissue are orthotopically exchanged between trunk regions of phenotypically indistinguishable embryos, the effects of dosage are clearly seen. Specifically, a foreign-crested host, an embryo grafted with two lateral folds from another mutant-pattern frog, maintains the graft pigment cells through the larval period (Fig. 8-6). At metamorphosis most of

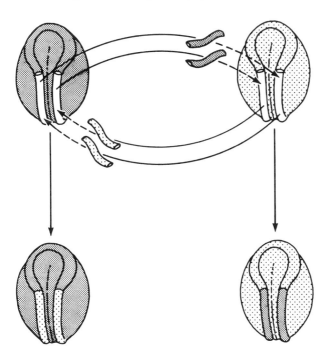

Foreign · Crested embryos

Fig. 8-6 Technique of bilateral homotransplantation of neural folds. Both lateral neural folds are reciprocally exchanged. Each member of the pair is thus both a donor and a host of neural fold material. (*From*: Volpe & Gebhardt, *J. Exp. Zool.,* **160**: 11, 1965.)

the host's trunk region originates from grafted neural folds, and the pigmentary pattern is characteristic of its genotype.

On the other hand, the chimeric-crest frog embryo bears only one mutant-pattern lateral neural fold allograft and the embryo invariably rejects it. As a consequence, graft pigment cells fail to persist beyond metamorphosis. Thus, instead of one side with host characteristics and the other with those of the donor, the frog's trunk

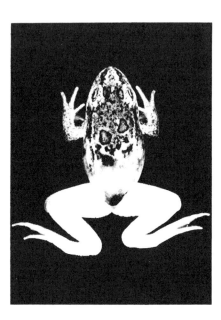

Fig. 8-7 External appearance of a foreign-crested host frog when the population of grafted cells falls below the critical concentration embodied in two complete lateral neural folds. Sites of rejection of graft cells remain devoid of pigment in the absence of repair by host pigment cells. (*From*: Volpe & Gebhardt, *J. Exp. Zool.*, **160**: 11, 1965.)

becomes populated on both sides by both kinds of pigment. In other words, the donor and host propigment cells intermix and disperse laterally over each side of the embryo's trunk. When sham operations are performed, or when the neural fold is removed and then replaced onto the same embryo as an autograft, the pigment pattern of the frog is not affected. Although cell derivatives of allotransplanted neural fold material may either stimulate or suppress the host's immunologically competent cells, the eventual rejection or persistence of the graft is primarily a function of graft cell dosage. Hence, the effects of dosage are clearly more significant than the status of the frog's immune response mechanism. Larvae that do not become tolerant to the double dose of transplanted neural fold tissue probably have not received sufficient donor tissue to induce tolerance (Fig. 8-7). This may be due to technical errors; tolerance is induced only when a sufficient antigen dosage is transplanted.

Histocompatibility after Transplantation of Nuclei
The Condition in Platanna (the South African Clawed Toad, Xenopus laevis)

Nuclear transplantation brings the nucleus and cytoplasm into association in a way that normal fertilization of the egg or artificial hybridization cannot achieve. When nuclei from cells of disaggregated embryonic tissues are injected into unfertilized eggs following the destruction of the pronuclei by ultraviolet irradiation (Table 8-1), many genetically identical toads may be obtained from a single donor embryo

(Simnett 1964). The genetic identity of the clone can be assessed by reciprocal grafting of skin or other tissues between members of a single clone and between members of different clones. The actions of histocompatibility loci result in acceptance between members of the same clone and rejection between those of a single and those of different clones (Table 8-1).

Table 8-1

Summary of grafting experiments on immature *Xenopus laevis laevis*
at environmental temperature 25°C.

Derivation of graft host	Derivation of graft donor	Designation	Reaction to graft	No. of operations
Fertilized egg	Same individual as host.	Autograft	Negative	36
Fertilized egg	Fertilized egg from same mating (sibling).	Homograft	Positive	36
Nuclear transplantation	Nuclear transplantation. Nuclei identical to host. Recipient egg cytoplasm identical to host.	Intraclonal graft	Negative	10
Nuclear transplantation	Nuclear transplantation. Nuclei different from host. Recipient egg cytoplasm identical to host.	Interclonal graft	Positive	8
Nuclear transplantation	Nuclear transplantation. Nuclei identical to host. Recipient egg cytoplasm different from host.		Negative	12

From: Simnett, Exp. Cell Res., **33**: 232, 1964.

The value of the nuclear transplant method for obtaining multiple genetically identical individuals of *Xenopus laevis* is indicated by the absence of subsequent allograft reactions in intraclonal grafts. This technique could conceivably provide clones from species in which no inbred strains have as yet been derived for use in experiments requiring permanent retention of transplanted tissue. When reciprocal skin grafts are exchanged between members of a single clone, allografts behave just like autografts. They become revascularized and survive without hemostasis or depigmentation. Moreover, allografts between toads produced by transplantation of nuclei from a single donor embryo into eggs laid by two different females are not rejected. Reciprocal grafts between clones, however, result in cessation of blood flow and death of graft melanocytes. Nuclear transplantation can, thus, be used to provide groups of isogenic individuals.

The appearance of the individuals resulting from nuclear transplants is entirely dependent upon the origin of the nucleus. Evidently, the cytoplasm does not significantly modify nuclear function as there is no difference in the appearance between toads derived from the same nucleus that is transferred and allowed to replicate in the cytoplasm of eggs produced by different females. Any genetic deviation from the nuclear parent, as determined by immunological techniques, is the result of a cytoplasmic effect in the association between nucleus and cytoplasm. For example, embryos from an intraspecific association, such as one resulting from nuclear transplantation between *Rana pipiens* and *Rana sylvatica*, undergo normal development. However, when nuclei of *Rana temporaria* are transplanted into egg cytoplasm of *Xenopus laevis* and subsequently transplanted back into *Rana* egg cytoplasm, gastrulation is not promoted for the duration of the interspecific association between *Xenopus* and *Rana*. This suggests that embryonic abnormalities in interspecific nucleocytoplasmic associations result from a permanent impairment of nuclear function, rather than from an incompatibility between nucleus and cytoplasm. On the other hand, no such impairment or modification of nuclear function is apparent when the nucleocytoplasmic association is intraspecific. Allografts exchanged between toads derived from normally fertilized eggs are rejected, confirming an immune mechanism that results from the integrity of the genes effecting genotype differences between host and donor.

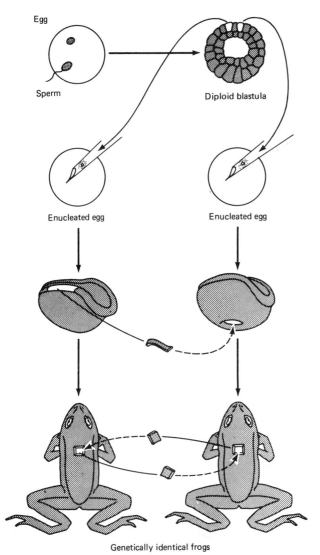

Egg

Sperm

Diploid blastula

Enucleated egg

Enucleated egg

Genetically identical frogs

Fig. 8-8 Successive operative steps. Several genetically identical embryos were produced by the technique of nuclear transfer. For illustrative purposes, only a pair of identical embryos is shown. When this pair reached the neurula stage of development, one lateral neural fold of one embryo was transplanted to the abdominal region of the other embryo. This was followed, when both embryos metamorphosed into juvenile frogs, by a reciprocal transplantation of pieces of dorsal skin. (*From*: Volpe & McKinnell, *J. Heredity,* **57**: 167, 1966.)

Production of Genetically Identical Leopard Frog, Rana pipiens

The survival and persistence of donor pigment cells is an almost invariant feature of grafts exchanged between members of the same isogenic group (Fig. 8-8). Pieces of allografted ventral skin between isogenic frogs blend so well that their borders are scarcely perceptible. As the host embryo grows into a feeding larva, the bulge at the graft area flattens, and the graft becomes the center of a circular patch of chromatophores, most of which are melanophores (Fig. 8-9). There are some instances where

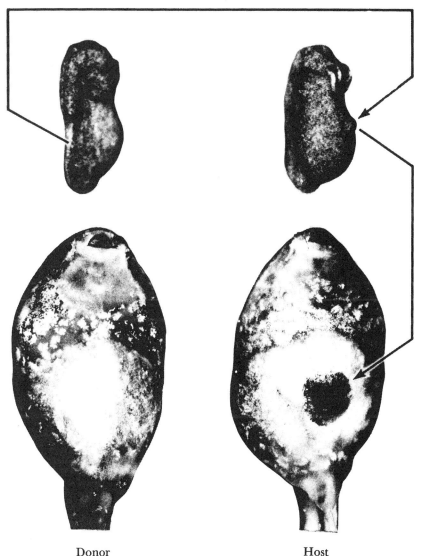

Donor   Host

Fig. 8-9 Postoperative appearance of donor and host at embryonic tailbud stage 17 (*top*); a conspicuous feature of the host embryo is the dome-shaped elevation in the ventral surface, the site of the neural fold implant. Self-differentiation of the neural fold graft is evident in the comparisons of donor and host at larval stage VIII[25] (*bottom*). The host larva bears ventrally a distinctive circular mass of graft pigment cells (particularly melanophores), surrounded by, but not invaded by, host guanophores. (*From*: Volpe & McKinnell, *J. Heredity*, **57**: 167, 1966.)

embryonic neural crest or subsequent skin grafts from donors of the same isogenic group do not survive. In these incompatible cases, it is likely that the host frog lacks one or more antigens possessed by the other clonal members. It is highly unlikely that a point mutation may have arisen in the chromosome bearing the histocompatibility gene, or that a small, nonlethal deletion of one histocompatibility locus has occurred in the chromosome. Without exception, however, skin grafts exchanged between members of different isogenic groups always deteriorate (Fig. 8-10).

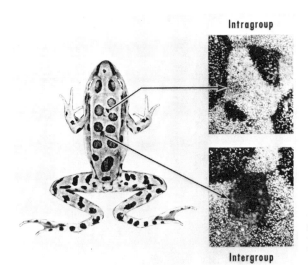

Intragroup

Intergroup

Fig. 8-10 A host frog carrying a successful skin graft from a member of the same isogenic group ("Intragroup" graft) and an unsuccessful skin graft from a member of a different isogenic group ("intergroup" graft.) (*From*: Volpe & McKinnell, *Heredity*, **57**: 167, 1966.)

TRANSPLANTATION IMMUNITY IN THE IMMUNOLOGICALLY COMPETENT TADPOLE

Introduction

Embryologic investigations involving transplantation have only recently taken into account certain immune aspects. Hildemann and Haas (1959) called attention to the importance of immune competence in developmentally immature animals. The larval anuran has since figured prominently in deciphering problems related to the maturation of the *self, not-self* recognition capacity and, ultimately, to an understanding of when the immune response develops. Once the response develops, it is as fully developed in larvae as it is in adults. The important distinction between inducing immunity and inducing partial tolerance depends also on when the antigen is administered.

The Bullfrog Tadpole

An autograft, or *self* tissue, is transplanted from a tadpole to itself and is always accepted; *not-self* tissue, an allograft, from a sibling tadpole is first accepted as *self*, but eventually is recognized as foreign and rejected by the host's immune system. It is obvious (from Fig. 8-11) that the tadpole has destroyed its posterior allograft but

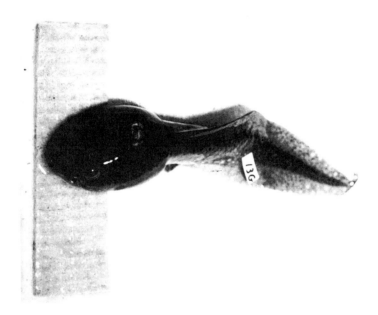

Fig. 8-11   Bullfrog larva showing fully viable, rectangular skin autograft anteriorly and a similar but pale homograft at survival end point posteriorly. Photograph taken 11 days after grafting at 25°C. (*From*: Hildemann & Haas, *J. Immunol.*, **83**: 479, 1959.)

the anterior autograft is well healed and shows no signs of incompatibility. The immune response provoked by foreign grafts is characterized by active leukocyte invasion, notably small lymphocytes. These cells infiltrate the area surrounding a foreign graft and mediate the host's rejection response. The graft area usually becomes inflamed and is characterized grossly by vasodilation, hemostasis, and, finally, the graft's destruction.

The bullfrog *Rana catesbeiana* develops its response to skin allografts during larval stages. Normally, larvae become competent to reject allografts at about forty days posthatching, when small lymphocytes appear in the peripheral blood. However, bullfrog tadpoles are partially tolerant to allografts during the period of development when small lymphocytes are not apparent in the peripheral blood (Table 8-2). Transplantation alloimmune responses can be abrogated in later adult anuran life by removing the thymus early in the tadpole's life. The thymus is the main generator of lymphocytes.

First-set allografts on larvae from two months to two years of age have the same median survival time of 11.8 ± 1.0 days. Therefore, once allograft responsiveness develops it is essentially the same regardless of the age of development, despite the profound physiologic changes occurring later in metamorphosis. Consequently, some of the newly-hatched larvae up to thirty-six days of age are immunologically immature and can thus be made partially tolerant to allografts during this period. During the transition period between tolerance and immunologic competence, strict *individual* immunologic specificity does not always occur. Some larvae, for example, will show

Table 8-2

Developmental appearance of blood cell types in relation to larval age
and immunological maturity

	Age of initial appearance in blood in days post-hatching	Immunological status of animals at age indicated
Undifferentiated stem cells	0—7	Homograft tolerant
Erythroblastic cells	8—11	Homograft tolerant
Mature nucleated erythrocytes	15	Homograft tolerant
Monoblasts and lymphoblasts	15	Homograft tolerant
Monocytes	20—22	Homograft tolerant
Large and medium lymphocytes	20—22	Homograft tolerant
Eosinophils	36	Homograft tolerant
Neutrophils	36	Homograft tolerant
Basophils	36	Homograft tolerant
Small lymphocytes	40—45	Transitional state or weak homograft reaction

From: Hildemann & Haas, 1961. In *Mechanisms of Immunological Tolerance* (Prague: Publishing House Czechoslovakia Academy of Sciences)

prolonged survival of skin allografts as a result of a previous tailbud allograft, even from a different donor.

The bullfrog's capacity for immunologic memory or anamnesis is confirmed by its accelerated rejection of second-set allografts in 5.1 ± 0.3 days at 25°C. As in the immunologic reaction of other poikilotherms, temperature greatly affects the immune response of amphibians. Allografts survive about three times as long at 15°C as they do at 15°C, and the second-set response, though prolonged, is also curtailed with respect to first-set grafts. The allograft rejection response of bullfrog larvae at 25 ± 1°C is characterized by the dissemination of pigment cells throughout the epidermis. Breakdown of the epidermis and invasion of the dermis by lymphocytes and fibroblasts begins during the first week. Prior to its destruction, the dermis appears as a thick, homogeneous, eosinophilic, almost acellular mass that is gradually replaced by a cellular connective tissue. During the early stages of rejection eosinophils become prominent in the epidermis, kidneys, and liver. Increased numbers of mitoses, large lymphocytes, and blast cells appear in the lymph glands, spleen, and liver before cellular infiltration of the allograft begins. It is, however, the small lymphocytes that predominate, indicating their important role in the rejection mechanism.

Second-set survival times are shorter, and the rejection is much more abridged with less congestion. Although the time of rejection is variable, once initiated the process goes to completion rapidly. Lymphocytic and fibroblastic reactions are more intense than in first-set rejection. Lymphoid follicles in the liver and intestinal wall are generally larger than in the first-set group. Again, small lymphocytes are quite prominent in lymph glands, spleen, liver, and intestine.

Leopard Frog Larvae

Leopard frog larvae, *Rana pipiens*, also regularly destroy skin allografts. Survival time of grafts from sibling larvae is longer than it is for grafts from nonsiblings.

Grafts between young feeding larvae survive longer than those between older larvae. The allograft rejection pattern is essentially the same for larvae of stage IV and older, hypophysectomized larvae and larvae immersed in thyroxine for two weeks after grafting. Thyroxine, the hormone that causes metamorphosis, obviously does not interfere with an immune response once it is developed. Second-set grafts from the same donor are destroyed at four to five days before first grafts.

LYMPHOID INVOLVEMENT IN TRANSPLANTATION IMMUNITY

Thymectomy-Rana

Removal of any of the lymphocyte-producing organs offsets the immune response; thymectomy is one such procedure. Cooper and Hildemann (1965) established the prime role of the thymus in anuran cellular immunity. When bullfrog larvae, *Rana catesbeiana*, are thymectomized during the first month of larval life, allograft survival is prolonged. Similarly, Du Pasquier (1965, 1968) observed that thymectomy during the larval life of the midwife toad *Alytes obstetricans* also produces a state of tolerance to cutaneous allografts. As the thymus undergoes its most pronounced differentiation, which presumably affects peripheral centers, its effects are greatest during larval life if it is removed early. Curtis and Volpe (1971) thymectomized the leopard frog, *Rana pipiens*, to determine the subsequent fate of tail-tip and dorsal skin allografts. The most successful thymectomies, i.e., those where no thymus tissue is found during a later autopsy of tadpoles, correspond with a prolonged survival of allogeneic grafts. After incomplete thymectomies, leopard frog tadpoles either reject allografts at the same rate as, or more slowly than, control unoperated tadpoles. By contrast, neither a complete nor a partial extirpation of the thymus late in larval life leads to a decline in immunological capacity as measured by allograft survival. The thymus, therefore, seems to exert its most profound effect during, or shortly after, the time in which it fully differentiates as a lymphoid organ. This corresponds roughly to the time when small lymphocytes appear in the circulation. When the thymus in anurans such as *Rana catesbeiana* and *Alytes obstetricans* is removed prior to one month of age post-hatching, subsequent allografts have a significantly prolonged survival time. In addition, thymectomy causes a curious runting syndrome like that seen in thymectomized mammals. In mammals this is further characterized by weight loss and diarrhea. No such pathologic sequelae occur in larvae tolerant to one antigen.

Thymus and Spleen Development in Xenopus

Horton (1969) correlated allograft responses of *Xenopus* larvae with their thymus lymphoid development and that of other organs. He found more small lymphocytes in those larvae with allografts than in autografts, although autografts do show some lymphocytic invasion. According to his view, the thymus is the only lymphoid organ actively producing fully mature lymphocytes. To assess whether the thymus in *Xenopus* influences the peripheral lymphoid organs, especially the spleen, Manning (1971) removed the thymus when small lymphocytes first appeared in it but before their appearance in peripheral lymphoid centers. Though the spleen is smaller at first in thymectomized larvae than it is in sham-thymectomized controls, as the tadpole develops the difference is no longer significant. Apparently, the thymus does not affect the development of splenic white pulp.

Thymectomy in Xenopus

Horton and Manning (1972) successfully thymectomized larvae at only eight days post-fertilization when the thymus is 0.1 mm in diameter and just beginning to display lymphoid differentiation. Surprisingly, an early thymectomy has no apparent effect on the growth and development of larval or young adult toads, nor do the lymphoid organs lack lymphoid elements. However, the normal extensive lymphocytic invasion of skin allografts does not occur. This indicates that an early thymectomy impairs the subsequent alloimmune response capacity to tissue alloantigens. Horton and Manning believe it unlikely that any prolonged or extensive passaging of cells through the thymus could have occurred before a thymectomy at eight days post-fertilization. It is further unlikely that sufficient thymic-dependent lymphocytes occur in thymectomized toadlets to account for subsequent allograft rejection, unless the special properties of such cells are established by an embryonic thymic influence. Perhaps, then, graft rejection in *Xenopus* involves cell cooperation between different lymphoid sources. A chronic allograft response following larval thymectomy can, consequently, be regarded as due to the removal of one of the cooperating populations. Alternatively, the response may simply be the result of a loss of a major source of small lymphocytes from the thymus.

Thymectomy in Urodeles

Although urodele amphibians exhibit a much slower rate of allograft destruction than larval anurans, their immune tissues seem to be, at least superficially, in number, type, and bodily distribution, as diverse as those of anurans. Thus, the rapidity of graft rejection cannot be viewed as dependent entirely upon the lymphomyeloid organs. However, these tissues in different species may have differences in morphology that account for different rates of allograft rejection. According to Hightower and St. Pierre (1971), the thymus of the salamander contains no cortex, medulla, myoid cells, or Hassall's corpuscles. Besides the remote morphologically qualitative deficit, other factors, such as the lack of strong histocompatibility differences advocated by Cohen (1969), may be operative. Bilateral thymectomy of salamander larvae during the first month post-hatching effectively abrogates their development of transplantation immunity to weak alloantigens (Cohen and Borysenko 1970). If the thymus is removed as late as two months post-hatching, allograft survival is still prolonged. Thus, there is a correlation between the time that thymectomy is successful in crippling the immune response, thymic development, and the age of the animal.

Charlemagne and Houillon (1968) thymectomized six-to-eight-week-old larvae of *Pleurodeles waltlii*, and at twelve to fifteen months post-thymectomy transplanted allografts from four different donors. Sixteen larvae tolerated all four grafts. Of the eight larvae that rejected the transplants, macroscopic observations after dissection revealed thymic remnants in three and no thymus in five. Some of the thymectomized larvae succumbed to the usual runting disease and died at approximately twenty months. On the other hand, thymectomies performed prior to metamorphosis have no effect on the rejection of allografts, since presumably peripheral seeding of the cells has already occurred.

Charlamagne and Houillon have also thymectomized eight-week-old larvae of *Triturus alpestris* just prior to their metamorhposis. One year to eighteen months later they grafted each adult with two skin allografts from different donors. Of the thirty-nine animals, thirty tolerated both allografts indefinitely (more than 200 days), but nine rejected them with normal delayed responses. Of the nine, four had thymic remnants but five had no thymus at all. No case of natural tolerance in *Triturus alpestris* was evident in several previous experiments involving the rejection of 542 grafts and 100 animals. It therefore appears that a complete larval thymectomy produces an indefinite tolerance to skin allografts in 60 to 70% of adult *Pleurodeles waltlii* and *Triturus alpestris*. On the other hand, transplant destruction that does occur in thymectomized larvae seems to correlate with an incomplete thymectomy and regeneration. Alternatively, other organs may be effecting rejection in the absence of the thymus.

Maturation of Transplantation Immunity in Turtles

Borysenko (1969) has been instrumental in focusing attention on the development of transplantation immunity in turtles. Skin allografts and xenografts transplanted to young snapping turtles, *Chelydra serpentina*, ranging in age from newly-hatched to six months, provide tests for assessing the degree of immunologic maturation. The snapping turtle's capacity to reject grafts matures immunologically several months after hatching. Newly hatched turtles require at least ninety days to reject grafts. When they are six months old, snapping turtles reject skin allografts and xenografts at about the same rate as adults. Skin xenografts are rejected faster than allografts at every age. Among siblings, there are instances of extended skin allograft survival during the early months post-hatching, suggesting tolerance induction. In older turtles, sibling allografts are rejected at nearly the same rate as nonsibling allografts.

In xenograft studies Yntema (1970) performed embryonic grafts in the turtles *Chelydra serpentina* (hosts) and *Chrysemys picta* and *Amyda ferox* (donors). Chromatophores in reptiles are derived from neural crest as in other vertebrates. Thus, somites and overlying ectoderm with or without adjacent neural tube are transplanted unilaterally and orthotopically in the anterior region of the carapace. With a *Chrysemys* donor, pigment cells form conspicuous red areas ventrally when neural crest is a part of the graft. The pigment fades gradually but persists for three or four years. When somites and adjacent ectoderm of *Chrysemys* carapace are used, the graft area is lightly pigmented at hatching and subsequently increases. *Chrysemys* grafts are either accepted or partially rejected. In cases of apparent tolerance, the graft region acquires host characteristics. By contrast, carapace rudiments derived from *Amyda* donors retain their own donor characteristics. When the turtles hatch, dark spots appear on a yellow background and scutes are absent. A few months after hatching, the graft area becomes necrotic; later, scutes with host characteristics or skin cover the graft area. The conditions that govern the induction of tolerance or immunity seem to apply to reptiles, although they, like fish, have been used less extensively than amphibians, birds, and mammals for tolerance studies.

SUMMARY

The anuran amphibian tadpole of the genera *Rana*, *Alytes*, and *Xenopus* and *Hyla* have figured prominently in understanding the concept of *self* vs. *not-self*, and when it develops. The ability of the immune system to recognize *self* is a property acquired by contacting antigenic determinants of *self*-tissues at some time during development. This was tested by removing the buccal component of the pituitary gland at a stage in development before the gland differentiates but after it is determined or possesses the ability to *self*-differentiate. Rapid allograft rejection always occurs once the tadpole's alloimmune response capacity is developed. The concept of tolerance induction first developed from studies in mammals as a result of certain crucial observations made in nature. Experimentally, tolerance is known to be inducible in most vertebrates; however, there is little information on fishes and reptiles.

BIBLIOGRAPHY

Billingham, R. E., Brent, L., and Medawar, P. B. 1953. Actively acquired tolerance of foreign cells. *Nature* **172**: 603.

Borysenko, M. 1969. The maturation of the capacity to reject skin allografts and xenografts in the snapping turtle, *Chelydra serpentina*. *J. Exptl. Zool.* **170**: 359.

Burnet, F. M., and Fenner, F. 1949. *The Production of Antibodies*. Melbourne: MacMillan.

Charlemagne, J., and Houillon, C. 1968. Effects de la thymectomie larvaire chez l'amphibien urodèle, *Pleurodeles waltlii* Michah. Production a l'état adult d'une tolérance aux homogreffes cutanées. Compt. Rend. Acad. Sci. **267**: 253.

Cohen, N. 1969. Immunogenetic and developmental aspects of tissue transplantation immunity in urodele amphibians. In *Biology of Amphibian Tumors*, ed. M. Mizell, pp. 153–168. New York: Springer Verlag.

Cohen, N., and Borysenko, M. 1970. Acute and chronic graft rejection: possible phylogeny of transplantation antigens. *Transplant Proc.* **2**: 333.

Cooper, E. L., and Hildemann, W. H. 1965. Allograft reactions in bullfrog larvae in relation to thymectomy. *Transplantation* **3**: 446.

Curtis, S. H., and Volpe, E. P. 1971. Modification of responsiveness to allografts in larvae of the leopard frog by thymectomy. *Develop. Biol.* **24**: 177.

Du Pasquier, L. 1965. Aspects cellulaires et humoraux de l'intolérance aux homogreffes de tissu musculaire chez le têtard *d'Alytes obstetricans*; rôle du thymus. C. R. Acad. Sci. Paris **261**: 1144.

Hightower, J. A., and St. Pierre, R. L. 1971. Hemopoietic tissue in the adult newt, *Notopthalmus viridescens*. J. Morph. **135**: 299.

Hildemann, W. H., and Haas, R. 1959. Homotransplantation immunity and tolerance in the bullfrog. J. Immunol. **83**: 478.

Horton, J. D. 1969. Ontogeny of the immune response to skin allografts in relation to lymphoid organ development in the amphibian *Xenopus laevis* Daudin. J. Exp. Zool. **170**: 449.

Horton, J. D., and Manning, M. J. 1972. Response to skin allografts in *Xenopus laevis* following thymectomy at early stages of lymphoid organ maturation. Transplantation **14**: 141.

La Plante, E. S., Burrell, R., Watney, A. L., Taylor, D. L., and Zimmerman, B. 1969. Skin allograft studies in the pouch young of the opossum. Transplantation 7: 67.

Manning, M. J. 1971. The effect of early thymectomy on histogenesis of the lymphoid organs in *Xenopus laevis*. J. Embryol Exp. Morph. 26: 219.

Mintz, B. 1962. Formation of genotypically mosaic mouse embryos. Amer. Zool. 2: 432.

Moore, J. A. 1942. An embryological and genetical study of *Rana burnsi*. Weed. Genetics 27: 408.

Owen, R. 1945. Immunogenetic consequences of vascular anastomoses between bovine twins. Science 102: 400.

Porter, R. P. and Gengozian, N. 1969. Immunological tolerance and rejection of skin allografts in the marmoset. Transplantation 8: 653.

Simnett, J. D. 1964. Histocompatibility in the platana, *Xenopus laevis* (Daudin), following nuclear transplantation. Exptl. Cell. Res. 33: 232.

Triplett, E. L. 1962. On the mechanism of immunologic self recognition. J. Immunol. 89: 505.

Volpe, E. P. 1964. Fate of neural crest homotransplants in pattern mutants of the leopard frog. J. Exp. Zool. 157: 179.

Volpe, E. P., and Gebhardt, B. M. 1965. Effect of dosage on the survival of embryonic homotransplants in the leopard frog, *Rana pipiens*. J. Exp. Zool. 16: 11.

Yntema, C. L. 1970. Survival of xenogeneic grafts of embryonic pigment and carapace rudiments in embryos of *Chelydra serpentina*. J. Morph. 132: 353.

Chapter 9

Characteristics of Transplantation Immunity

INTRODUCTION

An animal's response to *self* and *not-self* develops phylogenetically, and within certain taxonomic groups the development of this response can be followed in ontogeny. Presumably it is among the vertebrates that differentiation is most complete. When immunologically competent cells, whether *in vivo* or *in vitro*, are confronted with foreign antigens, cells of the immune system recognize differences and the antigens are destroyed. There are complex host regulatory influences on the efficiency of antigen disposal, but the basic control is at the genetic level. It is programmed within the genes of immunocompetent cells which antigens they will respond to, even those from close relatives. Histocompatibility genes determine how animals react to closely related cell and tissue antigens. Assuming maximum recognition of such foreign antigens, events occur leading to the destruction of foreign cell or tissue transplants. These involve primarily the activities of various immune cells.

Let us examine briefly what happens if a tissue graft represents the source of antigen. Once a technically successful graft is performed, it acts as a trigger that sets the mechanism of the immune system in motion; later the graft is destroyed. Briefly, this involves the host's recognition of the foreign transplant by lymphocytes and phagocytic cells producing a pronounced inflammatory reaction; finally graft destruction is probably effected by a combination of unknown cell activities and their products, lymphokines, and perhaps even antibody. After an encounter with a graft, followed by its destruction, lymphocytes are capable of reproducing themselves and they, or their offspring, will respond to a second encounter with the same antigen that evoked the first response; this is *anamnesis*, or *memory*. When animals respond to the first graft and finally destroy it, they are then usually capable, within certain time limits, of responding to that same antigen faster than they did upon first contact. Immune cells "remember" that they have "seen" the antigen previously and they can therefore respond quicker, obviating the need for restimulating a new population of cells initially by antigen. A first graft is referred to as the *first-set graft* and a second from the same donor is the *second-set graft*.

There is a trend now to think of immunologic memory in broader, less strict terms because of newly available information from studies of a number of animal groups. According to the classical approach, if an experimenter wants to test whether the host developed memory to a first-set transplant, it is necessary to wait for a short period after rejection of the first graft before performing the second graft. In most animals that have been studied a great deal (e.g., mouse strains) and that differ at strong histocompatibility loci (H-loci), rejection of first-set grafts is rapid or acute and that of a second graft is even faster than the first. There are certain mouse strains and other animal species, however, where the time of second-set graft destruction is longer than the time required for rejection of the first graft. Hosts that show faster rejections of second-set grafts than first-set grafts have developed positive memory and those with longer rejection times, negative memory. Actually both kinds of memory responses are represented throughout the animal kingdom in various phyla.

The graft rejection response is specific. In addition to first- and second-set grafts from the same donor, one can simultaneously test the capacity of a host to respond specifically to another graft, independent in origin from either of the other two grafts. Such a graft is often referred to as the *third man* graft, and it's destruction usually occurs at a time independent of either the first or the second graft. In the absence of specificity a host would not be able to distinguish so sharply between antigens from any of the three grafts. Another test, cellular in nature, is useful for showing incompatibility between a host and several potential donors and is performed in the following way. Lymphocytes from an intended host are injected subcutaneously into a panel of recipients, one of which will be the donor. Of the four, the one that gives the minimal skin response is the best donor. Actually, the fact that a given host will not destroy an autograft but will reject a graft derived from a different but closely related donor is evidence for the earliest known specificity, even without a test from a third independent graft. Differentiating between *self* and *not-self* is specific. The metabolic events of autografts and allografts are different from each other. This can be easily determined by measuring uptake of a labelled precursor (Fig. 9-1).

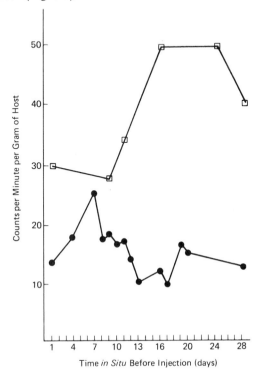

Fig. 9-1 Illustration of the average C^{14} uptake by groups of autografts (□) and homografts (●) at different days post implantation in *Rana pipiens*. (*From*: Staggers, *J. Exp. Zool.*, **153**: 149, 1963.)

Counts per Minute per Gram of Host

Time *in Situ* Before Injection (days)

When a foreign graft is transplanted it heals initially, is temporarily recognized as *self*, and enjoys all the priviledges of nourishment as if it were an autograft. However, the persistent immune surveillance system of every animal host recognizes the graft's foreign antigens and cells are soon mobilized to the graft site to effect its destruction. Along with the molecular events accompanying graft rejection (i.e., lymphokines or antibody) in any animal, there are also external, often quantifiable, visible signs of graft destruction: the survival of pigment cells in invertebrates, fishes, amphibians, and reptiles, is the gross, easily observable criterion of graft viability. In birds and in mammals, it is the condition of the feathers and hair. Once mammalian and avian grafts are destroyed they are movable as a cicatrix, but in the primitive vertebrates, grafts are gradually resorbed by the host; certain reptiles may be an exception. Except for the higher teleosts and mammals, this chapter considers one kind of graft rejection response, the chronic rejection pattern. It is slower than the acute response, found throughout the animal kingdom, and may represent an evolutionary relic. A preponderance of primitive animals possess this characteristic.

Transplantation Reactions in Fishes

Agnathans
  The hagfish

A description of allograft rejection in the hagfish merits considerable coverage. This animal, the most primitive of vertebrates, is so classified because of certain morphological features. The Pacific hagfish, *Eptatretus stoutii*, belongs to the class of cyclostome or myxinoid fishes. Hagfish probably evolved from the ostracoderm group of jawless Devonian fishes, which also lacked paired fins and may have been the first chordates. Hagfishes lack jaws and stomach, have a persistent notochord and cartilaginous skeleton, and possess at least four hearts. They possess only one nostril, whose sense of smell is powerful enough to offset their poor if not nonexistent vision; apparently their sense of touch is also well developed. Hagfish are extremely important to comparative immunology because of the work of Hildemann and Thoenes (1969), who settled a controversy over the exact point in evolution when vertebrate cell-mediated immune reactions appeared. Prior to their dedicated work, it was assumed that vertebrate immunity in its simplest form was first apparent in the lamprey, a close taxonomic relative of the hagfish. Such a contention only fostered the notion then of a gap in the evolution of cellular immunity among the annelids, echinoderms, and the lampreys. Immunologists trained as biologists realized that such an interruption was unlikely.

In contrast to teleost fishes or anuran amphibians, for example, the allograft rejection response of hagfishes is chronic, a condition more like certain other primitive fishes, apodan and urodele amphibians, certain reptiles, and some mammals. There is a dearth of information on birds. Despite the prolonged time required for rejection, there are the usual microscopic sequelae which characterize cell-mediated immunity. There is consistent lymphocyte infiltration, hemorrhagic inflammation, and, like other primitive vertebrates, pigment cell destruction. In fact, hagfishes, like the annelids and echinoderms (the only invertebrates so far studied) and all other vertebrates show persistent immunological memory to transplantation antigens. This is readily demonstrable by both positive and negative memory responses to second-set grafts.

Despite their primitive status, under proper laboratory conditions hagfish destroy allografts. Hildemann and Thoenes persisted, and in spite of many technical and logistic problems, successfully performed allografts on hagfishes. Skin allografts were usually transplanted just behind the head, and as a means of comparision they made

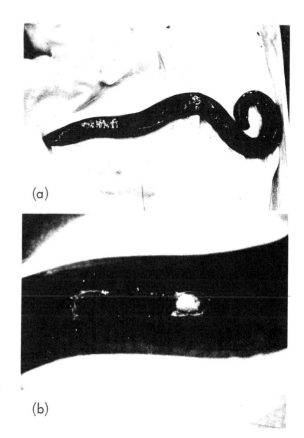

(a)

Fig. 9-2 Views of adult hagfish with skin grafts. (a) Entire hagfish showing grafts in anterior-dorsal position several centimeters behind the head. (b) Close-up view of fully viable autograft (*left*) and blanched allograft (*right*) at survival end point showing complete pigment cell destruction. (*From*: Hildemann & Thoenes, *Transplantation*, **7**: 506, 1969.)

(b)

companion autografts, which of course are never destroyed (Fig. 9-2). Both autografts and first-set allografts of skin require ten to fourteen days to heal with sufficient firmness at 18–19°C. At this time both grafts appear alike, i.e., like autogenous skin with no signs of incompatibility. There is a compact, continuous layer of dermal melanophores and, until healing is complete, only a slight inflammation in the form of hyperplasia appears in association with autografts at their contact zone with the host (Fig. 9-3).

At twenty-five to thirty days post-grafting, signs of beginning rejection occur in some first-set allografts. These signs are (1) envelopment of the graft by an unpigmented layer of hyperplastic host tissue resulting in a cloudy appearing graft; (2) vasodilation and hemostasis resulting in sluggish blood flow with some redness that

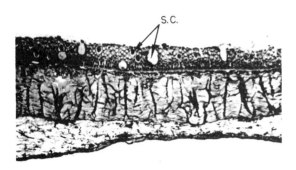

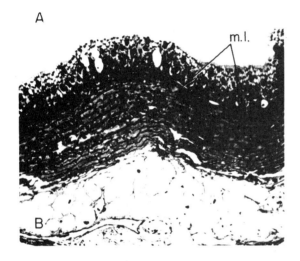

Fig. 9-3 Cross section of fully viable autograft at 80 days showing structure of normal skin. Note abundance of two types of secretory or mucous cells, *s.c.*, in epidermis. The dermal pigmentation (melanophores) lies in a layer, *m.l.*, just beneath the epidermis. This is more easily seen in (b) than in (a). The relatively thick dermis reveals mainly collagen, fibroblasts, and smooth muscle cells. A zone of areolar connective tissue extends from the vascular deep dermis to the collagen covering the underlying striated muscle. (H & E stain.) (*From*: Hildemann & Thoenes, *Transplantation*, **7**: 506, 1969.)

outlines an otherwise difficult to see capillary network; and (3) slight melanophore or pigment cell granulation. As shown in Fig. 9-2, allografts become pale or blanched and histologically show the following characteristics. Once rejection ensues, mononuclear cells infiltrate the graft dermis. Dermal melanophores are destroyed and the epidermis shows atrophy. Epidermal destruction is best represented by the disappearance of mucous cells (Fig. 9-4).

The median survival time of destroyed first-set grafts on hagfish is about seventy-two days, and for second-set grafts from the same donor, it is about twenty-eight days at a temperature of 18–19°C (Fig. 9-5). If second-set transplants are grafted immediately after first-set graft destruction they are rejected at an even faster rate, in approximately fourteen days. In classic immunologic terms the challenged host exhibits memory in its reaction to the second-graft, rejecting it more rapidly. Quite the opposite can also occur in hagfish. Rejection of second-set grafts is occasionally prolonged, a phenomenon known as *negative memory*. Negative memory seems to occur in taxonomic groups that possess weak histocompatibility antigens. Absence of recognizably strong, antigens that result in prompt second-set graft rejection effectively inhibit active cellular immunity and, thus, prolong graft acceptance.

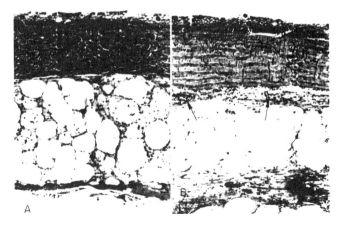

Fig. 9-4 (a) Cross section of first-set allograft at zero survival end point at 134 days after grafting. (b) Similar cross section of second-set allograft with late zero survival end point at 100 days after grafting. Note destruction of dermal melanophore layer persistence of lymphocyte infiltration, especially in second-set graft (*arrows*). Compare with Fig. 9-3. (H & E stain) (*From*: Hildemann & Thoenes, *Transplantation*, **7**: 506, 1969.)

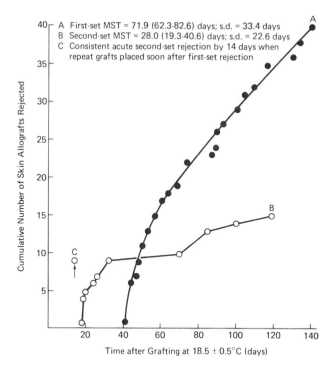

Fig. 9-5 Cumulative distributions of skin allograft survival times in Pacific hagfish. A. An MST of 72 days was determined for 40 single, first-set allografts with confidence limits as indicated. B. An MST of 28 days was found for 15 single, second-set allografts made while first sets were still viable but had presumably sensitized their recipients; unusual time-mortality distribution reflects prolonged or enhanced survival of some repeat grafts. C. Acute second-set rejection of 9 grafts occurred by 14 days when repeat grafts placed at 0–56 days after completion of first-set rejection. (*From*: Hildemann & Thoenes, *Transplantation*, **7**: 506, 1969.)

The Lamprey

Skin allograft rejection is certainly evident in a close relative of the hagfish, the lamprey, *Petromyzon marinus*. According to Perey et al. (1968), larvae of the sea lamprey, or ammocetes, show chronic or slow reactions to allografts at temperatures of about 20°C. As the authors used no rigid criteria for assessing graft rejection, a clear comparison of survival time of their first- and second-set grafts, to test for memory, cannot be made. Although survival times range from seven to 252 days, the rejection is no doubt immune, for it is accompanied by inflammation and the infiltration of lymphoid cells into the graft-host contact zones.

Chondrichthyes

In the cartilaginous fishes that have been studied there is chronic, or slow, rejection of first-set allografts. Other, more typical manifestations of immunity are also readily demonstrable. For example, autografts or *self* antigens are never destroyed. In their study of the stingray, *Dasyatus americana*, Perey's group found that the onset of its first-set graft rejection occurs by twenty-one days; second-set grafts have a curtailed survival of less than twelve days and more severe inflammatory reactions take place. Anamnesis is clearly indicated by these findings. Borysenko and Hildemann (personal communication) describe the progressive development of skin allograft immunity in the horned shark, *Heterodontis francisci*. Although the kinetics of its first-set rejection parallel those of the stingray, a defective immune system is not suggested by either animal's slow rejection of first-set grafts. The progressively decreasing survival time of successive skin allografts culminates in the vigorous, acute destruction of a fourth-set graft.

Osteichthyes
  Introduction

Because the bony fishes are easy to maintain in the laboratory, especially as pets, they are subjects of many studies of transplantation immunity. A detailed description of transplantation immune reactions found in poikilothermic vertebrates best begins with a brief mention of Hildemann's work with the goldfish in 1957. This investigation was a catalyst that initiated a new, secondary thrust for comparative immunology during the twentieth century. Based on the criteria Hildemann established then, significant information has become available through him directly, or indirectly through his students. In addition to maintenance methods for goldfish, he measured the median survival times (MST) and determined the nature of inflammatory reactions to scale allografts. The length of time required to reach the end points of both first- and second-set graft rejections varies inversely with temperature. Second-set scale allografts have a survival time that is approximately one-half to two-thirds that of primary grafts from the same donor at any given temperature. His gross criterion for allograft rejection, i.e., survival of pigment cells, is best illustrated by survival of melanocytes in another teleost, *Fundulus heteroclitus* (Fig. 9-6–9-11).

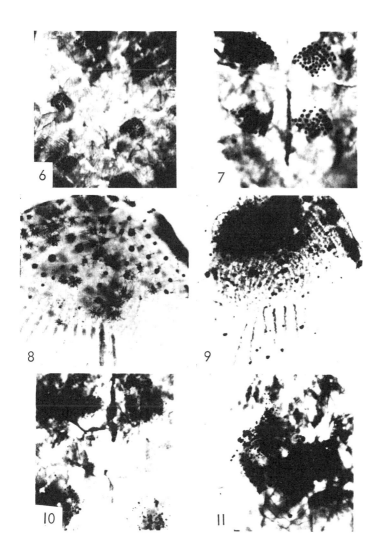

Fig. 9-6 Six scale homografts on the first day after transplantation. (*6×*).

Fig. 9-7 Four scale homografts, 1 day after transplantation, on either side of the linea alba showing the pattern of vascularization and the expanded melanocytes. (*12×*).

Fig. 9-8 Appearance of a single scale 3 days before the onset of the homograft reaction showing expanded melanocytes. (*50×*).

Fig. 9-9 Appearance of a single scale after the onset of the homograft reaction showing only the remaining melanin granules. (*25×*).

Fig. 9-10 Four scales after onset of homograft reaction. The melanocytes have completely broken down leaving only the melanin granules. (*12×*).

Fig. 9-11 Appearnce of a single scale graft after the onset of the homograft reaction. (*25×*). (*From*: Cooper, *Transplantation*, **2**: 2, 1964.)

Table 9-1

Comparative skin allograft survival times among diverse fishes

Class and (order)	Species	Median survival times and ranges (days)		Interval between first-set and second-set grafting (days)	Water temperature (°C)
		First-set	Second-set		
Agnatha (Myxiniformes)	Hagfish (*Eptatretus stoutii*)	71.9 (41–140)	28 0 (18–119)	30	18.5±0.5
(Petromyzontiformes)	Lamprey (*Petromyzon marinus*)	~38 (21– > 291)	~18 (7– > 252)	39	18–21
Chondrichthyes (Rajiformes)	Stingray (*Dasyatus americana*)	> 31 (< 31–53)	< 12 (?)	53	18–28
(Squaliformes)	Horn Shark (*Heterodontis francisci*)	41.1 (27–48)	16.7 (15–22)	60	22.0±1.0
Osteichthyes (Acipenseriformes)	Paddlefish (*Polyodon spathula*)	42–68 (21– > 76)	~12 (?)	68	18–26(1st set) 6–13(2nd set)
(Clupeiformes)	Arowana (*Osteoglossum bicirrhosum*)	17.9 (13–25)	5.1 (3–7)	30	25.0±0.5°C
(Cypriniformes)	Goldfish (*Carrasius auratus*)	7.2 (6–11)	4.7 (4–6)	25	25.0±0.5°C
(Perciformes)	Blue Acara (*Aequidens latifrons*)	7.2 (6–11)	4.5 (3–6)	25	25.0±0.5°C

(*From*: Hildemann, Transpl. Proc., **2**: 253, 1970.)

Chondrostean and Holostean

As Table 9-1 reveals there is indeed a dearth of information on allograft reactions in chondrosteans. Apparently chronic graft rejection reactions occur similar to those already described in more primitive fishes. However, one important environmental variable was neglected: they were maintained at wide temperature ranges and observations of grafts were infrequent, rendering the data unclear. Yet what was observed falls into a pattern of a seemingly progressive differentiation from chronic to acute (long to short rejection times) rejection times.

The paddlefish (a chondrostean) and the arowana are both primitive freshwater bony fishes, by morphologic criteria. However, their evolutionary antecedents and geographical origins are quite different. The paddlefish, *Polyodon*, is a specialized chondrostean fish from a temperate climate. By contrast, according to Greenwood et al. (1966), the genus *Osteoglossum* (the arowana) belongs to the superorder *Osteoglossomorpha*. Herein are "fishes of ancestry at or near the holostean level of organization in which all contained members have retained numerous primitive characteristics of the jaw suspension and shoulder girdle, and have developed complexly ornamented scales." Apparently this superorder, one of three such divisions at this taxonomic

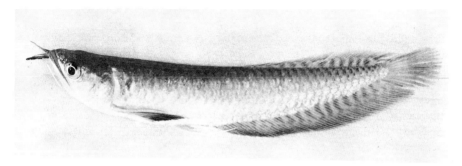

Fig. 9-12 An *Osteoglossum bicirrhosum*. (×2/3). (*From*: Borysenko & Hildemann, *Transplantation*, **8**: 403, 1969.)

level, probably reached their evolutionary end and were not involved in the ancestry of other teleosteans. Thus, any information on the immune responses of this group is intriguing when compared to the fishes in general. They fill an important gap in the field of comparative transplantation immunology. The Amazonian species known as the arowana (*Osteoglossum bicirrhosum*) will be discussed (Fig. 9-12).

For the arowana, the same criteria for establishing immunity to allografts are as applicable as in any other primitive vertebrate. Borysenko and Hildemann (1969) maintained a constant temperature of 25°C; the destruction of pigment cells provided a sensitive indicator of allograft rejection. The median survival time of first-set allografts is 17.9 days, a time considerably longer than that for most advanced teleosts, which is 7.2 days. To test for memory, second-set grafts were performed after rejection

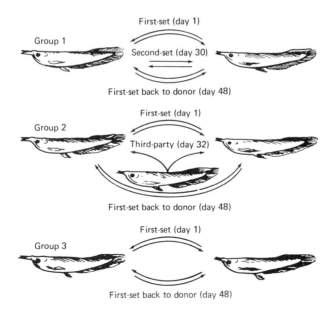

Fig. 9-13 Schema of scale allotransplantation experiments. (*From*: Borysenko & Hildemann, *Transplantation*, **8**: 403, 1969.)

of first-set grafts. The memory, or anamnestic response, is, however, prompt and at 5.1 days is acute.

The third-party graft is a convenient tool in transplantation immunology for testing the degree of genetic relatedness between hosts and donors (Fig. 9-13). If a host has destroyed a first-set graft at a hypothetical time $2 \times A$, a second-set survival time for a graft from the original donor, assuming faster second rejection or positive memory, should be shortened by one-half to time A. Now, to test for the relationship of the donor of the second graft and another donor in a population, one makes a transplant from the new unidentified individual. An equal survival time of A indicates antigen sharing. The results with arowana were different. Third-party survival times ranged from 4.3 to 15.4 days, i.e., $A - 2 \times A$. This suggests diverse histocompatibility genes and antigens in this species.

Higher Teleosts

Whole integument or scale allografts in fishes are more advantageous than comparable skin grafts in birds and mammals, especially for quantitative studies; there are still many species of fishes that await investigation even by the beginner in transplantation immunology. Because scales from fish are easily plucked and do not require cutting, an individual scale becomes a single transplant. These are merely inserted into another pocket from which a scale has been previously plucked and there it readily takes up residence in the new host site; there is no need for sutures or bandages. Scales usually possess chromatophores; the color is of course species specific. Melanophores, black pigment cells, are easily counted, thus making it possible to quantitate graft rejection. When scale allografts are well healed or belong to permanently healed autografts, they spread in a luxuriant manner and are easily counted (see Figs. 9-6 to 9-11). On the other hand, the fate of chromatophores is inevitable and they are doomed if they belong to allografts. Once the host's immune response is in motion and the grafts destroyed, the scale appears faded and peppered with spilled melanin granules—in quantitative terms, a zero survival.

Regardless of which vertebrate is examined, a transplanted graft must heal before the immune system can recognize that it is different. In fish, after scale transplantation, capillary blood flow is restored in first-set allografts by inosculation of the original graft and host vessels within seventy-two hours after transplantation. Such definitive circulation persists for only a few days; then blood flow ceases (hemostasis) and graft breakdown, of course, is the consequence. Circulation to second grafts, because the host is already primed, is sluggish and of short duration prior to rejection. Such second-set characteristics, if they involve a mammalian graft, are referred to as a *white graft reaction*.

Scale allograft reactions in all fishes elicit overt inflammation characterized by a cloudy epithelial hyperplasia at the graft-host contact zone. Only goldfish and carp scale allografts, however, produce conspicuous vascular damage that results in extravasation of blood. With regard to second-sets, the inflammatory response is more intense, accentuated, appears earlier, and develops more rapidly. The rapidity of the secondary response of these teleosts confirms their capacity for anamnesis, a third characteristic of immunity, typical of teleosts and other vertebrates. In most fishes, scleroprotein constitutes most of the organic matter of scale plates; it elicits late inflammatory reactions associated with gradual erosion and digestion of allograft scale plates. Thus, there is first a breakdown of soft tissues followed by erosion of scale plates. Actually, scale plates, i.e., scleroprotein, are antigenic, since accelerated reactions to second-set scale plate grafts do occur. Such vigorous allograft reactions exhibit the extremely fine sensitivity and highly developed alloimmune capacity typical of teleosts (Table 9-1). The median survival times of 8.6 ± 0.5 days and 6.0 ± 3 days for first- and second-set grafts on black-spot barbs, for example, are characteristic of the survival times for mammalian and avian skin allografts exchanged across distant genetic barriers.

Another important result of goldfish transplantation immune studies is the discovery that strong skin transplantation immunity can be developed by either a subcutaneous or an intramuscular immunization with blood leukocytes. However, no such response to transplantation antigens develops if goldfish are injected by the intraperitoneal route. Apparently the intraperitoneal space has no adequate filtering organs capable of capturing antigens on cells. Of secondary importance is the possible interrelationship between the synthesis of serum antibodies and graft rejection. If an animal has destroyed an allograft, are antibodies present against cells derived from the donor of the graft? Isohaemagglutinin titres determined before and after immunization with scale allografts reveal no correlation between serum antibody concentration and the degree of transplantation immunity. Thus, haemagglutinating antibodies are distinct from the cell-bound or cytophilic antibodies presumed to participate in scale allograft breakdown in goldfish. This conclusion may require reexamination.

Comment

In broad terms, the fishes possess two fundamental types of allograft reactions. The more primitive fishes show a prolonged, chronic, rather sluggish reaction to first-set allografts. It is not until we study the holosteans or their near relatives that we see acute second-set reactions. Thus, two generalizations emerge as a result of transplantation studies among the fishes. The more primitive fishes show chronic rejection of first-set allografts, and there is both positive and negative memory to second-set grafts. Memory may be weaker, however, and short-lived, since it seems to require a shorter time to develop. There seems to be a second trend among the primitive bony fishes. Although there is chronic rejection of first-set allografts, second-sets are rejected in an acute fashion. Perhaps at the level of holosteans, memory is sharper and better developed. Another crucial factor is the number of histocompatibility antigens within a population to which a host can react. In the holosteans, specifically within the arowana population, the evidence suggests the presence of a large number of histocompatibility antigens. It is clear that both responses are present in all major taxonomic groups; yet the significance or efficacy of the way in which a host fish handles a closely related cell or tissue antigen is unknown.

CHRONIC GRAFT REJECTION IN URODELE AMPHIBIANS

Introduction

The existence of two types of immune responses to skin allografts provides a criterion for classifying two groups of amphibians. The urodeles and the legless apodans exhibit chronic rejection, while the anurans exhibit more rapid acute rejection. The cell response to allografts is relatively weak in younger urodeles, in which the immune capacity has not differentiated to its fullest capacity. On the other hand, adult urodele and apodan cell responses nearly parallel those in mammals; the same infiltration into the grafts by lymphocytic and granulocytic cells occurs after grafting. Because the urodeles, unlike fishes or larval and adult amphibians, display a prolonged rejection of allografts, embryologists once attributed their precocious rejections to poor technical procedures. Such explanations have since been disproved by the immunologic and embryologic expertise of Cohen.

Histopathology of Graft Rejection in Adult Urodeles

Cohen (1966a, b) allografted dorsal pigmented skin to the throat and flank of adult *Diemictylus viridescens* collected in the field and maintained at $23 \pm 0.5°C$. A long latent period of about sixteen days occurs; the latent period is a time when allografts are grossly and histologically indistinguishable from autografts. There is an initial dilation of blood vessels in allografts, followed by restoration of blood circulation in both autografts and allografts between ten and eleven days after grafting. In general, *Diemictylus viridescens* begins to reject first-set allografts approximately seventeen days post-grafting, a typical chronic response. Certain events occur so that the response is characterized by secondary vessel dilation, hemostasis at about the twentieth day, hemorrhage by about the twenty-third day, and eventual melanophore death at the fortieth day. Whereas these times seem definite, these events may vary with respect to time of onset, intensity, and duration. At the histologic level, secondary vessel dilation is accompanied by an increased infiltration of small lymphocytes into the graft prior to its actual destruction. Finally, hemostasis, hemorrhage, and melanophore death are paralleled by stronger lymphocyte infiltration and death of integument glands. Though circulation is reestablished in 58 % of second-set transplants, these grafts, if performed twenty-eight days after the rejection of first-set grafts, elicit a clear anamnestic response. By contrast, second-set transplants grafted only ten days after first-set rejection are not rejected in a shorter time. Instead such grafts often survive for a few days longer than first-set grafts. Apparently, though the graft is destroyed by gross and even microscopic criteria, a longer residence succeeds in establishing and perhaps maintaining the initial state of immunity.

Tissue Antigen Recognition in Adult Urodeles

Antigen recognition in outbreeding, field-collected salamanders is important to phylogenetic and immunologic concepts because they, according to Cohen's interpretation, do not possess a major histocompatibility gene complex. Furthermore they lack lymph nodes, and their spleen, like that of other vertebrates, is unessential for graft rejection. These two characteristics alone however do not explain entirely the salamanders' skin allograft rejection pattern. Cohen defines the newt's rate of antigen recognition as the time required for a first graft to be in residence in order for a host to become immunologically capable of rejecting a subsequent second- and third-set graft at an accelerated rate. It appears that most newts must be exposed to a sensitizing first-set skin allograft for more than ten days before they reject second-set grafts more rapidly. Shorter exposure times seem to prime some hosts so that, although they reject second-set grafts in an accelerated fashion, survival of third-set grafts is prolonged. Longer exposure times of fifteen to thirty days for the test graft correlate with a more rapid rejection of second-set grafts and with an increased number of third-set grafts that are rejected significantly more rapidly than second sets.

TRANSPLANTATION REACTIONS IN ADULT REPTILES

Introduction

Although the immune response to skin allografts of fishes, amphibians, and reptiles has not been studied as extensively as it has been in birds and mammals, allograft immunity in poikilotherms is a reality. Usually allografts are exchanged between members of the same genus and species, but xenografts can be transplanted between two closely related animals that are of different genus and species. Among the invertebrates and poikilotherms, (the earthworm, urodele amphibians and reptiles, and adult birds and mammals), skin xenografts are rejected more rapidly than allografts. The reptiles served as subjects for sporadic studies of transplantation reactions that were usually devoted to biologic phenomena other than those characterized as immune. Early investigators were interested primarily in the fate of pigment cells after grafting skin between two lizards. May (1923), for example, attributed the pigment cell destruction to technical failure. Pigment cell breakdown is, however, today used by comparative immunologists as a gross criterion for assessing the survival time of a graft; it becomes, therefore, a measure of the host's immune reaction against the graft.

Since May's early work, knowledge of reptilian transplant immunity has increased considerably. Not only is pigment cell breakdown now viewed as a necessary criterion for assessing an immune reaction, but the reptilian host's immune reaction is known to be as temperature-dependent as it is in all other poikilothermic vertebrates. Furthermore, the law of recognition and acceptance of *self* tissue and rejection of *not-self* has been demonstrated to prevail among the reptiles. Studies of the turtle, *Chelydra serpentina*, have pointed out the role of lymphoid organs in regulating the immune response, and such findings have contributed to our knowledge of the ontogenesis of immunity. Though the turtle has yielded much of the present information on the various parameters involved in the reptile's allograft destruction, the chameleon, *Anolis carolinensis*, the iguana, *Ctenosaura pectinata*, and the yucca night lizard, *Xanthusia vigilis*, have also proved convenient, easily husbanded reptiles for study. Allograft rejection times of various reptiles are summarized in Table 9-2. By comparison, transplants survive longer in reptiles than in anuran amphibians but for approximately the same time as urodeles. Perhaps the greatest contribution reptilian studies could offer is to relate, either morphologically or functionally, the immune system of reptiles to that of birds, thereby providing another physiologic link between classes. We know from the fossil record that the present-day birds and also mammals probably evolved from ancestral reptiles.

The Chronic Response in Turtles

Though the turtle has more centers of lymphoid activity than most poikilotherms, it still exhibits chronic rejection of allografts. Thus, we are still unable to correlate precisely the machinery of the immune system (cells, tissue, and organs) with certain gross manifestations of immune responses. There might seem to be a purely physical reason for this—the turtle's thick dermal pad may retard the rate of lymphoid cell

Table 9-2

Skin allograft rejection in reptilia

Order	Genus and species	Temperature (°C)	MST* (and/or range)	
			First-set	Second-set
Chelonia	Chelydra serpentina (snapping turtle)	25	47 (41–70)	25 (20–32)
Squamata	Anolis carolinensis (chameleon)	23.5	60–90	—
	Cnemidophorus sexlineatus (race runner lizard)	—	> 26	—
	Ctenosaura pectinata (iguana)	25	48–87	30–86
	Calotes versicolor (bloodsucker lizard)	29–33	> 45	—
	Xanthusia vigilis (yucca night lizard)	20	21–245	—
	Thamnophis sirtalis (garter snake)	25	41 (31–53)	25 (21–29)
Crocodilia	Caiman sclerops (caiman)	25–27	> 65 (25– > 110)	—

*MST: mean or median survival time, in most cases representing zero end point or total allograft rejection.
(*From*: Borysenko, Transpl. Proc., **2**: 299, 1970.)

infiltration and thereby retard the entire rejection process. However, turtle skin may be actually no thicker than rabbit skin, yet rabbits reject first-set grafts within a week. Furthermore, six-month-old and one-year-old snapping turtles reject skin allografts from donors thier own age at about the same time as adults, even though such grafts are much thinner than those of large adult turtles. Thus, the rate of rejection, apparently, is not dependent on the physical thickness of the transplant, nor is it dependent upon age. Reptiles are the first group of animals in the evolutionary scale to show shedding of a rejected transplant, a gross criterion reminiscent of the process in birds and mammals. Certain microscopic changes are in progress when severe hemorrhaging appears grossly; this is followed one week later by complete graft destruction. The graft soon falls off as a dark scab leaving only a small collagen pad. Hemorrhaging and scab formation are easily observed gross changes (Fig. 9-14).

A second untenable explanation for the snapping turtle's slow allograft response is that it has a phylogenetically primitive or deficient immune system that renders it immunologically incapable of acute or rapid rejection of skin grafts. If this should prove to be true it would be restricted and peculiar to cell-mediated immunity as revealed by graft rejection. The turtle's immunoglobulin-producing capacity is as advanced as that in birds. There is, however, much experimental support for the hypothesis that the turtle's chronic rejection results from sharing of histocompatibility genes between certain turtle populations. For example, two-year-old animals bearing

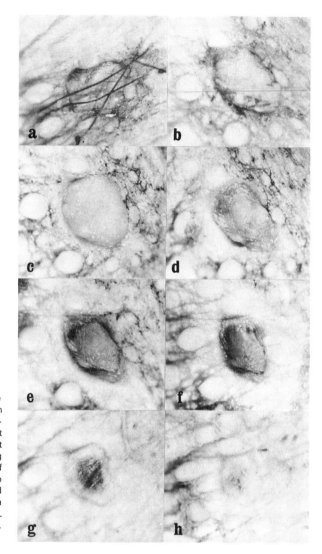

Fig. 9-14 A series of photographs showing the healing, survival, and rejection of a typical skin allograft at 25 1 C. (a) Day 1, the graft immediately after the operation. (b) Day 17, the graft has healed firmly in place. (c) Day 22, the graft looks quite healthy. (d) Day 34, hemorrhaging in periphery of the graft, making the beginning of graft rejection (Event 1). (e) Day 37, scab beginning to form. (f) Day 44, scab is well formed (Event 2). (g) Day 48, scab sloughed, leaving a wound. (h) Day 54, wound at graft site healed. (*From*: Borysenko, *J. Exp. Zool.*, **170**: 341, 1969.)

xenografts that were transplanted during embryo periods reject third-party xenografts that survive much longer than those on previouly ungrafted turtles. This reflects a tolerance to skin xenografts from turtles unrelated to the orginal donor. One hypothetical explanation of this tolerance is the histocompatibility (H) gene-sharing between the donor species. Determination of the number of H genes that are in fact shared is difficult, as it requires laboratory conditions suitable for mating. If one could be certain of the genetic background of the turtles studied, one could define the number of shared genes. It is only among mammals that rigid laboratory inbreeding has yielded strains of mice, for example, with well-known genetic backgrounds that are easily analyzed by transplantation studies.

Histopathology

As Borysenko (1969) demonstrated clearly, the snapping turtle's response to skin allografts can be divided into two major phases: a latent phase and a rejection phase. The latent phase involves graft healing and adjustment to the new host. Certainly at this time the antigens in the graft will soon be recognized. The end of the latent phase cannot be determined grossly, since no obvious changes occur until the graft is near the end of the rejection phase. However, in the latter part of the latent phase, a marked dermal thickening in autografts, allografts, and xenografts occurs. The latent phase also involves several morphological changes due to the ongoing healing and adjustment. First of all, mononuclear cells migrate to the wound and sites of inflammation and are usually there up to three days after transplantation. Specifically, the cells are large and small lymphocytes, monocytes, and plasma cells. Although neutrophils also appear, studies of the turtle's peripheral blood reveal that they may be naturally scarce. It is interesting that autografts, too, show distinct mononuclear infiltrates, which undoubtedly means that such cells are responding to the presence of a wound and are thereby participating in general, nonspecific reactions. The final rejection phase follows and is characterized by lymphoid cell invasion, vascular breakdown, and, finally, necrosis of foreign tissue. Although vasodilation and hemostasis are usually reported as indicators of the rejection phase, these criteria are difficult to observe grossly in adult snapping turtles.

Importance of Temperature in Turtles

Borysenko (1969) has demonstrated that the immune response of the snapping turtle is as temperature-dependent as it is for other poikilotherms. At 25°C ± 1° there is a ten-to-fifteen-day period during which skin allografts are indistinguishable from autografts. Despite some minor mononuclear cell infiltrations, autografts remain unchanged grossly and histologically. Subsequent to this ten-to-fifteen-day period, allografts on both one- and two-year-old turtles and on fully mature turtles are rejected at 25°C ± 1°. Graft rejection is preceded by substantial melanophore death, but followed by little or no scab formation. However, at 10°C ± 1° snapping turtles do not react immunologically to skin allografts. Neither gross nor histological evidence of skin allograft or xenograft incompatibility appears. Evidently, the low temperature either inhibits the rejection process or decelerates it markedly. One interesting event that occurs in both allografts and autografts at this temperature is aggravated vasodilation of the vessels in the grafts at one to three weeks after transplantation. Similarly, no grossly observable reaction to skin xenografts from either painted or Blanding turtles seems to occur at 10°C ± 1°. Moreover, histological analysis indicates no abnormal lymphoid cell infiltration. At 25°C ± 1°, one- and two-year-old snappers do reject xenografts from adult painted turtles. Borysenko also noted that when the animals are transferred to 25°C ± 1°C after fifty days, they develop loose xenografts at eighteen to twenty-six days and lose the grafts at twenty-three to twenty-nine days after transfer. Raising the temperature thus seems to augment or release a brooding latent reaction. At a temperature of 33°C ± 1° snappers reject allografts at about twenty-four days, which is significantly faster than those at 25°C ± 1°C.

Squamata
  The Lizards
    The Mexican Iguana

The iguana is suitable reptile for studies of allograft reactions, since it, like the turtles and snakes, is a representative modern reptile. Transplants are relatively easy to perform and skin allografts and autografts behave like those of other vertebrates: the autografts heal permanently, while the allografts heal initially but are later rejected. Allograft rejection is chronic and characterized by a breakdown of melanophores. Furthermore, the inflammatory response accompanied by lymphocytic infiltration is usually observed in destroyed grafts. Cooper and Aponte (1968) suggested that a chronic rejection response in the Mexican iguana, *Ctenosaura pectinata*, may be the result of too low a temperature (25°C) during experimentation, since other reptiles have been maintained at temperatures as high as 40°C. This conclusion may be untenable; further analysis is required, since we know that in certain homothermic mammals, chronic rejection is not temperature dependent. Of particular interest in the iguana is the phenomenon of negative memory. As has been noted, in most mammals, birds, anuran amphibian larvae, and certain teleost fishes, the specific response to a second-set transplant from the orginal donor is an accelerated rejection of the second grafts, revealing positive memory. This, however, does not occur in the iguana, or in earthworms, mice, outbred Syrian hamsters, salamanders, or in legless, apodan amphibians. Survival time of most second-set grafts is longer than it is for first-set grafts. It appears that those animals that usually exhibit a chronic rejection of first-set grafts have a significant majority of second-sets that survive longer than the initial grafts. Here, too, we must infer that the iguana is no different from any other animal in that weak H-loci seem to govern the degree of compatibility between donors and hosts.

The Garden Lizard

In their studies of the garden lizard, Manickavel and Muthukkaruppan (1969) observed that autografts and allografts heal well and become fully vascularized during the first week after grafting. In addition, host epithelium extends over the open wound at the edges of allograft and autograft host contact zones. In allografts, however, by the ninth day after grafting, dilation of blood vessels begins, and by the fifteenth day the stellate portions of the melanophores disrupt, leaving loose, dark melanocyte granules. Two weeks later disruption is more intense, leaving increased numbers of granules so that only a few intact melanophores remain. Total dissolution of all pigment cells, reflecting complete graft destruction, occurs about forty-five days after grafting.

According to Manickavel and Muthukkarupan (1969), the time sequence of skin allograft rejection is similar to that which occurs in the snapping turtle. Whereas Cooper and Aponte (1968) define the final stage of the iguana's rejection as sloughing of dead allografts or actual dislodging of the outer keratin layer, Manickavel defines the final stage of the lizard's rejection as the changes in melanophores in whole mount preparations of scales. This method, i.e., the enumeration of melanocyte numbers, is similar to the one used to calculate the survival time of fish scale allografts.

The Cellular Response in Snakes
Introduction

Up to now we have only dealt with the gross manifestations of allograft survival in vertebrates that show both chronic and acute rejection reactions. There are certain gross characteristics peculiar to each animal group; usually, in the case of fishes, amphibians, and reptiles, one of them is the survival time of pigment cells. Then there is sloughing of destroyed grafts, first recognizable among the reptiles. At both the gross and microscopic level we know of the inflammatory response characterized by hemorrhaging and finally, microscopically, the presence of a variety of immune cells within the graft area.

Cell Responses

Snakes also exhibit a latent phase and a rejection phase after transplantation of integument allografts. Though the latent phase in snakes involves an initial period of in-

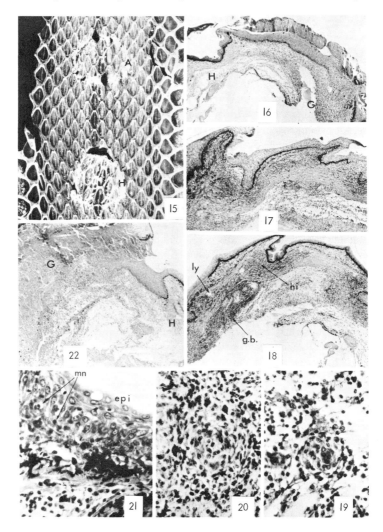

flammation and wound healing, common responses of other animals, wound healing in snakes is accompanied by a shedding cycle in which newly formed layers of epithelial cells close the surface wounds at graft-host contact zones. This is well illustrated in Figs. 9-15–9-22 of Tereby (1972). Both autografts and allografts are histologically similar during the latent phase, for a similar proportion of granulocytes, monocytes, macrophages, and lymphocytes appear in the imprints of each. Imprints are made by blotting a graft on a slide and staining it routinely with a common blood stain.

The rejection phase in the snake begins with the appearance of additional mononuclear cells after about the eighth day. Because more cells appear in imprints obtained from allografts than from autografts, it is unlikely that imprints reveal only those leukocytes that may escape from injured blood vessels. Instead, differential cell counts indicate that mononuclear cell infiltrations associated with the allograft rejection phase are characterized by the presence of a large proportion of lymphocytes. No change in the number of lymphocytes appears in the imprints of autografts. The pattern of distribution of these cells that infiltrate grafts is found in Fig. 9-23 and the cell types themselves in Figs. 9-24–9-45. Note that these cells are certainly representative of those that make up the machinery of the immune system and are there precisely because of the presence of an antigen.

Plasma cells appear during the late stages of rejection. They regularly synthesize antibody to soluble and particulate antigen and their presence here suggests the role antibody may play in graft rejection. They have the characteristic round, eccentric nucleus, clumped chromatin pattern reminiscent of a clockface, and the basophilic cytoplasm with a clear Golgi area. They are equipped for active protein synthesis, i.e., antibody and its secretion. Large lymphoid cells resembling blasts are also present late in the allograft rejection phase. In addition, some mitotic figures are found. After the third or fourth week, macrophages appear in secretions of allografts more commonly than they did in imprints, which only provide an assessment of loosely

Fig. 9-15 Day 16. Homograft, *h.*, and autograft, *a.* A positive print was obtained when the shed skin from a shedding cycle was used as a negative. The ability of donor epithelium to participate in the shedding cycle of the host showed that homologous epithelial cells were viable and able to divide. (×*2.1*)

Fig. 9-16 Day 20 in animal 29–27–1. Host skin, *h.*, and homograft, *g.*, are separated by a graft-host junction. The wound at the graft-host junction has been repaired by an infiltration of fibroblasts and loose connective tissue. Dark staining mononuclear cells have infiltrated into the connective tissue. The infiltration does not extend into surrounding host skin. (×*33*)

Fig. 9-17 Day 20 in animal 29–27–1. Semisagittal section of two scales which show a heavy infiltration of mononuclear cells into the superficial papillary layer of the dermis. No gross signs of rejection were evident in this animal. The epithelium is markedly thickened compared to surrounding host epithelium in Fig. 9-16.

Fig 9-18 Day 20 in animal 32–31–1. Cross section of two scales showing an extensive mononuclear infiltration in the hinge regions, *hi.*, of the scales and in the graft bed, *g.b.* The clear areas in the scales represent lymphatic spaces lined by endothelium, *ly.*

Figs. 9-19–9-20 High power magnification of two regions in the graft bed in animal 29–27–1. Reticular-like tissue accumulates around the blood vessels (Fig. 9-19). In Fig. 9-20 this tissue has been infiltrated with mononuclear cells.

Fig. 9-21 Day 28 in animal 59–56–1. This homograft showed a diffuse infiltration of mononuclear cells, *m.n.*, which have invaded into the epithelium, *epi.* In contrast to the animal in Fig. 9-22, necrotic changes were not yet evident.

Fig. 9-22 Day 28 in animal 53–51–1. A homograft, *g.*, which showed necrotic changes beginning on day 25. Surrounding host epithelium is seen growing into the inflammatory site to undermine the graft. (×*33*) (*From*: Tereby, *J. Morphol.*, **137**: 149, 1972.)

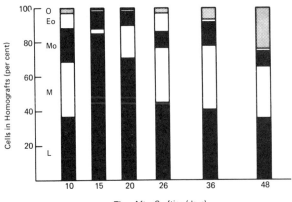

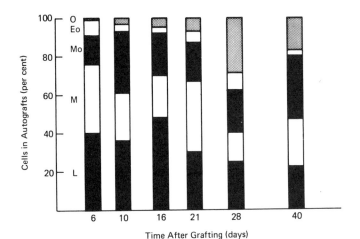

Fig. 9-23 (a) Per cent cells in imprints from homografts taken from animal 88–87–1. L, lymphocytes; M, macrophages; Mo, monocytes; Eo, eosinophils; O, other cells. (b) Per cent cells in imprints from autographs taken from animal 115–116–1. L, lymphocytes; M, macrophages; Mo, monocytes; Eo, eosinophils; O, other cells. (*From*: Tereby, 1972, *J. Morphol*, **137**: 149–160.)

> **Fig. 9-24** A group of macrophages. Pigment granules have been phagocytized by the cells. (×295)
>
> **Fig. 9-25** A large fibroblast-like cell. Many of these cells show clear vacuoles and phagocytic activity. (×650)
>
> **Fig. 9-26** Three erythroblasts. In this animal, the blood was invaded by erythroblasts and immature erythrocytes during the homograft reaction. (×650)
>
> **Fig. 9-27** Monocytes. The cytoplasm contains fine granules which are barely resolved by the microscope. (×650)
>
> **Fig. 9-28** Lymphocyte. (×712)
>
> **Fig. 9-29** Lymphocyte. (×650)
>
> **Fig. 9-30** Macrophage. The cytoplasm stains poorly and the nucleus contains a characteristic clear vacuole. (×650)
>
> **Fig. 9-31** Disrupted pigment cell with pigment granules. (×650)
>
> **Fig. 9-32** Myelocyte. The granules stain in shades of purple and red and appear in several sizes. (×650)
>
> **Fig. 9-33** Macrophage. The cytoplasm stains poorly and the nucleus contains a characteristic clear vacuole. (×650)
>
> **Fig. 9-34** Unknown binucleated cell possibly related to the cell type in Fig. 9-35. (×650)

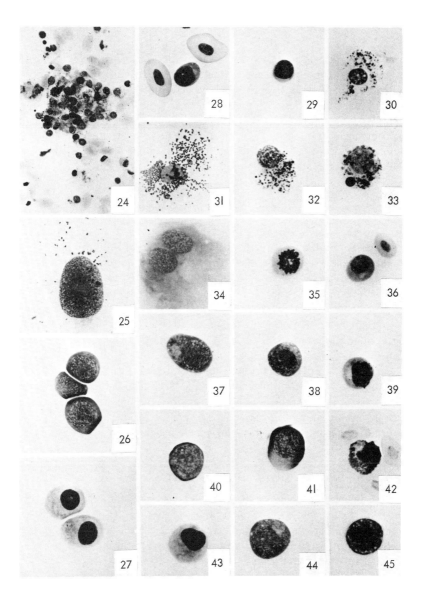

Fig. 9-35 Mitotic figure of a lymphoid cell. (×*650*)

Fig. 9-36 Mature plasma cells. The nucleus contains a clumped chromatin pattern and is placed at the periphery of the cell. The cytoplasm is intensely basophilic with a clear area. (×*650*)

Figs. 9-37–9-38 Immature plasma cells. The chromatin pattern is dispersed, and the cytoplasm gives a suggestion of a clear area. (×*650*)

Fig. 9-39 Mature plasma cell. The nucleus contains a clumped chromatin pattern and is placed at the periphery of the cell. The cytoplasm is intensely basophilic with a clear area. (×*650*)

Figs. 9-40–9-41 Blast cells. A technique artifact produced the localized basophilia in Fig. 9-41. The significance of blast cells in homografts is now known. (×*650*)

Fig. 9-42 Basophil. (×*650*)

Fig. 9-43 Monocytes. The cytoplasm contains fine granules which are barely resolved by the microscope. (×*650*)

Fig. 9-44 Blast cell. (×*650*)

Fig. 9-45 Eosinophil. (×*650*)

adhering cells. This suggests that they are capable of rapid movement into the graft itself. The cellular condition in snakes thus reflects the condition in all vertebrates and in one invertebrate (the earthworm) and indicates unequivocally that the response is immune. In mammals, allograft rejection has been transferred adoptively by populations of these very same cells derived from lymph nodes, now seen infiltrating the allografts. Thus, memory resides within the immune cells. As in other poikilotherms, the response is also dependent on temperature, and we infer that genes completely control the hosts' response to allografts or to closely related xenografts.

A FINAL COMMENT ON CHRONIC ALLOGRAFT REJECTION

We have seen a possible trend in vertebrate responses to skin allografts. Either a graft is destroyed in a rapid manner or it requires a longer period for destruction. The trend in evolution seems to be from chronic to acute rejection patterns. Strong histocompatibility gene barriers are characteristic of diverse species of vertebrates. These include teleost fishes, frogs, mice, and men. There appears to be a single, complex genetic locus that accounts for acute allograft rejection in most species. This locus is designated B in chickens, Ag-B in rats, H-2 in mice, and HL-A in humans. The Syrian hamster was once thought to be a natural quirk, since it showed chronic allograft rejection. Actually this pattern in hamsters is typical and it served as a first model of weak histocompatibility reactions. Chronic skin allograft rejection, which is under the control of weak histocompatibility loci, is also characteristic of various breeds of pigs, urodele amphibians, apodan amphibians, and earthworms. To account for such a response in any of the vertebrate groups, or even in an invertebrate, the earthworm, Hildemann and Cohen (1967) have proposed six rules that are generally applicable.

1. The later the time of onset of graft rejection, the greater is the interval between onset and complete rejection;

2. The longer the median or average survival time, the greater is the range or spread in survival times of individual grafts;

3. Multiple histocompatibility differences will exhibit additive or augmentative effects leading to curtailed allograft survival whenever the ratios between the constituent median survival times are not large (3:1 or less);

4. The "strength" of histoincompatibility is a function of the interallelic combination rather than the H-locus involved;

5. Allograft survival times on females are usually shorter than on males of the same strain;

6. Where only very weak histocompatibility differences exist, small grafts are likely to be rejected eventually, while large grafts may survive indefinitely under the same conditions.

We have seen that genes determine the presence or absence of histocompatibility between donors and recipients of tissue transplants. Cohen and Borysenko (1970) hypothesize that the presence and molecular structure of transplantation antigens, as can be determined by histocompatibility genes, have evolved. This evolution is reflected in the rapidity of skin allograft rejection. As shown in Fig. 9-46 Cohen and Borysenko conclude that among the ectothermic or poikilothermic vertebrates there is a trend based primarily upon the rapidity of graft rejection. Acute or rapid rejection

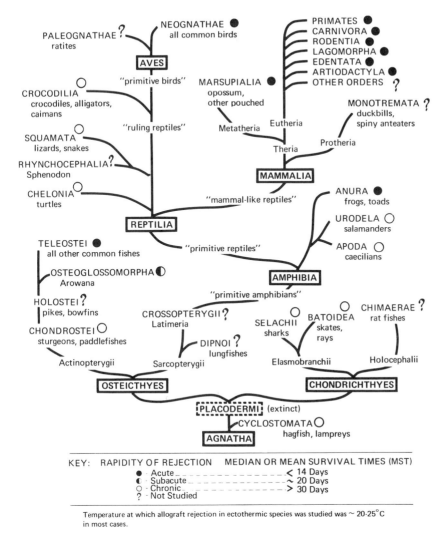

Fig. 9-46 Evolutionary trends in rapidity of allograft rejection in vertebrates. (*From*: Cohen & Borysenko, Transpl. Proc., **2**: 333, 1970.)

arose from chronic or slow rejection at least four times: once in the evolution of the fishes and again in the anurans, birds, and mammals, or lines leading to them. Acute rejection, as in higher teleosts and anurans, is characteristic of modern avian and mammalian species. Confirmation of these apparent trends in evolutionary schemes greatly depends upon more detailed and temperature-controlled studies of transplantation immunity in paleognathus birds and the metatherian and protetherian mammals. Moreover, some transplantation studies are lacking data about other critical evolutionary links such as the dipnoi, holostean fishes, primitive anurans and sphenodons, and living reptiles whose origin is traceable to a primitive reptilian ancestor. Only when new studies are carried out to fill the gaps in these areas will the picture presented by Cohen and Borysenko become more representative.

BIBLIOGRAPHY

Borysenko, M. 1969. Skin allograft or xenograft rejection in the snapping turtle, *Chelydra serpentina.* J. Exp. Zool. **170**: 341.

Borysenko, M., and Hildemann, W. H. 1969. Scale (skin) allograft rejection in the primitive teleost, *Osteoglossum bicirrhosum.* Transpl. **8**: 403.

Cohen, N. 1966a. Tissue transplantation immunity in the adult newt, *Diemictylus viridescens.* I. The latent phase: healing, restoration of circulation, and pigment cell changes in autografts and allografts. J. Exp. Zool. **163**: 157.

————. 1966b. Tissue transplantation immunity in the adult newt, *Diemictylus viridescens.* II. The rejection phase: first and second-set allograft reactions and lack of sexual dimorphism. J. Exp. Zool. **163**: 173.

Cohen, N., and Borysenko, M. 1970. Acute and chronic graft rejection: Possible phylogeny of transplantation antigens. Transpl. Proc. **2**: 333.

Cooper, E. L., and Aponte, A. 1968. Chronic allograft rejection in the iguana, *Ctenosaura pectinata.* Proc. Soc. Exptl. Biol. and Med. **128**: 150.

Greenwood, P. H., Rosen, D. E., Weitzman, S. H., and Myers, G. S. 1966. Amer. Mus. Nat. Hist. Bull. **131**: 1.

Hildemann, W. H. 1957. Scale homotransplantation in goldfish (*Carassius auratus*). Ann. N. Y. Acad. Sci. **64**: 775.

Hildemann, W. H., and Cohen, N. 1967. Weak Histocompatibility: Emerging Immunogenetic Rules and Generalizations. In Histocompatibility Testing. Eds. E. S. Curtoni, P. L. Mattiuz, R. M. Tosi. Baltimore: Williams and Wilkins Co.

Hildemann, W. H., and Thoenes, G. 1969. Immunological responses of Pacific hagfish. I. Skin transplantation immunity. Transplantation **7**: 506.

Manickavel, V., and Muthukkaruppan, V. R. 1969. Allograft rejection in the lizard, *Calotes versicolor.* Transplantation **8**: 307.

May, R. M. 1923. Skin grafts in the lizard, *Anolis carolinensis.* Brit. J. Exp. Biol. **1**: 539.

Perey, D. Y. E., Finstad, J., Pollara, B., and Good, R. A., 1968. Evolution of the immune response. VI. First- and second-set skin homograft rejections in primitive fishes. Lab. Invest. **19**: 591.

Tereby, N. 1972. A light microscopic study of the mononuclear cells infiltrating skin homografts in the garter snake, *Thamnophis sirtalis* (Reptilia: Colubridae). J. Morph. **137**: 149.

Chapter 10

Genetic Control and Transplantation Immunobiology

Introduction

The immune response is controlled by the genetic background of the host. Knowing the genetic constitution, we can often predict the outcome of an induced immune response once an animal is immunized. As a consequence of the genetic background, one can adoptively confer a state of immunity on a nonimmune animal in the laboratory without the recipient having been previously immune, or one can produce the reverse, allogeneic disease, because the genetic constitution of the host and donor differ significantly. There is a wealth of literature on how numerous strains of animals react to countless numbers of antigens; however, within the scope of this book, only those aspects of transplantation biology which have been studied from the comparative viewpoint will be emphasized.

Transplantation Immunity and the Genetic Background

Genetic Laws

As long as we deal with outbred animal populations it is difficult to assess the purity of genetic influences on recognition and destruction of closely related cell or tissue antigens. Yet, if we are at all concerned about the relevance of findings in vertebrates other than humans, it is probably information derived from outbred strains that is most applicable. Whereas there are certain advantages to the use of outbred populations, the value of inbred laboratory animals should not be discounted. Inbred animals have been maintained under controlled breeding conditions; they are the offspring of siblings bred with each other. Such brother-sister matings result in genetic homogeneity. The genetic condition of highly inbred strains of laboratory animals approaches, and in fact, mimics the genetic constitution of nature's own inbred animals or identical twins.

In order to indicate the genetic relationship between donors and recipients of experimental tissue grafts, certain terms are strictly applicable. Table 10-1 summarizes the terminology used when denoting the classification of transplants involving donors and recipients. This terminology has been largely derived from studies of mice; however they are general terms expressing principles applicable to all animal groups. The prefixes auto-, *iso- (syn)*, *homo- (allo)*, and *hetero- (xeno)* denote the kind of

Table 10-1

Terminology used in Tissue Grafting

Old noun	Old adjective	New noun	New adjective	Definition
autograft	autologous	none	none	Recipient receives graft of his own tissue
isograft	isologous	syngraft	syngeneic	Recipient receives graft from a genetically identical or near-identical donor of the same species (identical twins or inbred animal)
homograft	homologous	allograft	allogeneic	Recipient receives graft from a genetically dissimilar donor of the same species
heterograft	heterologous	xenograft	xenogeneic	Recipient receives graft from a donor of another species

(*From*: Weiser, R. S., Myrvik, Q. N., Pearsall, N. N. 1969. *Fundamentals of Immunology for Students of Medicine and Related Science*)

graft; these are combined with nouns and suffixes. The older adjectives had the suffixes *-ologous*, but the new adjectives end in *-geneic*. The prefixes in parentheses are preferred. Autograft, literally a *self* graft, involves the exchange of a transplant from an animal to itself. *Self* tissue evokes no antagonism; it heals and is accepted permanently. A syngraft is exchanged between siblings, nature's inbred strain or identical twins, leading to no response between donor or host. Inbred strains will accept syngeneic transplants exchanged between donor and host; this evokes no response, provided the animals are truly inbred. In fact, in order to test the efficacy of inbreeding either in the laboratory or in a natural population, exchanging tissue grafts such as skin and waiting for the outcome is a convenient method.

Because allografts are exchanged between donor and host of the same genus and species that are not inbred, the host, once the graft is healed, recognizes the donor antigens and the immune system is promptly set into motion. The most extreme, but initially successful, transplant involves an exchange of xenografts. The terminology here however must be used with caution. According to some authors, xenografts are not defined as they are in Table 10-1, which states that xenografts are exchanged between members of a different species, implying they are of the same genus. Sometimes, xenografts are exchanged between two closely related members of a different genus and species.

The genetic basis for acceptance or rejection of transplants was derived from early detailed studies involving mouse tumor grafts. The results are relevant however, to the transplantation of normal tissues. If we begin with two animals of a particular strain that differ by a single gene and mate them, we arrive at an F_1 that possesses genes from each parent. Mating the F_1 parents produces F_2 offspring with four possible genotypes. Twenty-five percent will either be homozygous for one histocompatibility gene A/A and 25% for A'/A'. Fifty percent are A/A'. These exist in the ratio 1:2:1. If grafts are transplanted from the P_1 they show several rejection patterns. F_2 A/A will reject grafts from A'/A' and the F_2 A'/A' will reject grafts from A/A

P_1. Instead of rejection, 75% of the F_2 will accept grafts from either the A/A P_1 or the A'/A' P_1.

Transplantation immunogenetics is a discipline based largely on the results of combined comparative studies involving fishes, amphibians, reptiles, birds, and mammals, including man. Isografts exchanged between animals within a highly inbred strain are accepted permanently. However, if grafts are exchanged between members of two different but highly inbred strains, the grafts are destroyed due to the presence of foreign transplantation antigens. These antigens are determined by histocompatibility genes located on the chromosome at histocompatibility loci (H loci).

Adoptive Transfer

At one time it was central to immunologic dogma that the immune response was due primarily to humoral events. Attempts to transfer certain cell-mediated responses by blood serum were, however, unsuccessful. Moreover, investigators observed that lymphoid cells accumulated around graft sites and that the regional lymph nodes draining such doomed grafts showed mitoses and large blast cells, changes indicating cell stimulation. Adoptive transfer is based on the hypothesis that a particular immune response is primarily cell-mediated, and that stimulated lymphocytes contain all the necessary information for transferring immune reactivity.

Testing this hypothesis involves transplanting a graft from one animal to another, allowing sufficient time for buildup of the immune response, and then removing lymph nodes from the putatively immune host. Nonimmune recipients are then injected with lymphocyte suspensions and the efficacy of the transferred immune state is tested. When the animal made immune by proxy is given a graft from the original donor, it promptly destroys the graft in an accelerated fashion. Grafts from other donors do not evoke this response. Thus, tissue transplant destruction is mediated primarily by cellular reactions, and its success depends on the genetic constitution of the animal. Except for earthworms, no other animals inferior to mammals and birds have been used to adoptively transfer cell-mediated immune responses.

Graft vs. Host Reaction

Although the host's immune system is capable of destroying a graft, in certain experiments the graft can also react against the host. This response is well studied and characterized in birds and mammals and to a limited extent in amphibians. It is referred to appropriately as the *graft-vs.-host* reaction (GVH), and in mammals it usually leads to the host's death preceded by certain pathologic sequelae. These are characterized by severe lymphoid atrophy, depressed serum immunoglobulins and immunity to microorganisms, and lesions of the viscera, skin, and joints. Although several different terms will be used the resulting syndromes are basically alike.

Various methods are available for inducing homologous or graft-vs.-host disease syndromes. Certain parameters however, are necessary for the development of the GVH syndrome. First, the graft, whether it be cells or a solid tissue, must contain immunologically competent lymphocytes. Second, the host and donor must differ genetically, since grafted lymphocytes must be confronted with foreign transplantation antigens. Finally, the host must be immunologically incompetent, unable to respond to the attacking lymphocytes insuring the graft's advantage against the host. In addition to natural immunologic immaturity, host unresponsiveness can be achieved experimentally by administering irradiation, which effectively damages cells of the immune system. Regardless of how the GVH reaction is induced, it results from an encounter between grafted immunologically competent cells and an immunologically incompetent host.

In runt disease, adult lymphoid cells are injected from strain A mouse into neonatal recipients of strain B. The term *runt* is used because the victim of immunologically competent lymphocytes becomes extremely small as a result of lymphocyte attack. Similar procedures are used for induction in birds by grafting or inoculating immunologically competent lymphocytes onto the chorioallantois membrane *in ovo*. Grafted cells react against the immunologically incompetent "fetal" bird, the spleen enlarges, and death of the host follows (Simonsen, 1957). The necessary condition in these two examples is that the recipients are neonatal animals. With advancing age, there is increased resistance by the formerly more vulnerable host, and the animals progressively lose the capacity to be attacked by grafted cells as the host becomes increasingly immunologically mature and capable of reacting against offensive donor cells.

Adult animals may be affected as a consequence of confrontation with immunologically competent cells. If large numbers of lymphoid cells from strain A adult mice are injected into another strain rendered immunologically tolerant of donor transplantation antigens, the recipients develop homologous disease, due to aggressive lymphocytes injected into a defenseless animal. In another, similar situation, if adult mice of one strain are injected with large numbers of lymphoid cells from several donors presensitized with recipient cells, they too, may show signs of homologous disease. This results from being overwhelmed by offending effector lymphocytes. F_1 hybrid disease develops by injecting large numbers of strain A cells into irradiated F_1 hybrids. Parabiosis intoxication is a lethal, wasting syndrome that develops in adult mice, rats, or salamanders after they are united by parabiosis with foreign allogeneic partners. The disease develops more readily if one of the parabionts is the parental strain. A final disease produced by allogeneic encounter between animals and lymphocytes is secondary or radiation disease. Animals will recover from irradiation by injecting isogeneic marrow; injections of allogeneic cells, however, leads to death.

TRANSPLANTATION AS A TOOL TO DETECT HISTOCOMPATIBILITY

Histocompatibility in Populations

Isolated populations are the raw material from which new subspecies or even new species arise. A limited number of genes exist in small isolated populations, but it is possible for different alleles to become established in otherwise similar populations of a given species. Several different and analyzable approaches exist for studying the genetic variability of an isolated population. For example, one can record the frequencies of polymorphic pigment patterns or blood group antigens. However, one of the most sensitive gross indicators of genetic differentiation in an isolated population is the transplantation test. In a genetically uniform population, members possess a majority of similar histocompatibility alleles, and the antigenic differences between them is small. In other words, the more uniform the population the longer allografts will survive after exchange among its members.

Transplantation is a tool in immunogenetics that is used to estimate the number of histocompatibility loci. This involves crossing a homozygous inbred strain, to permit the successful exchange of tissue grafts, with individuals of a second unrelated strain. Grafts survive in those hosts which possess a histocompatibility gene also present in the homozygous inbred strain. The actual number of histocompatibility loci in common is estimated from the percentage of transplants that are accepted. The presence of diverse transplantation antigens in large populations is revealed by making third-party grafts using donors different from those that gave the original second-set grafts. They are destroyed at varying times dependent upon what common antigens exist between the host and the two donors.

The number of histocompatibility loci controlling the presence of tissue antigens is at least 16 for the rat (Billingham et al. 1962), 14–17 for the mouse (Barnes and Krohn 1957, Prehn and Main 1958), and more than 12 for the teleost fish, *Xiphophorus maculatus*. There is limited information available for other vertebrate phyla, but demonstration of complete allograft rejection strongly supports the view that a large number of histocompatibility genes are present in most vertebrates. According to Kallman's (1964a) estimate for example, the presence of sixteen histocompatibility genes would result in forty-three million possible different genetic combinations. On the basis of this astronomical prediction, the possibility of selecting at random two individuals from a large interbreeding population that would allow one of them to accept the other's graft is indeed small. In higher teleosts and amphibians the "uniqueness of the individual" enunciated by Medawar (1957) is as highly developed as it is in birds and mammals. In many instances transplants will never survive longer than three to four weeks, except for chronic rejectors (see Chap. 9).

Kallman's work (1964b) with *Xiphophorus couchianus*, the Monterrey platyfish, and two subspecies supports the value of transplantation techniques for immunogenetic analysis of populations. *Xiphophorus couchianus* is restricted to three isolated spring systems in the Huasteca Canyon near Monterrey, Mexico. Another subspecies, the northern platyfish, is found in three small lagunas near Cuatro Ciènegas, Mexico. Varying degrees of genetic homozygosity exist within each of the two subspecies populations. Since many allotransplants are accepted, the antigenic differences between individuals of the same population is evidently small. Furthermore, transplants that survive several weeks or months suggest that a few weak histocompatibility genes are present. Members of one species react vigorously against heterotransplants from the other, since each has developed different histocompatibility alleles.

Transplantation in Fishes: Tools for Immunogenetics
  Introduction

The works of Kallman and Harrington (1964) and Harrington and Kallman (1968) are of continued importance in extending our understanding of the genetic control of transplantation immunity. Certain species of fish may in fact be ideal models for studying immunogenetics. Within a sexually reproducing fish population, its members share a common gene pool from which countless numbers of genetic recombinations can be obtained by cross fertilization; this insures high genetic variability. Thus, sexual reproduction among animals and plants is proof of the adaptive advantage of this mechanism. The heterozygous condition may be more superior in fitness for the environment than the homozygous one, since such individuals often show greater adaptability to environmental variables. By contrast, in uniparental reproduction, species or races of fish, for example, are prevented from acquiring new genotypes through recombination because of other mechanisms of reproduction such as parthenogenesis, gynogenesis, and self-fertilizing hermaphroditism. Despite the negative aspects of uniparental reproduction, there is at least one advantage: favorable gene combinations can be maintained and rapidly passed on to future generations. The resulting offspring from these types of reproduction are members of clones that have identical genotypes, as is easily proven by the results of tissue transplantation experiments.

Gynogenesis

Several unisexual reproductive conditions exist in fish that render them useful for transplantation immunology. In gynogenesis, an all-female species reproduces by mating with males of related species; there are no male traits observable in laboratory stocks or in natural populations. *Mollienesia formosa* reproduces by gynogenesis; the sperm merely stimulates the egg's development without contributing any genetic material to the zygote. When *Mollienesia formosa* females are mated to males of *Mollienesia sphenops*, *Mollienesia latipinna*, or a number of other related species, they produce female offspring phenotypically indistinguishable from the *Mollienesia formosa* parent. This is diagrammed as it occurs in the same or a closely related genus (Fig. 10-1). The descendants of each female constitute a clone, and therefore all members possess identical genotypes. This is easily confirmed by exchanging transplants (isografts). Grafts exchanged between the descendants of a given female survive permanently regardless of the species from which the "male parent" was taken. Transplants between unrelated fish are rejected. According to Kallmann (1962),

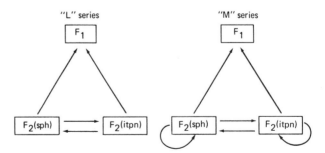

Fig. 10-1 Demonstration of maternal inheritance in *P. formosa* collected from the Rio Guayalejo. Wild-caught gravid females "L" and "M" produced F_1 broods in the laboratory. Part of each brood was mated with *P. sphenops* and part with *P. latipinna* males, producing F_2 broods. Tissue transplants are indicated by arrows pointing from donors to hosts. Each arrow represents five transplants except the intergeneration studies where each arrow represents one or two transplants (for a total of six). Sib transplants were carried out only for the F_2 progeny of the "M" series. All tissue transplants shown in this figure were accepted. Transplants from the F_2 fish to their male parents were uniformly rejected and are not shown in the figure. (*From*: Darnell, et al., *Evolution*, **21**: 168, 1967.)

grafts made among the descendants from three *Mollienesia formosa* females are successful if host and donor belong to the same clone. They are rejected within two weeks if host and donor are from different clones. As can be seen in Figs. 10-2 and 10-3, transplants are successful when performed between members of the same clone.

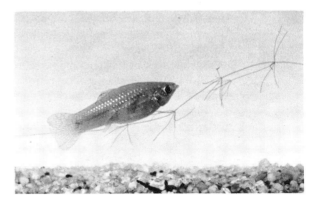

Fig. 10-2 A *Mollienesia formosa* female with a dorsal fin transplant above its anal fin. The transplanted fin is distorted and smaller than a fin in its normal position. *Intra*-clone graft. (Photographed 12 months after the operation, *courtesy* Dr. Klaus Kallman.)

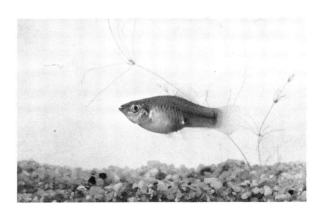

Fig. 10-3 A *Mollienesia formosa* female with a heart transplant implanted into the area above the anal fin. Notice that the transplanted heart bulges slightly from the body surface. *Intra*-clone graft. (Photographed 12 months after the operation, *courtesy* Dr. Klaus Kallman.)

Homozygous Clones from Self-fertilizing Hermaphrodites

Kallmann and Harrington (1964) tested the idea that a species or race of self-fertilizing hemaphrodites should consist of clones, i.e., with all members being homozygous and possessing identical genotypes. They used the transplantation test on *Rivulus marmoratus* (from the east coast of Florida) to determine whether fish that had descended from the same wild-caught progenitor possess identical genotypes. Fins, spleens, and hearts were transplanted in thirty-six different host-donor combinations involving six different lines (sib to sib, parent to offspring, offspring to parent). Only two transplants failed to survive, probably due to technical reasons; thus the information supports theoretical prediction, that these fish are largely homozygous. Kallman (1970) also observed true parthenogenesis in the mosquito fish, *Gambusia affinis*. Transplants taken from the offspring of, and grafted onto, a virgin female survived. By contrast, control grafts among sexually-produced siblings of *Gambusia affinis* from the same population as the virgin female survive for only five to twelve days, as do grafts from biparental offspring to either parent.

Adult Urodele and Larval Anuran Amphibian Populations

Most animals show prompt acute skin allograft rejection that reflects a diversity of transplantation antigens unique to donor and host. These are controlled by loci analogous to the H-2 loci in mice, and they dictate the fate of allotransplants. When individuals of a population are derived from the same sex, by uniparental reproduction, usually no paternal genes are present to diversify the gene pool; thus the populations are essentially inbred. The results from transplantation immunity tests bear out this theoretical view.

The urodele, or tailed amphibians, however, are different. Cohen and Hildemann (1968) investigated at least fifteen urodele species representing nine genera and four families. Despite the presence of an organ system capable of a vigorous alloimmune response to certain tissue antigens, chronic graft rejection commonly occurs in urodeles. The authors attribute this to four immunogenetic explanations: 1) the absence of a major "H-2 type" of complex histocompatibility locus as defined for the mouse; 2) a cumulative interaction of weak transplantation antigens; 3) antigen sharing; 4) genetic control of the immune response itself.

Among many amphibian populations, there are at present no appropriate mating studies available, although the leopard frog may be an exception (Nace and Richards, 1969). Thus we can make no firm deductions concerning the number of histocompatibility loci, the number of alleles per locus, or allele frequencies within populations as has commonly been done for fishes and mammals. The more characteristic chronic rejection pattern in *Diemictylus*, the newt, and several other genera of urodeles is not attributable to a physiologically or anatomically deficient immune system. This is revealed by the many instances of acute and subacute skin allograft rejection in intrapopulation transplants. Third-party test grafting reveals widespread sharing of histocompatibility genes among newts in the same population.

In the absence of any strong histoincompatibility in *Diemictylus* populations, the high incidence of acute rejection in different populations is tentatively explained by the additive or synergistic effects of certain multiple weak histocompatibility alleles. Allele frequency differences plus additive effects of multiple histocompatibility differences may account for the increased incidence of earlier rejections. Prolonged or indefinite survival may represent sustained enhancement or actual tolerance with respect to the weakest histocompatibility antigens that segregate in these populations. Alternatively, nearly complete antigen sharing may be operative.

Geographically isolated populations of bullfrog tadpoles from Southern California provide a test system for immunogenetic analyses of amphibian populations (Hildemann and Haas, 1961). Single skin allografts exchanged between pairs of unrelated tadpole siblings are not destroyed until at least nine days at 25°C. In a second experiment, pair combinations are changed so that each tadpole serves as both donor and recipient of two successive allografts. Accelerated rejection within seven days or less invariably occurs when the same donor provides both grafts. Thus, accelerated rejection of a second graft from a different donor indicates that both donors share one or more strong histocompatibility antigens absent from the recipient.

In one population, approximately 10% of randomly selected tadpoles share antigens, but 56% of known siblings from the same population reject second test allografts by accelerated reactions. Such a five-to-six-fold increase in common histocompatibility antigens among siblings is highly significant. Thus, many histocompatibility alleles at various loci are apparently segregating in wild bullfrog populations. Since all tadpoles reject all allografts, then every tadpole has at least one antigen different from those occurring in any other tadpole. This implies that the percent of antigen sharing is a measure of genetic diversity in populations.

Parthenogenesis in Turkeys

Naturally occurring parthenogenesis occurs in the eggs of Beltsville white turkeys (Healey et al. 1962, Poole et al. 1963). First discovered in 1952 in a population of birds of a selective breeding program, 121 parthenogens hatched from 10,000 eggs. The stimulus for parthenogenesis, although unknown, may be an avian virus. All parthenogens are male that have a diploid number of chromosomes, possibly established either by chromosomal doubling in the haploid gamete or by nondisjunction at the second maturation division. The male parthenogens inherit all genetic material from the dam, their mother, and thus cannot exceed her genetic endowment. Grafts of wattles and skin in control normal populations and from dam to parthenogen are rejected. Grafts from parthenogens to their dams, including second sets, survived permanently. Thus, no histocompatibility factors are present in the offspring that are not also present in the dam, as confirmed by the above transplantation experiments.

SUMMARY

The remarkable amount of work in the field of transplantation immunology has been in large part due to dedicated investigators seeking to decipher the mechanisms underlying transplant rejection. The rejection of allografts results primarily from the genetic background of donor and host. If the host possesses transplantation antigens that are absent from the donor, the resulting graft will be destroyed. It is the immune system that effects the destruction. Whether graft rejection is rapid and acute or long and chronic also is a reflection of the genetic constitution. Large numbers of strong histocompatibility gene-controlled differences lead to acute rejection, but relatively few differences produce chronic destruction. Genetic analysis is rather easy even in wild-caught populations of fishes, amphibians, birds, and mammals. Unlike the long-developed, sophisticated inbreeding techniques for mammals from which we know most about the numbers of histocompatibility loci, certain fish populations are unique in that they can exist naturally as clones; nature has bred many of them already in the wild. They are usually derived by uniparental reproduction from the mother, and transplants within such clones are therefore readily accepted. Any deviations from this prediction are directly referable to genetic changes within the single parent, and not to the combined effects of both parental contributors. Estimations of the numbers of histocompatibility loci would be performed differently on animals derived from biparental reproduction.

BIBLIOGRAPHY

Barnes, A. D., and Krohn, P. L. 1957. The estimation of the number of histocompatibility genes controlling the successful transplantation of normal skin in mice. Proc. Roy. Soc. London B **146**: 505.

Billingham, R. E., Hodge, B. A., and Silvers, W. K. 1962. An estimate of the number of histocompatibility loci in the rat. Proc. Nat. Acad. Sci. **48**: 138.

Cohen, N., and Hildemann, W. H. 1968. Population studies of allograft rejection in the newt, *Diemictylus viridescens. Transplantation* **6**: 208–217.

Harrington, R. W., and Kallman, K. D. 1968. The homozygosity of clones of the self-fertilizing hermaphoditic fish, *Rivulus marmoratus* POEY (Cyprinodontidae, Atheriniformes). *Am. Nat.* **102**: 337.

Healey, W. V., Russell, P. S., Poole, H. K., and Olsen, M. W. 1962. A skin grafting analysis of fowl parthenogenesis: Evidence for a new type of genetic histocompatibility. Ann. N. Y. Acad. Sci. **99**: 698.

Hildemann, W. H., and Haas, R. 1961. Histocompatibility genetics of bullfrog populations. *Evolution* **15**: 267.

Kallman, K. D. 1962. Population genetics of the gynogenetic teleost, *Mollienesia formosa* (GIRARD). *Evolution* **16**: 497.

———. 1964a. An estimate of the number of histocompatibility loci in the teleost *Xiphophorus maculatus. Genetics* **50**: 583.

———. 1964b. Genetics of tissue transplantation in isolated platyfish populations. Copeia **3**: 513.

———. 1970. Genetics of tissue transplantation in teleostei. Transpl. Proc. **2**: 263.

Kallman, K. D., and Harrington, R. W. 1964. Evidence for the existence of homozygous clones in the self-fertilizing hemaphroditic teleost *Rivulus marmoratus* (POEY). Biol. Bull. **126**: 101.

Medawar, P. B. 1957. *The Uniqueness of the Individual.* London: Methwen and Co., Ltd.

Nace, G. W., and Richards, C. M. 1969. Development of Biologically Defined Strains of Amphibians. In *Biology of Amphibian Tumors*, ed. M. Mizell, p. 409. New York: Springer-Verlag.

Poole, H. K., Healey, W. V., Russell, P. S., and Olsen, M. W. 1963. Evidence of heterozygosity in parthenogenetic turkeys from homograft responses. Proc. Soc. Exp. Biol. Med. **113**: 503.

Prehn, R. T., and Main, J. M. 1958. Number of mouse histocompatibility genes involved in skin grafting from strain Balb/cAn to strain DBA/2. J. Nat. Cancer Inst. **20**: 207.

Simonsen, M. 1957. The impact on the developing embryo and new-born animal of adult homologous cells. Acta Path. Microbiol. Scand. **40**: 480.

Chapter 11

Invertebrate Humoral Immunity

INTRODUCTION

The diverse environments inhabited by invertebrates are replete with microorganisms which prey on them and pose a threat to their existence. Yet the animal kingdom contains innumerable invertebrates, which manage to survive despite the potentially hazardous effects of pathogenic microorganisms. That invertebrates reproduce their kind in large numbers partially accounts for their successful population of the world. A built-in protective defense or immune system is another important reason for their ability to survive.

The concept of invertebrate humoral immunity is rooted in studies of any invertebrate that possesses a fluid-filled coelomic cavity. The microorganisms that attack the invertebrate are neutralized by the synthesis of substances within the coelomic fluid. By most criteria these substances are physically unlike vertebrate immunoglobulins; nevertheless they provide invertebrates with part of the necessary machinery for fighting pathogens. In their actions, these substances lack the specificity of vertebrate immunoglobulins. Invertebrates do clear insulting pathogens (antigens), and after clearance, substances that destroy the antigen are formed. The clearance, synthesis, and ultimate removal of antigen constitutes the invertebrate's humoral response.

To distinguish between vertebrate and invertebrate humoral responses, Chadwick (1967) proposes a new terminology. She suggests that the term *insect immunogen* replace *antigen*, and that *naturally occurring bactericidal substance* or *specific inducible substance* be substituted for *antibody*. Such distinctions are probably more useful and instructive than defining invertebrate immunity entirely in terms that have been derived from exhaustive vertebrate research; these new terms, however, have not been widely accepted. Regardless of terminology, the invertebrate immune response must be considered in light of vertebrate antigen-antibody reactions, for there are no existing terms that are used exclusively for invertebrates. The choice of antigen, the route of immunization, times of booster injections, and the methods for detecting substances in the coelomic fluid are important parameters in the induction of an invertebrate's humoral immune response. However, the most fundamental variable, to which much attention should be devoted, is the mode of laboratory maintenance. Experimental subjects must be in excellent health before being injected with antigens, or, for that matter, being subjected to any experimental procedure.

LYSINS, BACTERICIDINS, AND AGGLUTININS IN THE SIPUNCULIDA

The habitat of *Sipunculus nudus* contains numerous ciliates and bacteria that occasionally penetrate the body cavity through breaks in the intestinal wall. Body cavity injections of crab blood containing large numbers of ciliate parasites, *Anophrys magii*, induce the synthesis of lysins specific for the ciliate (Bang 1966). Within one to two days after injection, the lysin develops in the plasma and the entire ciliate disintegrates within fifteen minutes (Fig. 11-1). As Fig. 11-2 indicates, the lysin can be in-

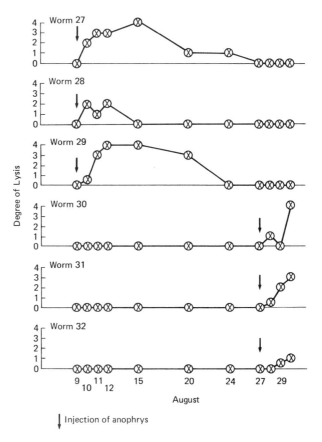

Fig. 11-1 Appearance of lysin after one injection of *Anophrys*. (*From:* Bang, *J. Immunol.*, **96**: 960, 1966.)

duced many times, even after several bleedings. The duration of the response lasts from five to seven days but apparently does not increase after repeated injections. High and persistent lysin titers are also found in animals infested with naturally occurring amoeboid flagellates. Spontaneous infections also stimulate lysin production. The lysin is characteristically destroyed if heated to 45°C for five minutes and is inactivated by ether. Like antibody, the lysin is a protective substance associated with a disease, and it is responsible for the sipunculid's defense.

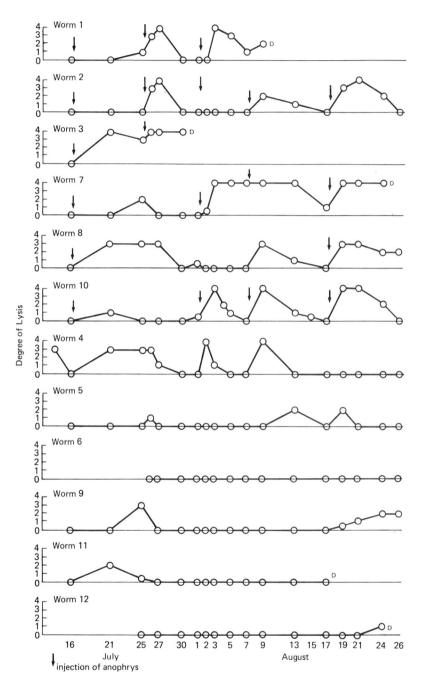

Fig. 11-2 Effect of repeated injections on appearance of lysin. (*From*: Bang, *J. Im-munol.*, **96**: 960, 1966.)

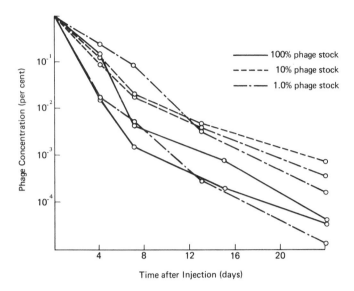

Fig. 11-3 Result of various phage concentrations. This figure shows the rate of disappearance of T_4 phage from the blood of sipunculids that have been injected with tenfold initial differences of concentration of phage, the highest concentration being 2.0×10^9 phage/ml. (*From*: Cushing, *Fed. Proc.*, **26**: 1666, 1967.)

Serum isolated from sipunculids is not capable of inactivating phage (Cushing 1967, Cushing et al. 1969). Sterile sipunculid sera retains the same lysin titer for fourteen days without killing T_4 phage. T_4 phage still persists for long periods of time even in the blood of another sipunculid, *Dendrostomum zostericolum*. It is cleared and disappears at a relatively steady rate that is independent of the length of time it persists in the blood, the size of the initial inoculum, or by previous injections of phage (Figs. 11-3, 11-4).

By contrast, Evans et al. (1973) induced a bactericidin in the sipunculid worm *Dendrostomum zostericolum* Chamberlain by intracoelomic injections of killed bacteria. Bactericidal titers in coelomic fluids from noninjected control worms were either low or nonexistent. The best response occurred after 4×10^8 bacteria per injection, producing bactericidal titers of up to 1:1280 within seven days. Whereas cross-immunization with another antigen leads to nonspecificity, injections of sterile sea water alone produce no response. As further evidence of an induced substance, coelomic fluids could be inactivated by heating at 50° or 56°C for twenty minutes. That the bactericidin is present in immune worms is confirmed by lack of restoration of activity by a pool of unheated coelomic fluid from nonimmunized worms. The bactericidin is of interest because its discovery increases the available information on invertebrate humoral immune substances.

Weinheimer et al. (1970) have further characterized sipunculid coelomic fluid by challenging *Dendrostomum zostericolum* with several other antigens. As shown in Table 11-1, a natural hemolysin and hemagglutinin for several species of foreign erythrocytes are found in it's coelomic fluid. The activity is not totally temperature dependent, since incubation of the coelomic fluid with a constant amount of sheep erythrocytes at 0°, 4°, and 25°C for a twelve-four period results in 100% hemolysis.

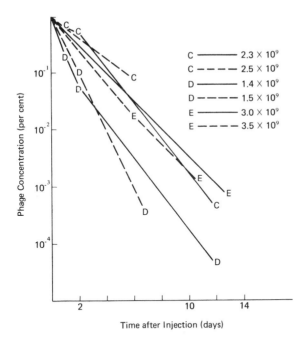

Fig. 11-4 Sipunculid—primary and secondary responses. Examples of the disappearance of T_4 phage from the blood of three sipunculids that received second injections of phage (*broken lines*) 12 days after an initial injection (*solid lines*). Letters stand for individual worms and numbers for initial phage titers and are placed along the lines at each sampling point. The results are characteristic of a variety of experiments showing that the reduction in phage titer is not enhanced by various manipulations. (*From*: Cushing, *Fed. Proc.*, **26**: 1666, 1967.)

However, only 60% lysis occurs for the same period of time at 37°C, indicating a heat-labile system. Although lysin activity is completely inhibited at 52°C, the hemagglutinin activity is not affected until heated above 70°C. Concentrations from 0.02 to 0.09 M of the chelating agent ethylene diamine tetraacetic acid (EDTA) do not alter

Table 11-1

Range of hemolytic and hemagglutinin activity of sipunculid coelomic fluid

Erythrocyte species	Titer*	
	Hemolysin	Hemagglutinin
Sheep	32	16
Rabbit	32	8
Calf	32	4
Horse	16	32
Dog	16	16
Turkey	32	16
Chicken	16	16

*Values are expressed in reciprocal of final dilution of coelomic fluid showing activity.
From: Weinheimer et al. Life Science, 9: 145, 1970.

the hemolysin. Chelating agents prevent the action of Ca^{++} and Mg^{++}; thus, contrary to some vertebrate immune reactions, divalent cations are not required for hemolysis in sipunculids. Apparently the sipunculid's lysin response is not analogous to the mammalian hemolytic response, which is mediated by complement that is dependent upon divalent cations.

The coelomic fluid of *Goldfingia gouldii*, an east coast sipunculid worm, does exhibit antibacterial activity against several marine bacteria (Krassner and Florey 1970). The activity is also heat labile and resistant to pepsin or lipase treatment and toluene extraction, but is unaffected by freezing and thawing. However, antibacterial activity stops after dialysis treatment and after trypsinization. In addition, *Dendrostomum pyroides* exhibits a similar type of antibacterial activity *in vitro*. Thus, nonspecific antimicrobial substances are common in sipunculids and constitute a formidable defense against bacteria.

THE ANNELIDA

Inducible immune substances may be a universal attribute of invertebrate immune responses; however, annelids may be an exception (Cooper et al 1969). Lack of induction may be due to such variables of immunization as choice of antigen, dosage, and route. After injecting the earthworm, *Lumbricus*, with various antigens, such as bacterial strains from it's slime and gut cavity, a gram-negative bacillus (EMB1) from the crustacean, *Panulirus argus*, and *Salmonella typhosa* H antigen, it seems to be incapable of synthesizing detectable humoral substances.

Lumbricus does possess a naturally occurring agglutinin (Cooper et al 1974), and the coelomic fluid of the earthworm *Eisenia* contains a protein factor that will lyse, nonspecifically, the cells of various vertebrates (Du Pasquier and Duprat 1968). At 1:3920, cytolytic activity occurs against sheep and human erythrocytes, a reaction that is substantial in contrast to the toad *Alytes*, which destroys erythrocytes at a dilution of 1:240. The Jerne plaque system suggests that chloragogue cells found in the coelomic fluid may be responsible for producing the lytic substance. Although this conclusion requires more investigation, microscopic examination reveals chlorogogue cells in the center of each plaque.

ANTIGEN CLEARANCE AND PHYSIOCHEMICAL ANALYSES IN THE MOLLUSCA

Pelecypoda
    Antigen clearance

Antigen clearance is an important demonstrable feature of invertebrate humoral immune responses, and our understanding of it is derived from numerous studies of the oyster, *Crassostrea virginica*. Twenty-eight days after a primary injection, the oyster's muscle, mantle, gill, and viscera contain T2 phage that persists up to fifty-six days (Fig. 11-5). However, after a secondary injection, T2 is absent from all tissues twenty-eight days later (Fig. 11-6). This is a hundred-fold difference in the primary and secondary clearance rate.

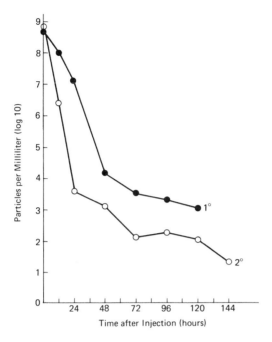

Fig. 11-5 Hemolymph clearance of T2 bacteriophage in oysters after primary intra-cardial injection compared to clearance of T2 in oysters given *Pseudomonas* P-35 bacteriophage 28 days before a "mock" T2 secondary injection. Shell intact. Temperature 25°C. (*From*: Acton & Evans, *J. Bacteriol.*, **95**: 1260, 1968.)

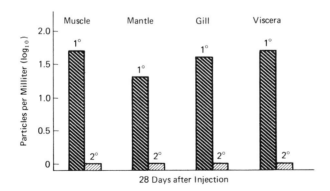

Fig. 11-6 Distribution and clearance of bacteriophage T2 in the tissues of oysters given primary and secondary intramuscular injections. Temperature 27 to 32°C. (*From*: Acton & Evans, *J. Bacteriol*, **95**: 1260, 1968.)

Physiochemical Analysis

Physicochemical analysis of oyster serum reveals no relationship between oyster hemagglutinin and vertebrate immunoglobulins. Oyster hemolymph migrates as a broad peak on cellulose acetate (pH 8.6, ionic strength 0.1) (Fig. 11-7). This mobility is

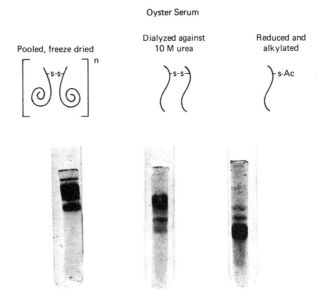

Fig. 11-7 Acrylamide gel electrophoretic patterns of whole oyster hemolymph, whole hemolymph dialyzed overnight against 10M urea and whole hemolymph totally reduced and alkylated. Gels were run for 4 hours at 3 *m*-amp per tube in 0.1 M sodium phosphate (pH 7.2) and 0.1 sodium lauryl sulfate. Drawings at the top of the figure are schematic representations of the probable state of the polypeptide chains under the specified experimental conditions. (*From*: Acton et al., *Comp. Biochem. Physiol.*, **29**: 149, 1969.)

comparable to the α-globulin of human serum. The hemagglutination activity and 98% of the oyster hemolymph proteins are completely removed by absorption with sheep erythrocytes. The hemagglutinin activity resides in a heterogeneous group of rapidly sedimenting molecules that constitute the essential components of the hemolymph. One major active component has a sedimentation coefficient of 33.4S, and several minor components have lower sedimentation coefficients (Fig. 11-8).

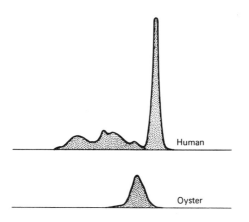

Fig. 11-8 Cellulose acetate zone electrophoresis of whole oyster hemolymph compared with whole human serum. Forty μ1 of oyster hemolymph was applied and 10μ1 of human. Samples were run in barbital buffer, pH 8.6, for 20 min at 250 V. (*From*: Acton et al., *Comp. Biochem. Physiol.*, **29**: 149, 1969.)

The oyster hemolymph protein differs markedly from the immunoglobulins of representative vertebrates. Untreated hemolymph contains four to five bands, but dialysis against 10M urea causes a partial breakdown to lower molecular weight components (Fig. 11-9). Reduction and alkylation yields nearly total dissociation to a single subunit. Dialysis against buffers with pH values below 7 and above 8 also produces dissociation similar to that achieved by 10M urea. According to Acton et al. (1969), the naturally occurring hemagglutinin factor of oysters is nondialyzable, inactivated by dialysis against 0.4M sodium citrate, but heat stable up to 56°C for thirty minutes.

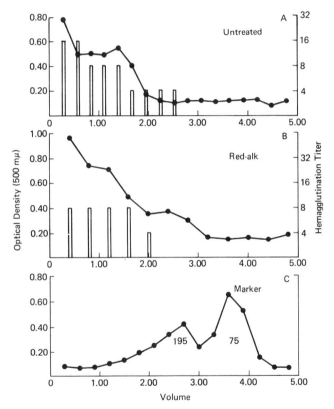

Fig. 11-9 Sucrose density gradient ultracentrifugation experiments showing the distribution of oyster hemagglutinin reactive against sheep erythrocytes. Vertical bars represent hemagglutinin titers. A. Whole oyster hemolymph; B, purified oyster hemagglutinin partially reduced and alkylated (RED-ALK); C, markers consisting of human 19S and 7S immunoglobulins. (*From*: Acton et al., *J. Biol. Chem.*, **15**: 4128, 1969.)

The molecules are dissociable into subunits consisting of single polypeptide chains with approximate molecular weights of 20,000. By using 5M guanidine-HCl, complete dissociation is achieved and reveals noncovalent linkage of the subunit (which possesses a relatively high histidine content), but no lysine is present. The sequence of the first two residues from the NH_2 terminus of the subunit is Thr-Ala. The carbohydrates are mainly mannose, galactose, and glucosamine, resulting in a total carbohydrate content of 13%. Such features are not characteristic of mammalian immunoglobulins. The hemagglutinins of another molluscan species, the Murray mussel, *Velesunio ambiguus*, have been analyzed. The hemagglutinins of neither mollusc contain cysteiene, methionine, or tyrosine, and both are rich in aspartic acid, phenylalanine, and glutamic acid, which are also features uncharacteristic of mammalian immunoglobulins.

Gastropoda

To further characterize molluscan hemolymphs, Pauley et al. (1971) studied the sea hare, *Aplysia californica*, a marine gastropod. Its hemolymph agglutinates marine bacteria and vertebrate erythrocytes with activity peaks exhibiting sedimentation coefficients of 18.5 S and 31.0 S. The activity resides in a heterogeneous group of molecules that have high molecular weights. A protein component is evidently present, since the hemolymph is sensitive to heat, pH extremes, and extraction with 2-mercaptoethanol, phenol, chloroform, and trichloracetic acid. Sephadex separation of the agglutinin reveals an estimated molecular weight in excess of 150,000, for the elution pattern on Sephadex G-50, G-100, and G-200 is equal to that of blue dextran, which has a molecular weight of 2×10^6 (Fig. 11-10).

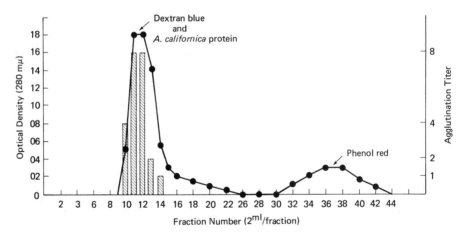

Fig. 11-10 Sephadex column chromatography of *A. californica* serum. Concentrated serum was separated by Sephadex G-200 column chromatography as outlined in the text. Collected fractions were assayed for agglutinating activity against *M. aquivivus* (62S). Line graph shows the optical density of each fraction as measured at 280 mm. Agglutinating activity is indicated by bar graphs. Agglutinating titer of concentrated control serum not subjected to column chromatography was 32. Blue destran was eluted in tubes 11 and 12, while phenol red was eluted in tubes 34–38. (*From*: Pauley, et al., *J. Invert. Pathol.*, **18**: 207, 1971.)

APPROACHES TO SPECIFICITY IN ARTHROPODA (INSECTA)

Lepidoptera
Specificity

The degree of humoral immune specificity is surprising in butterflies and moths. Injection of homologous endotoxin into the wax moth, *Galleria mellonella*, results in subsequent protection against *Pseudomonas aeruginosa* but not against some other

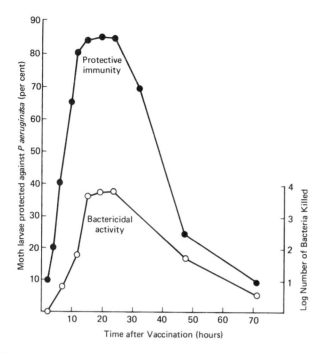

Fig. 11-11 Parallel development of protective immunity and bactericidal activity against *P. aeruginosa* in actively immunized wax moth larvae. (Larvae vaccinated at zero time.) (*From*: Chadwick, *Fed. Proc.* **26**: 1675, 1967.)

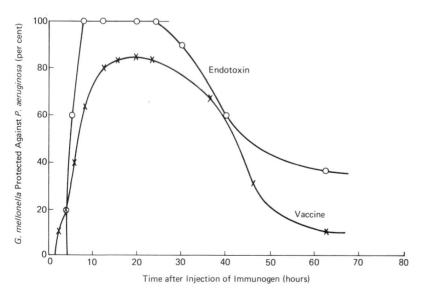

Fig. 11-12 Development of protective immunity to *Pseudomonas aeruginosa* in *Galleria mellonella* following injection of larvae with formolized vaccine or with endotoxin. (*From*: Chadwick, *In Vitro*, **3**: 120, 1967.)

pathogenic gram-negative species. It may be that endotoxin is the component in *Pseudomonas aeruginosa* vaccine that is responsible for protection against closely related but homologous organisms. After injecting wax moth larvae with a heat-killed vaccine of *Pseudomonas aeruginosa*, specific bactericidal activity in the hemolymph develops. This activity parallels protective immunity in the wax moth and is comparable to the endotoxin response (Figs. 11-11 and 11-12).

Gel Filtration of Hemolymph

By using gel filtration, Hink and Briggs (1968) found that the hemolymph of normal and immunized *Galleria mellonella* larvae contains a bactericidal substance that has properties in common with normal serum. Fractions of normal and immune sera also exhibit bactericidal activity, as Figs. 11-13 and 11-14 indicate. Two peaks

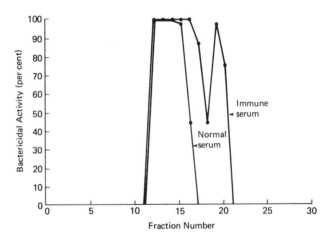

Fig. 11-13 Bactericidal activity of 1.0 ml fractions of normal and immune sera fractionated on a 274 × 10 mm bed of Bio-Gel P-2. Immune serum fractions incubated with forty-one bacteria and those from normal serum with thirty-three bacteria. The curves through fraction 18 represent Factor A, the curve from fraction 18 to 21 represents the smaller Factor B. (*From*: Hink & Briggs, *J. Insect Physiol.*, **14**: 1025, 1968.)

of activity occur in immune serum, but only one occurs in normal serum. In immune serum there is an active substance that is absent from normal serum. The substance present in both types of sera, A, has a larger molecular weight than factor B, present only in immune serum. Factors A and B also seem to exhibit varying degrees of specificity *in vivo* and may be more active against homologous than heterologous organisms. The relative amounts of factors A and B may depend on the type of antigen. Furthermore, factors A and B may be produced only in response to injection of *Pseudomonas aeruginosa*. Other antigens may lead to the production of other factors with different properties.

Factors A and B are both nonproteins with much lower molecular weights than vertebrate antibodies, and thus they are not analogous substances. However, they resemble antibodies, since factor B is formed and the activity of factor A increases after antigenic challenge. Also, passive immunity is conferred on recipient larvae by injection of a bactericidal factor from immune serum. This implies that the activity of factors A and B also operates *in vivo* and, undoubtedly, plays an important role in the insect's immunological response.

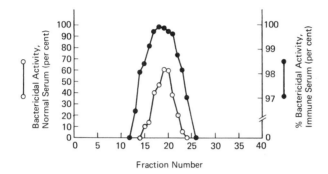

Fig. 11-14 Bactericidal activity of 1.0 ml fractions of normal and immune sera fractionated on a 272 × 10 mm bed of Bio-Gel P-100 overlaid with 10 mm of Bio-Gel P-2. (*From*: Hink & Briggs, *J. Insect. Physiol.*, **14**: 1025, 1968.)

To further understand the immune response of *Galleria* larvae, Hink and Briggs (1969) ligatured instar larvae with nylon thread, divided them by weight into two equal halves, and then immunized them with a lethal dose of *Pseudomonas aeruginosa* (OSU strain 216). Nonimmunized halves of larvae are vulnerable to a 100% bacteremia, but in the treated halves, no bacteremia develops. Second-challenge dosages to test for a secondary response are lethal to unimmunized larvae. Immunity seems to develop in the posterior portion of larvae, for larvae that are immunized in the posterior half and challenged twenty-four hours later develop no bacteremia. Of those immunized and challenged in the anterior half, 63% die from bacteremia.

Hemiptera

The choice of antigen and the experimental techniques used for detection of induced substances are crucial. The large milkweed bug, *Oncopeltus fasciatus* (Dallas), responds to a single injection of *Pseudomonas aeruginosa* (Schroeter) Migula vaccine by producing lytic substances that provide increased resistance to bacterial infection (Fig. 11-15). The acquired resistance that is mediated by lytic substances is detectable four hours after vaccination, reaches a maximum level by twenty-four hours, and disappears within five days. Since a weak transitory resistance and low titres of lytic substances to *Pseudomonas* infection can also be provoked by the injection of heterologous substances, the response is not specific. According to Gingrich (1964), immunity can be passively transferred, for normal insects innoculated with immune serum exhibit a resistance equal to that of immunized bugs. The lytic substances resist exposure to 75°C, 1N HCL, and 1N NaOH for one hour and retain activity after storage at −20°C for at least six months. Thus its activity is strong.

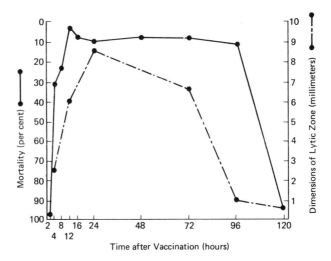

Fig. 11-15 The relationships between the degree of immunity in vaccinated *O. fasciatus* adults and the demonstrable lytic activity of their immune sera. Immunity expressed as percent mortality among groups of vaccinated insects after challenge with lethal doses of *P. aeruginos*; lytic activity represented by dimensions of lytic zone produced by immune serum in agar-well diffusion tests. (*From*: Gingrich, *J. Insect. Physiol.*, **10**: 179, 1964.)

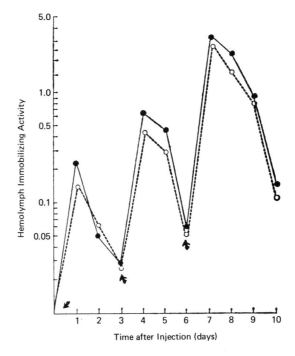

Fig. 11-16 Titer of immobilizing activity of cockroach hemolymph after repeated injections of *Tetrahymena pyriformis S*. Units of activity are expressed as the reciprocal of the minimum amount of hemolymph protein (micrograms) which in the standard assay effects immobilization of washed ciliates (*see text*). Arrows indicate time of injection of 250 μg (dry weight) of ciliates. Each assay was made in pooled diluted hemolymph from three animals. Closed circles and solid line represent data obtained from injection of living ciliates; open circles and dotted line represent data with heat-killed ciliates. (*From*: Seaman & Robert, *Science*, **161**: 1359, 1968.)

210

Orthoptera

The immune response capacity of the American cockroach, *Periplaneta americana*, to the ciliated protozoan, *Tetrahymena pyriformes* S, has been studied by Seaman and Robert (1969). This ciliate occurs in adult female cockroaches, is easily removed, and can be isolated into axenic cultures. Most ciliates injected into the hemocoels of adult males die. That these cannot be recovered from the hemolymph suggests that the male produces an immunological substance against the ciliates. As these findings suggest, the immune response of insects may be hormonally controlled (Fig. 11-16).

The immune capacity of the cockroach resides in a protein. Seaman and Robert (1969) ran disc electrophoretic patterns of ammonium-saturated material on 7.5% polyacrylamide gel at pH 9.5 toward the anode and at pH 4.3 toward the cathode at 5 ma per column. As Fig. 11-17 illustrates, the protein is detected by staining with aniline black. Two basic proteins with identical mobilities appear in samples from normal and immunized roaches. However, five acidic protein bands can also be separated from normal hemolymph. Three additional bands (1A, 2A, and 1E) of acidic proteins are apparent in the immune fraction. That activity which immobilizes the ciliates is obtained from the C band of the immune hemolymph, but the C band of normal male hemolymph shows no activity. The hemolymph from immune roaches confers protection on others injected with it.

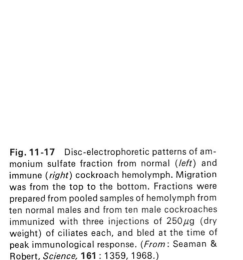

2A
1A
A
B
C
D

1E

E

Fig. 11-17 Disc-electrophoretic patterns of ammonium sulfate fraction from normal (*left*) and immune (*right*) cockroach hemolymph. Migration was from the top to the bottom. Fractions were prepared from pooled samples of hemolymph from ten normal males and from ten male cockroaches immunized with three injections of 250 μg (dry weight) of ciliates each, and bled at the time of peak immunological response. (*From*: Seaman & Robert, *Science,* **161** : 1359, 1968.)

Crustacea

The crayfish, *Cambarus virilis*, will clear human serum albumin (HSA I[131]) antigen from the circulation, but it shows no acquired specific humoral responses to it (Teague and Friou, 1964). Second and third injections of the same antigen lead to no accelerated removal. The degradation of HSA I[131] antigen is nonspecific, not acquired, and, hence, nonimmune. Because of its rapid degradation, perhaps its antigenic activity is reduced in the crayfish. Crayfish challenged with the bacteriophage ϕX174, a larger, more complex molecule composed of protein and a single-stranded deoxyribonucleic acid, do not exhibit an immediate rapid clearance. Thus, there is a need for employing different kinds of antigens when testing arthropods for humoral immunity.

By contrast, McKay and Jenkin (1969) conclude that the crayfish *Parachaeraps bicarinatus* produces an adaptive immune response. The response they discovered is similar in some respects to that of vertebrates: its expression and duration is dependent on the dose of antigen, the time of second challenge after the initial immunizing dose, and the environmental temperature. However, since a variety of vaccines derived from gram-negative bacteria are able to increase the crayfish's resistance to subsequent *Pseudomonas* infection, its immunity appears to be relatively nonspecific. Moreover, immunity can also be induced by treating crayfish with lipopolysaccharides

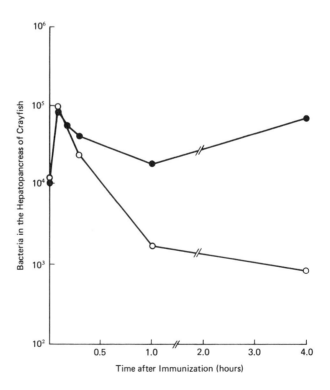

Fig. 11-18 Fate of *Pseudomonas* CP in the hepato-pancreas of the crayfish (*Parachaeraps bicarinatus*).

●————● Normal crayfish
○————○ Immunized crayfish

(*From*: McKay & Kenkin, AJEBAK, **48**: 599, 1970.)

from gram-negative bacteria unrelated to the pathogen. It is important that a similar nonspecific immunity can be likewise induced in vertebrates. For example, mice treated with endotoxin are subsequently able to resist a variety of bacterial and viral infections (Rowley 1956, Landy and Pillomer 1956).

With regard to the distribution of antigens in tissues, the hepatopancreas is a likely site wherein phagocytosis occurs to a high degree. One week after an initial injection of 10^6 *Pseudomonas*, crayfish are challenged via the ventral sinus. In the hepatopancreas of immune crayfish (Fig. 11-18), following the initial rapid uptake there is a pronounced decrease in viable bacteria, suggesting a memory response at the cellular (phagocytic) level, i.e., increased uptake after a second challenge. By contrast in normal crayfish, after a brief period the number of bacteria increase in the hepatopancreas and are associated with a rapid rise in bacteria of the haemolymph, leading ultimately to death due to persistent bacteraemia (Fig. 11-19).

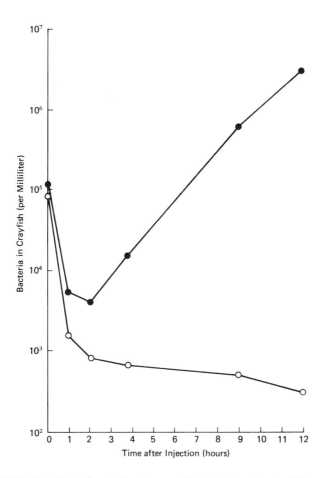

Fig. 11-19 Growth in vivo of *Pseudomonas* CP in the hemolymph of the crayfish (*Parachaeraps bicarinatus*).

●————● Normal cryfish
○————○ Immunized crayfish

(*From*: McKay & Jenkin, AJEBAK, **48**: 599, 1970.)

The West Indian spiny lobster, *Panulirus argus*, possesses an interesting, naturally occurring hemolysin that is apparently specific for sheep erythrocytes. Figure 11-20 illustrates the typical dose response curve that results from the addition of increasing amounts of lobster hemolyph to a constant amount of sheep erythrocytes (Weinheimer etal. 1969). As can be seen, with each increase in the volume of hemolymph there is a corresponding increase in the percentage of hemolysis of sheep erythrocytes.

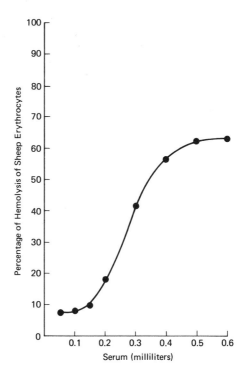

Fig. 11-20   Dose response curve; percentage of hemolysis of sheep erythrocytes plotted as a function of the volume of lobster hemolymph. (*From*: Weinheimer, et al., *Proc. Soc. Exp. Biol. Med.*, **130**: 322, 1969.)

Evans et al. (1968) immunized the Indian spiny lobster, *Panulirus argus*, with intracardial injections of 10^9 cells of various live and heat-killed bacteria in 0.9% sodium chloride solution. According to their results, the most effective antigen is the gram-negative bacillus, EMB-1, isolated from the normal intestinal flora of healthy *Panulirus argus*. A bactericidin is present and usually detectable in the hemolymph within twelve hours after injection and reaches a peak level within twenty-four to forty-eight hours (Fig. 11-21). This bactericidin is less specific than mammalian antibody, as Fig. 11-22 reveals, for heterologous bacteria produce similar results. On the other hand, secondary bactericidal responses are more intense than the primary ones, as illustrated in Fig. 11-23. Evans et al. believe the lobster's "immunologic memory" is indicated by its more intense tertiary responses than its secondary responses. In addition, residual titers persist for many days or weeks without additional antigenic

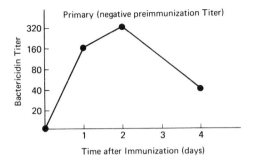

Fig. 11-21 Primary response curve of hemolymph bactericidin following immunization with gram-negative bacillus, EMB-1 (*From*: Evans et al., *Proc. Soc. Exp. Biol. Med.*, **128**: 394, 1968.)

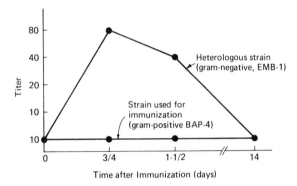

Fig. 11-22 Nonspecific response induced by gram-positive bacillus, BAP-4. (*From*: Evans et al., *Proc. Soc. Exp. Biol. Med.*, **128**: 394, 1968.)

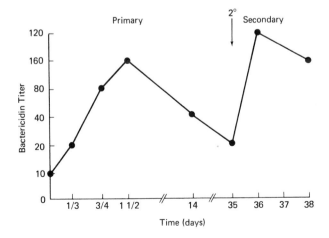

Fig. 11-23 Bactericidal response of spiny lobster; 35-day interval between primary and secondary antigen injections. (*From*: Evans et al., *J. Bacteriol*, **98**: 943, 1969.)

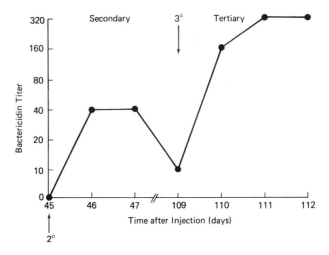

Fig. 11-24 Secondary and tertiary bactericidal responses; secondary at day 45; tertiary at day 109. (*From*: Evans, et al., *J. Bacteriol.*, **98**: 943, 1969.)

stimulation (Fig. 11-24), and similar results have been obtained with the California spiny lobster, *Panulirus interruptus*.

After partial characterization, Cornick and Stewart (1973) determined that the natural agglutinin of the North American lobster's hemolymph is similar in many respects to that of other invertebrates. It is inactivated by temperatures of between 56° and 65°C like the spiny lobster (Tyler and Scheer 1945), the American oyster, the Murray mussel, and the crayfish; the sea hare differs with an inactivation temperature of 65°–70°C. Calcium stabilizes agglutinin activity with increasing temperatures in the lobster just as it does in the oyster. Furthermore, in serum dialyzed against calcium, agglutinin activity is low and essentially unchanged over a pH range of 6.0–9.0 (titer 16). If calcium is removed by dialysis, the activity increases to a titer of 64 at pH levels on both the acidic and basic sides of the physiological pH, 7.6.

In order to demonstrate an erythrocyte receptor site for the agglutinin, Evans et al. performed blocking experiments similar to those of McDade and Tripp (1967) using various saccharides. A known volume of saccharide at a concentration of 0.10 g/ml in 0.85% NaCl solution was added to 0.025 ml of hemolymph dilutions in microtiter plates. Hemagglutination tests were performed using erythrocytes of several different species. The chemical nature of the antigenic reactive site differs, but generally, D-glucosamine blocks or inhibits adsorption of the agglutinin to erythrocytes of most species tested. Agglutinins are known to enhance phagocytosis in the lobster, and because of their association with hemocytes, they may well be responsible for agglutinin production, confirming lobster hemocytes as examples of primitive receptor cells.

It is not surprising that the crayfish, *Procambarus clarkii*, possesses a hemolymph agglutinin. The titers against three marine bacteria and two vertebrate RBC range from 2–4 to 8–16, and they are higher against chicken RBC than any other cells. According to Miller et al. (1972), the crayfish agglutinin is active over a wide range of pH (~5–10) but totally inactivated at acid (pH 1.6) and alkaline (pH 11.0)/extremes.

Normal agglutination titers are unaffected by dialysis, freezing and thawing, and storage at low temperatures. Furthermore, the agglutinin is stable at 50°C/30 minutes, partially inactivated at 60°C/30 minutes, and totally inactivated at 70°C/30 minutes. TCA and phenol extraction are the only chemical tests that completely inactivate the agglutinin. The agglutinin is stable to dialysis; thus it is probably a macromolecule. By means of Sephadex G-200 molecular sieve chromatography, the molecular weight of the agglutinin is estimated to be greater than 150,000.

Limulus polyphemus, the horseshoe crab, evolved from ancestors of the primitive arthropods, and for this reason it is of much interest for comparative immunology. Marchalonis and Edelman (1968a) isolated and partially characterized the agglutinin from the hemolymph by a variety of methods including starch gel electrophoresis, amino acid analysis, two-dimensional high-voltage electrophoresis of tryptic peptides, and immunological analysis. With regard to structure, by means of electron microscopy, Fernández-Morán et al. (1968) found that the agglutinin consists of uniform ring-shaped structures with a diameter of about 100Å. Each particle contains a well-defined, dense central core 20–40Å in diameter. Close examination of single molecules suggests a hexagonal shape, but occasionally, elongated structures are observed, probably corresponding to a side view of a stack of 100Å rings (Fig. 11-25).

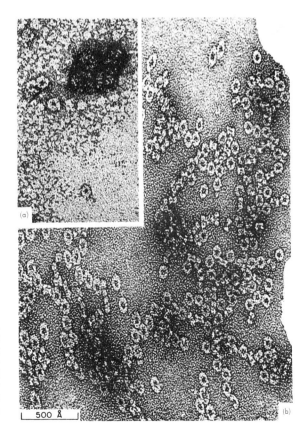

Fig. 11-25 (a) Hemolymph of *Limulus polyphemus* stained with uranyl acetate showing, in addition to hemocyanin molecules, typical ring structures about 100Å in diameter. (b) Hemagglutinin isolated from *Limulus polyphemus* stained with uranyl formate showing uniform 100Å particles with same kind of ring structure (×*300,000.*) (*From*: Fernandez-Moran, et al., *J. Mol. Biol.*, **32**: 467, 1968.)

500 Å

ARTHROPODA AND ECHINODERMATA COMPARED

Two important agglutinins from two key animals in evolution are considered together, These are the horseshoe crab, *Limulus polyphemus*, and the starfish, *Asterias forbesi*. Both purified and nonpurified agglutinins from *Limulus* and *Asterias* were inactivated at temperatures between 65° and 70°C or by addition of EDTA; addition of Ca^{++} ions to the EDTA-inactivated agglutinins does not reestablish the agglutinating activity. It is interesting though that agglutinating activity is specific. For example, absorption with horse cells reduces the titer to horse cells but does not affect the agglutinating activity for sheep or rabbit cells; the reverse is also true. Thus, the agglutinins seem, at least in part, specific for each separate erythrocyte population.

With regard to physicochemical analysis, the sedimentation velocity obtained for *Limulus* (5mg/ml) agglutinin is 12.6S and that of *Asterias* (4mg/ml), 6.5S. Both purified agglutinins show a single precipitin band during immunoelectrophoresis, when each is developed against rabbit antiwhole hemolymph or rabbit antisera against whole coelomic fluid of the respective species. At pH 8.6, the electrophoretic mobility of purified *Limulus* agglutinin is cathodal but *Asterias* agglutinin is anodal. Furthermore, when each of the purified agglutinins is reacted against the respective rabbit antiserum, each shows a single line on double diffusion in agar, but there are no cross reactions between the purified agglutinins of *Limulus* and *Asterias*.

With regard to amino acid composition, both proteins contain cystine residues. The N-terminal amino acid analysis reveals that the *Limulus* agglutinin has a single leucine residue. The *Asterias* protein by contrast contains multiple N-terminal residues of aspartic acid, glutamic acid, serine, and threonine. By means of circular dichroic

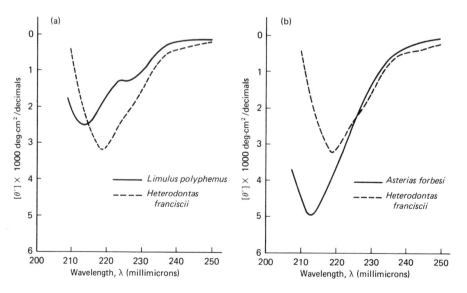

Fig. 11-26 Comparative circular dichroic spectra of purified invertebrate agglutinin and shark immunoglobulin. *Limulus* agglutinin (——) and 18.5S *Heterodontas* immunoglobulin (----) (a); *Asterias* agglutinin (——) and 18.5S *Heterodontas* immunoglobulin (----) (b). (*From*: Finstad, et al., *J. Immunol.*, **108**: 1704, 1972.)

spectra, analyses yield dissimilar spectra for the purified *Limulus* and purified *Asterias* agglutinins with θ' values of -2475 at 214 nm and -4950 at 213 nm, respectively. Both spectra differ grossly from the typical spectra of vertebrate immunoglobulin. For example, the 18.5S immunoglobulin of *Heterodontas franciscii*, the shark, reveals a θ' value of -3200 at 217 nm (Fig. 11-26). The *Limulus* and *Asterias* proteins possess typical ultraviolet spectra with an absorption maximum at 276 nm.

The *Limulus* agglutinin subunit apparently has a molecular weight of approximately 25,000, and that of *Asterias* agglutinin, approximately 30,000 (Fig. 11-27).

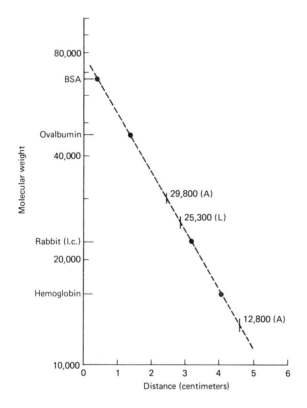

Fig. 11-27 Molecular weight determinations of *Limulus* (L) and *Asterias* (A) subunits by sodium dodecyl sulfate-15% acrylamide gel analysis. (*From:* Finstad, et al., *J. Immunol.*, **108**: 1704, 1972.)

The disulfide linked heavy-light chain pairs of vertebrate immunoglobulins are different from the subunit organization defined in invertebrate agglutinins. Agglutinins are composed of noncovalently linked subunits with molecular weights of approximately 25,000 to 30,000. Of importance for future studies are the biologic specificity of these molecules. Furthermore, it will be informative to study the comparative amino acid sequences and molecular structure of the combining sites to determine possible relationships between the agglutinins and immunoglobulins.

Table 11-2

Comparison of the physicochemical properties of invertebrate hemagglutinine and fibrinogen

	Horseshoe Crab HA	Oyster HA	Snail HA	Murray Mussell HA	Sea hare HA	Starfish HA	Crayfish HA	Spiny lobster HA	Spiny obster fibrinogen
Molecular Weight	400,000	–	100,000	–	>150,000	–	>150,000	400,000	420,000
$S^\circ_{20,w}$	13.5	33.4	5.3	28	18.5,31	6.5	–	10.3	14.5
$D^\circ_{20,w}$	–	–	–	–	–	–	–	2.4	2.9
Subunit Mol. Wt.	22,500	20,000	–	–	–	30,000	–	68,500	70,000
Carbohydrate (%)	–	8.8	7	–	–	–	–	4.6	3
Amino-Terminal Residues	Leucine	Threonine	–	–	–	Threonine, Serine, Aspartic acid Glutamic acid	–	Phenylalanine	Leucine
Calcium Dependency	+	+	–	–	0	+	–	+	+

From Acton and Weinheimer Contemporary Topics in Immunobiology **4**: 271, 1974

PHYSICAL AND CHEMICAL STUDIES OF HEMAGGLUTININS

Comparison of Hemagglutinins

Hemagglutinins represent an important factor in invertebrate humoral immunity. They seem to be related chemically and may actually represent primitive receptor molecules. Other closely related hemolymph factors include inducible bactericidins, naturally occurring hemolysins, and clotting factors. Finally, hemagglutinins may have evolved from a common ancestral gene (Acton and Weinheimer 1974). In addition to biological properties described in earlier sections, there are sufficient physico-chemical properties that can be enumerated. First, hemagglutinin molecules tend to aggregate or dissociate depending on the pH and Ca^{++}-ion concentration; however, such fragility makes it difficult to determine their molecular weight. Second, sedimentation of hemagglutinin molecules usually depends upon concentration (Table 11-2). Third, hemagglutinin molecules (e.g., in oyster) do not readily dissociate into respective subunits, and they require strong denaturing solvents for dissociation to occur. Moreover, thiol-binding reagents must be components of the dissociating solvents in order to inhibit disulfide interchange and subsequent aggregation. Notwithstanding these technical difficulties, the hemagglutinin molecules of horseshoe crabs, oysters, and spiny lobsters possess a remarkable degree of similarity with regard to amino acid composition and peptide maps. Calcium is important in stabilizing the molecules, which show greater effectiveness in a pH range of 7 to 8, an additional common property. There is some known specificity for N-acetylated amino sugar, a component of certain cell membranes.

Carbohydrate Composition of the Hemagglutinins

Acton and his colleagues (Acton et al. 1973) have been instrumental in analyzing hemagglutinin structure in the oyster, starfish and spiny lobster subunit, especially with respect to their carbohydrate moieties (Table 11-3). Both subunits have common

Table 11-3

Carbohydrate composition of hemagglutinin subunit

	Oyster		Lobster	
	%	Moles per subunit*	%	Moles per subunit*
Fucose	0.6	0.8	0.1	0.4
Mannose	3.7	4.2	2.9	10.9
Galactose	1.5	1.1	0.6	2.4
Glu NH$_2$	2.7	3.0	0.8	3.0
Sialic Acid§	0.2	0.1	0.2	0.5
Total CHO//	8.8	9.2	4.6	17.2

*Molecular weight of subunit = 20,000
†Molecular weight of subunit = 68,000
‡Glucosamine as free base
§Sialic acid as N-acetylneuraminic acid.
//Total carbohydrate as sum of monosaccharides.
From: Acton and Weinheimer Contemporary Topics in Immunobiology **4**: 271, 1974

components such as fucose, mannose, galactose, glucosamine, and sialic acid. There is a difference however if the two subunits are compared on a molar basis. The spiny lobster hemagglutinin contains approximately twice as much total carbohydrate as the oyster hemagglutinin. The molar quantities of the mannose and galactose are almost proportional to the molecular weights of the subunits and account for most of the difference in total carbohydrate content. The ratio of galactose to mannose is approximately 1 : 4 in both subunits.

Significance of Invertebrate Humoral Immunity

General Considerations

Invertebrate humoral immunity involves the presence of biologically active molecules that occur naturally or that may be induced. These molecules are able to act on the antigens responsible for their induction in several ways, notably by their lytic or agglutinating properties. In this respect they resemble the action of vertebrate antibodies. Invertebrate humoral factors differ, however, in lacking the high degree of specificity that characterizes vertebrate antibodies. A resolution of the problem of homology rests on more detailed primary data on molecular structure. According to Weinheimer (1970b) the hemagglutinins, bactericidins, and erythrocyte hemolysins of the spiny lobster are apparently separate entities. This suggests a progression from primitive to advanced among the invertebrates in the presence, numbers, and kinds of separate humoral substances. Comparing the oyster with the spiny lobster, for example, it will be seen that oysters possess hemagglutinins but lack hemolysins, bactericidins, and clotting factors. The earthworm may lack bactericidins but not clotting factors, and in a close relative, the sipunculid worm, it only lacks clotting factors. Arthropods are relatively advanced when compared with annelids and molluscs; thus, primitive creatures may lack the complexity of hemolymph components operative in arthropods.

Comparisons with Vertebrate Complement

Despite the important differences in invertebrate humoral substances and vertebrate antibody, both groups of molecules possess the common property of providing immune defense mechanisms. In vertebrate animals, antigens stimulate antibody synthesis, and the resulting antibody binds to antigen forming complexes. Under certain conditions these antigen-antibody complexes can bind to complement or to certain cells, setting in motion a whole array of inflammatory reactions. The complement system alone can be activated by by-passing the need for antigen and antibody. *Complement* is a system of proteins that mediates a number of reactions such as cell lysis, chemotaxis, agglutination, and phagocytosis. There is some resemblance of the vertebrate complement system to several effector mechanisms that sequester infectious agents in invertebrates (Gigli and Austen 1971). Day et al. (1970) have found in some invertebrate species hemolymph activities that resemble those mediated by the terminal components of the vertebrate complement system. This represents, at least for now, the most striking similarity between invertebrate and vertebrate immune components.

Evolution of Genes Coding for Hemagglutinins

At the present time, what is known about the genes that code for antibody is far less speculative than our knowledge of genes that are coded for invertebrate humoral substances. Because there are similarities between the respective hemagglutinins, it is possible to speculate that they had common origins and that such molecules were the primitive receptor units that evolved in invertebrates. The receptor would be localized on the surface of immunocytes and would serve as a recognition unit for foreign antigens. Acton and Weinheimer (1974) believe that a precursor gene may have coded for a molecule with a molecular weight of about 20,000. They believe that by fusion, contiguous gene duplication, and possible translocation, genes evolved that coded for hemagglutinin molecules of about 69,000 molecular weight (e.g., the spiny lobster). Such genes could have undergone considerable mutation, producing the well-known molecules with diverse functions (e.g., hemolysins, bactericidins, and clotting factors). As an alternative hypothesis, they propose that many genes that coded for invertebrate hemolymph factors were lost when vertebrates evolved. It is relevant that a hemagglutinin occurs in the lamprey, one of the most primitive jawless fishes; its hemagglutinin differs from its immunoglobulin (Marchalonis and Edelman, 1968a, b).

SUMMARY

The criteria for adaptive immunity have been defined on the basis of the vertebrate responses. Thus, the classical vertebrate immunologist often concluded that invertebrates show no adaptive immunity. However, unlike vertebrate antibody, precise distinctions between the invertebrate's naturally occurring substances and the induced substances still remain obscure. The conceptual and technical approaches to understanding humoral synthesis in invertebrates is limited. An encompassing definition that considers both vertebrates and invertebrates should be the following: First, an animal should reach a stage of altered characteristics after antigen presentation. Second, the antigen should induce the formation of a humoral component. Finally, the antigen should also become sequestered by the component. The examples given in this chapter show instances of induced invertebrate humoral immunity that fulfill these criteria; but there is a distinct lack of data on this topic.

BIBLIOGRAPHY

Acton, R. T., and Weinheimer, P. F. 1974. Hemagglutinins: Primitive Receptor Molecules Operative in Invertebrate Defense Mechanisms. In *Contemporary Topics in Immunobiology*, IV 271, ed. E. L. Cooper. New York: Plenum Press.

Acton, R. T., Weinheimer, P. F., and Niedermeier, U. 1973. The carbohydrate composition of invertebrate hemagglutinin subunits isolated from the lobster *Panulirus argus* and the oyster *Crassostrea virginica*. Comp. Biochem. Physiol. **44**: 185.

Acton, R. T., Bennett, J. C., Evans, E. E., and Schrohenloher, R. E. 1969. Physical and chemical characterization of an oyster hemagglutinin. *J. Biol. Chem.* **244**: 4128.

Bang, F. B. 1966. Serologic response in a marine worm, *Sipunculus nudus*. J. Immunol. **96**: 960.

Chadwick, J. S. 1967. Serological responses of insects. *Fed. Proc.* **6**: 1675.

Cooper, E. L. Acton, R. T., Weinheimer, P., and Evans, E. E. 1969. Lack of a bactericidal response in the earthworm, *Lumbricus terrestris*, after immunization with bacterial antigens. J. Invert. Pathol. **14**: 402.

Cooper, E. L., Lemmi, C. A. E., and Moore, T. C., 1974. Agglutinins and cellular immunity in earthworms. Ann. N. Y. Acad. Sci. **234**: 34.

Cornick, J. W., and Stewart, J. E., 1973. Partial characterization of a natural agglutinin in the hemolymph of the lobster, *Homarus americanus*. J. Invert. Pathol. **21**: 255.

Cushing, J. E. 1967. Invertebrates, immunology and evolution. *Fed. Proc.* **6**: 1666.

Cushing, J. E., McNeely, D. S., and Tripp, M. R. 1969. Comparative immunology of sipunculid coelomic fluid. J. Invert. Pathol. **12**: 4.

Day, N. K. B., Gewurz, H., Johannsen, R., Finstad, J., and Good. 1970. Complement and complement-like activity in lower vertebrates and invertebrates. J. Exp. Med. **132**: 941.

Du Pasquier, L. and Duprat, P. 1968. Aspect humoreaux et cellulaire d'une immunité naturelle non spécifique chez l'oligachète *Eisenia foetida* sur (Lumbricidae). C. R. Acad. Sci. Paris **266**: 538.

Evans, E. E., Cushing, J. E., and Evans, M. L. 1973. Comparative immunology: Sipunculid bactericidal responses. *Inf. and Immunity* **8**: 355.

Evans, E. E., Painter, M. L., Evans, M. L., Weinheimer, P., and Acton, R. T. 1968. An induced bactericidin in the spiny lobster, *Panulirus argus*. Proc. Soc. Exptl. Biol & Med. **128**: 394.

Fernández-Morán, H., Marchalonis, J. J., and Edelman, G. M. 1968. Electron microscopy of a hemagglutinin from *Limulus polyphemus*. J. Mol. Biol. **32**: 467.

Finstad, C. L., Litman, G. W., Finstad, J., and Good, R. A. 1972. The evolution of the immune response. XIII. The characterization of purified erythrocyte agglutinins from two invertebrate species. J. Immunol. **108**: 1704.

Gigli, J., and Austen, K. F. 1971. Phylogeny and function of the complement system. Ann. Rev. Microbiol. **25**: 309.

Gingrich, R. E. 1964. Acquired humoral immune response of the large milkweed bug, *Oncopeltus fasciatus* (Dallas), to injected materials. J. Insect. Physiol. **10**: 179.

Hink, W. F., and Briggs, J. D. 1968. Bactericidal factors in haemolymph from normal and immune wax moth larvae, *Galleria mellonella*. J. Insect. Physiol. **14**: 1025.

————. 1969. Immune responses of ligatured *Galleria mellonella* larvae. J. Invert. Pathol. **13**: 308.

Krassner, S. M., and Florey, B. 1970. Antibacterial factors in the sipunculid worms, *Golfingia gouldii* and *Dendrostomum pyroides*. J. Invert. Pathol. **16**: 331.

Landy, M., and Pillamer, L. 1956. Increased resistance to infection and accompanying alteration in properdin levels following administration of bacterial lipopolysaccharide. J. Exp. Med. **104**: 53.

Marchalonis, J. J., and Edelman, G. M. 1968a. Isolation and characterization of a haemagglutinin from *Limulus polyphenus*. J. Mol. Biol. **32**: 453.

————. 1968b. Phylogenetic origins of antibody structure. III. Antibodies in the primary immune response of the sea lamprey, *Petromyzon marinus*. J. Exp. Med. **127**: 891.

McDade, J. E., and Tripp, M. R. 1967a. Mechanism of agglutination of red blood cells by oyster hemolymph. J. Invert. Pathol. **9**: 523.

McKay, D., and Jenkin, C. R. 1969. Immunity in the invertebrates. II. Adaptive immunity in the crayfish *Parachaeraps bicarinatus*. Immun. **17**: 127.

Miller, V. H., Ballback, R. S., Pauley, G. B., and Krassner, S. M. 1972. A preliminary physicochemical characterization of an agglutinin found in the hemolymph of the crayfish *Procambarus clarkii*. J. Invert. Pathol. **19**: 83.

Pauley, G. B., Granger, G. A., and Krassner, S. M. 1971. Characterization of a natural agglutinin present in the hemolymph of the California sea here, *Aplysia californica*. J. Invert. Pathol. **18**: 207.

Rowley, D. 1956. Rapidly induced changes in the levels of nonspecific immunity in laboratory animals. Brit. J. Exp. Path. **37**: 223.

Seaman, G. R., and Robert, M. L. 1968. Immunological response of male cockroaches to injection of *Tetrahymena pyriformis*. Science **161**: 1359.

Teague, P. O., and Friou, G. J. 1964. Lack of immunological responses by an invertebrate. Comp. Biochem. Physiol **12**: 471.

Tyler, A., and Scheer, B. T. 1945. Natural heteroagglutinins in the serum of the spiny lobster, *Panulirus interruptus*. II. Chemical and antigenic relations to the blood protein. Biol. Bull. **89**: 193.

Weinheimer, P. F. 1970. Immunophylogeny. A review of immune-like mechanisms of invertebrate species. Alabama. J. of Med. Sci. **7**: 451.

Weinheimer, P. F., Acton, R. T., Cushing, J. E., and Evans, E. E. 1970. Reactions of sipunculid fluid with erythrocytes. Life Sci. **9**: 145.

Weinheimer, P. F., Evans, E. E., Strand, R. M., Acton, R. T., and Painter, B. 1969. Comparative immunology: Natural hemolytic system of the spiny lobster, *Panulirus argus*. Proc. Soc. Exp. Biol. and Med. **130**: 322.

Chapter 12

Antibody Synthesis

INTRODUCTION

Antibodies or immunoglobulins are among the most interesting products of differentiated cells. This claim is based on two fundamental properties related to antibody synthesis. First, the exquisite specificity of the host response, both to the antigen that induces the antibody and to the final antibody that sequesters the inducing antigen. Second, the cells of the immune system, once they have been primed by a given antigen, are, upon second challenge, fully capable of responding in a specific, heightened manner. In other words, the cells or their descendants "remember" that they have "seen" the antigen previously and the entire sequence of events requires no initial tooling up again. Once differentiation of the primed cell proceeds, the cell "knows" and is therefore ready for a more rapid second encounter with the same antigen, and except for closely related antigens, there is almost no cross-reactivity.

The simplest processes by which antigen induces the formation of antibody is analogous in many respects to a stimulus response situation. For example, the antigen acts as a stimulus, and immune cells of varying kinds give a response. Since the immune response is multifaceted, one can expect to define the entire series of events at various points in the immune response continuum. Although there are still unclear areas about the precise role of certain cells, we are safe in assuming that most lymphocytes and plasma cells synthesize and secrete antibody, which, except for cell-bound antibody, is released into the serum. It is the antigen-sensitive cell, the recognizing cell, or the receptor cell that is thought to be the first cell involved in setting the immune response in motion. In fact, in any stimulus response system (especially obvious in animal sense organs) there must first be receptor cells (e.g., taste, smell, sight, hearing) that pulse the environment for the correct stimuli. So, too, must the receptor cell of the immune system sense appropriate antigens. Antigen stimulates the synthesis of antibody; when interpreted from the viewpoint of development and differentiation, the response antigen $\longrightarrow$ antibody is one of the better known and better defined inducer $\longrightarrow$ product situations.

There is still controversy regarding the role of phagocytosis by macrophages in the scheme of antibody synthesis. If we assume that lymphocytes sense antigen, then a second appropriately equipped cell, the phagocytic cell, must be ready to degrade the antigen, receive information, and somehow communicate it to the effector cell, another lymphocyte or plasma cell, that finally synthesizes and secretes the antibody.

We know the respective functions for each cell type, but the crucial findings and interpretations will unite isolated observations to form a chain of events from contact with antigen to antibody synthesis.

ANTIGEN ELIMINATION

Introduction

It is at this point in the pathway leading to antibody synthesis that macrophages and phagocytosis are particularly important. Because macrophages are strategically located throughout the body, they are able to make contact with and to capture antigen. Phagocytosis represents one facet of the immune response that is found throughout the animal kingdom; to it are gradually added, in evolution, several other immunocyte types with varied functional roles, notably antibody synthesis. Any vertebrate, for example, is amply equipped, by means of the various cells, tissues, and organs throughout the entire body, for capturing and trapping antigen.

The blood circulates throughout the body, and it, like other tissues, contains a multiplicity of cell types, at least two of which, the monocytes and neutrophils, function primarily in phagocytosis. One can easily envision how constant blood flow not only nourishes the body but provides an ever-present phagocytic surveillance mechanism. Regardless of the level of phylogeny, all vertebrates and invertebrates possess an array of phagocytic cells, thereby fulfilling the basic primeval necessity for a system capable of eliminating antigen. This portion of the immune response fits broadly into the inductive period. In addition to phagocytosis, pinocytosis is as efficient in leading to removal of soluble antigens. During the first hour antigen is eliminated from the blood, and if we searched from this time on through the fourth to the seventh day, we would find the antigen localized in the cells and tissues.

During the inductive period antigen is broken down or degraded by enzymatic hydrolysis and digestion. Therefore this period requires that several factors be operative to insure optimum degradation. Certainly a host animal must possess the necessary enzymes to react with an antigen. Presumably under the usual circumstances, i.e., when an animal is confronted by an antigen in nature, it is equipped with the required enzyme for antigen degradation. This may not be the case, however, in experimental conditions where various animals are often barraged with an array of antigens, e.g., synthetic haptens for which they may not possess the required enzymes.

The final phase of antigen removal, should it occur at all, may require extensive time, from weeks or months to years. However, there is a second major burst of antigen elimination different from the first and reflecting antigen removal from the blood. This period of antigen removal is partially due to the combination of newly formed antibody molecules with the antigen, promoting a second burst of phagocytic activity, digestion, and antigen removal.

Disappearance of Antigen from the Blood Stream
Sharks

The mammal has been the usual subject for numerous studies on the relationship between antigen elimination and immune responses. Because of the shark's phylogenetically more archaic and simpler physiology, it offers an interesting and contrasting

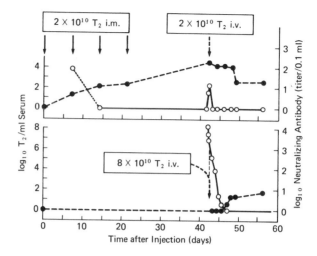

Fig. 12-1 (*upper panel*) Phage and neutralizing natibody levels in the serum of sharks previously immunized with phage. The injection for clearance administered i.v.; (*lower panel*) Phage and neutralizing antibody levels in the serum of normal sharks following i.v. injection. (*From*: Sigel et al., *Proc. Soc. Exp. Biol. Med.*, **128**: 911, 1968.)

model, when compared to amphibians or mammals, for analyses of antigen elimination (Sigel et al., 1968). The lemon shark, *Negaprion brevirostris*, eliminates a bacteriophage antigen from its circulation fairly rapidly after an intravenous injection, so that by day 2, the amount of free phage is reduced by four logs and by day 5 no phage is detectable (Fig. 12-1). The upper panel of Fig. 12-1 shows the condition of sharks previously immunized with T_2 phage by four weekly intramuscular injections. Antibody titer increases slowly, with the highest titer at day 42. When given a second intravenous injection of 8×10^{10} pfu of the bacteriophage, there is essentially no detectable phage, presumably due to its combination with existing antibody. If phage is injected by the intramuscular route it is eliminated as rapidly as after an intravenous injection, with no antigen present by day 4. After a second intramuscular injection, no phage occurs at any time. It is obvious that the route of antigen entrance is important to the resulting response, for an animal is not immune immediately after antigen entrance. As antigen disappears, antibody becomes obvious.

Mammals

If we administer an antigen intraveneously, it is eliminated from the host animal in a characteristic pattern. After injection, most antigenic material is rapidly catabolized. We see the following pattern of elimination of I_{131} trace-labeled rabbit γ-globulin (I*RGG), bovine γ-globulin (I*BGG), and bovine serum albumin (I*BSA) from the circulation of rabbits (Fig. 12-2, Dixon 1957). All three antigens equilibrate during the first two days. This form of antigen catabolism, which occurs prior to the appearance of significant amounts of antibody, is nonimmune catabolism. When antibody begins to appear about the fourth day after injection of I*BGG and the eighth day after injection of I*BSA, these antigens are rapidly catabolized and soon disappear from the circulation by immune catabolism. Free antibody then appears in the serum.

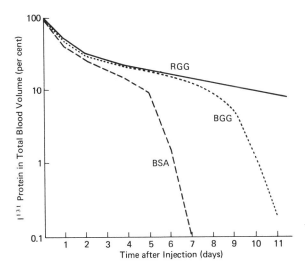

Fig. 12-2 Disappearance of I^{131} proteins from the blood of rabbits. (*From*: Dixon, *J. Cell. Comp. Physiol.*, **50**: 27, 1957.)

At the time that free antibody appears in the serum, antigens disappear from the tissues; both events are referable of course to the animal species receiving the antigen. Comparing the elimination of the bacterial antigen, *Salmonella typhimurium* from mice and rats, we find characteristic differences. With low challenge doses, most of the recovered organisms are equally distributed between the liver and spleen, although the peritoneal cavity yields some organisms; however, none are recoverable from the blood (Fig. 12-3). The blood of mice shows a low number of organisms up to

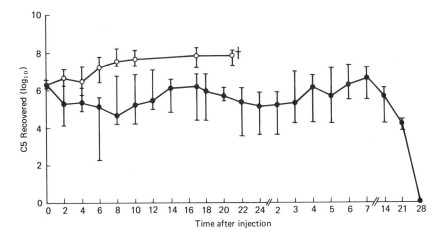

Fig. 12-3 Log_{10} average recovery from blood, peritoneum, liver and spleen of live *Salmonella typhimurium* C5 injected intraperitoneally; 1.1×10^7 C5 into rats (●———●), 2.0×10^7 C5 into mice (○———○). The vertical bars represent the range of variation obtained. (*From*: Ielasi & Kotlarski, AJEBAK, **47**: 689, 1969.)

day 5, which then declines to approximately 10 % of the total organisms. With a higher challenge dose the distribution is essentially similar; however, rats show a low level of persisting bacteremia, whereas mice show a higher level of bacteremia, which increases rapidly until death (Fig. 12-4).

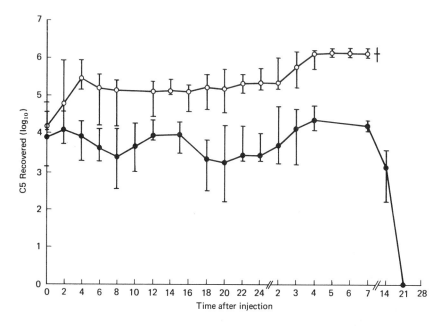

Fig. 12-4 Log_{10} average recovery from blood, peritoneum, liver and spleen of live *Salmonella typhimurium* C5 injected intraperitoneally; 6.6×10^4 C5 into rats (●———●), 6.7×10^4 C5 into mice (○———○). The vertical bars represent the range of variation obtained. (*From*: Ielasi & Kotlarski, AJEBAK, **47**: 689, 1969.)

Effects of Dose

Antigen elimination is different for a normal, unimmunized animal and one that has been immunologically suppressed. Tolerance to BSA is readily demonstrable in adult mice. Marchalonis (1971) extended this observation to adult toads and found that high doses of soluble BSA induce no antibody. In fact, the toads are specifically suppressed and are unable to form antibodies to BSA even when it is administered with adjuvant to provide maximal stimulation of the immune system. Their response to BSA is specific, since he observed no immune response to an unrelated antigen, human γG immunoglobulin. Now we can compare the kinetics of clearance of radioactively-labelled BSA antigen from normal controls and previously immunologically suppressed toads (Fig. 12-5). Suppressed toads, given high doses of labelled BSA, always exhibit nonimmune metabolic clearance or elimination when challenged with an immunogenic dose. By contrast, control nonsuppressed toads eliminate the antigen in a nonimmune metabolic fashion for approximately eight days and then switch to a rapid immune clearance of antigen due to the presence of antibody. Actually, at twenty-two days post-injection, control nonsuppressed toads possess no detectable I^{125}-labelled BSA and exhibit antibodies demonstrable at titers ranging from 64–256.

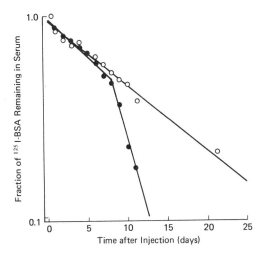

Fig. 12-5 Kinetics of elimination of ^{125}I-labelled bovine serum albumin (BSA) from the blood of immune (●———●) and tolerant (○———○) *B. marinus*. Animals were rendered tolerant by injection of 250 mg BSA in saline. Controls (immune) were given only diluent. Both groups were challenged with an immunogenic dose of soluble BSA containing a trace amount of the radioiodinated antigen. Seven animals were included in each group. The scale of the ordinate is logarithmic. (*From*: Machalonis, *Am. Zool.*, **11** : 171, 1971.)

Adult anuran amphibians
  Antigen Localization

The jugular bodies of anuran amphibians have been the subject of many studies involving antigen localization, particularly in the toad, *Bufo marinus*. Antigen localization is followed by proliferation of antibody-forming cells and then the appearance of antibody. Kent et al. (1964) were among the first to be concerned with the histologic changes in jugular bodies following administration of the antigen, BSA. By means of an immunofluorescent technique, they demonstrated the presence of antibody-forming cells in the jugular bodies after antigen localization. Using another antigen, I^{125} trace-labelled flagella from *Salmonella adelaide*, Diener and Nossal (1966) extended this earlier work. They found antigen localized in the jugular bodies and spleen (Figs. 12-6 to 12-8). Five days later, pyroninophilic cells began to proliferate in these same organs. Both the phagocytic antigen-trapping cells and the first pyroninophilic blasts are scattered randomly throughout the jugular bodies (Figs. 12-9 to 12-11). Like the jugular bodies of bullfrogs, as Cooper (1967) also noted, those of *Bufo* contain no clear-cut separation into cortex and medulla, nor are there any germinal centers.

The jugular body contrasts somewhat with the spleen; it is roughly divided into red and white pulp. Antigen is trapped in the red pulp of the spleen. However, although antigen concentrates around islands of white pulp one day after injection, it never appears *within* the white pulp. The kidney is probably the toad's major antigen-sequestering organ; it is likewise important as a site for antibody synthesis. After antigenic stimulation, both focal and diffuse collections of lymphoid and pyroninophilic cells are found in the kidney after antigenic stimulation. According to Diener and Nossal (1966), the absence of immunologic memory in the toad may be due to the absence of an efficient antigen-trapping net and pronounced germinal

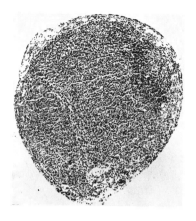

Fig. 12-6 Jugular body of *Bufo marinus*; note the absence of circular sinus, germinal centers and differentiation into cortex and medulla. (Toluidine Blue × 33.)

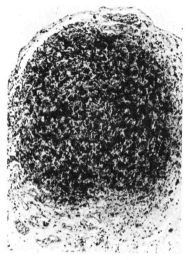

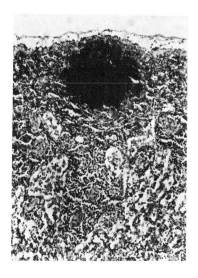

Figs. 12-7–12-8 Comparison in antigen localization pattern between toad jugular body and rat lymph node, 1 day after injection of [125I] flagella. Autoradiographs exposed 60 days. (12-7) Toad jugular body. Note wide, random scattering of label. (12-8) Rat lymph node. Note characteristic follicular localization. (Methyl green-pyronin. ×58.) (*From*: Diener & Nossal, *Immunol.*, **10**: 535, 1966.)

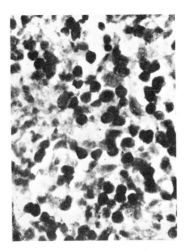

Fig. 12-9 Autoradiographs of section of jugular body 7 days after injection of [^{125}I] flagella. Pyroninophilic cells are scattered at random. (Methyl green pyronin. ×*290.*)

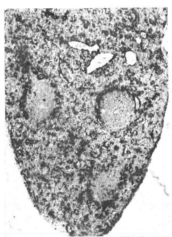

Fig. 12-10 Autoradiograph of spleen of *Bufo marinus* 24 hours after injection of [^{125}I] flagella. Note label scattered throughout red pulp and selective accumulation around the borders of the white pulp islands. (Methyl green-pyronin. ×*27.*)

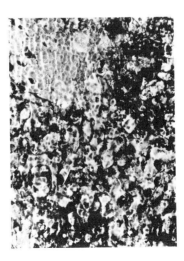

Fig. 12-11 Toad spleen section 24 hours after injection of colloidal carbon. The white pulp (*top left corner*) is relatively spared. The red pulp shows carbon-retaining cell bodies and cytoplasmic processes. (Toluidine blue. ×*53.*) (*From*: Diener & Nossal, *Immunol.,* **10**: 535, 1966.)

centers in lymphoid nodules. Yet, absence of this precise arrangement into follicles does not preclude a primary immune response *in vivo* as, for example, in *Xenopus*, a supposedly more primitive amphibian.

Mammalian Macrophages

Understanding the role of macrophages in the induction of an immune response depends upon understanding how they react with either soluble or particulate antigens. This period constitutes a portion of the initial response to an antigen. Macrophages can interiorize a variety of soluble and particulate molecules, which, once within the phagocyte, may fuse with primary and secondary lysosomes, thereby initiating the process of intracellular digestion. A well-defined purified enzyme used as antigen reacts in the following way with mouse macrophages: when mouse macrophages are exposed as monolayers to horseradish peroxidase (HRP), the level of cell-bound HRP diminishes exponentially with a half-life of seven to nine hours, regardless of the amount of enzyme initially interiorized (Fig. 12-12). At twenty-four to thirty hours HRP is detectable within membrane-bound granules where degradation by lysosomal hydrolases occurs. Eventually there is no detectable enzymatic activity (at 68 hours).

There is some indication that macrophage lysosomes are incapable of distinguishing between two different antigens for internal sequestration. Normal mouse macrophages that have ingested I^{125}-labelled human serum albumin and unlabelled ferritin

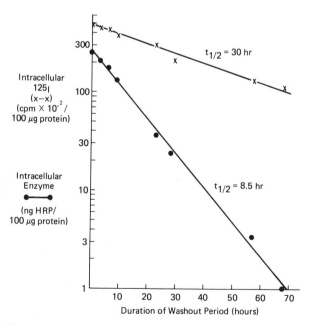

Fig. 12-12   The fate of HRP pinocytosed by macrophages 2 × 10⁶ cells were exposed to 1 mg/ml HRP-¹²⁵I (0.1 mCi/mg) for 2 hours. The cultures were washed eight times at room temperature and received an additional wash of 30 min at 37°C to remove all dish-bound enzyme. Fresh 20% NBCS-medium 199 was added and both intracellular enzymatic activity (●——●) and radioisotope (x——x) assayed over the next 68 hours. Each point is the mean of duplicate cultures. (*From*: Steinman & Cohn, *J. Cell. Biol.*, **55**: 186, 1972.)

can be shown by electron microscopic autoradiography to situate both antigens within the same lysosomes. Regardless of their inability to distinguish between antigens, Ada et al. (1967) showed that during the primary response, thirty minutes after antigen injection, littoral macrophages near the medullary sinus of lymph nodes show antigen at various stages of ingestion (Fig. 12-13). During the secondary response, thirty minutes after injection, antigen is found around the paranuclear region of medullary macrophages (Fig. 12-14). These observations stress the importance of macrophages in capturing antigen during the immune response.

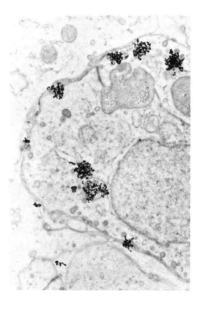

Fig. 12-13 Primary response, 30 min after injection. Part of a littoral macrophage near the medullary sinus showing antigen at various stages of ingestion. Arrow indicates clump of label not apparently associated with either vacuole or dense body. Bundle of collagen fibrils can be seen encloistered by cell cytoplasm; the scaling membranes display a tight junction of "intermediate" type where they run in apposition. (Magnification ×10,000.)

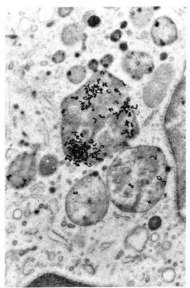

Fig. 12-14 Secondary response, 30 min after injection. Paranuclear region of medullary macrophage; the fusing of dense bodies can be seen (arrow). (Magnification ×14,260.) (From: Ada et al., Cold Spring Harbor Symposia on Quantitative Biology, XXXII, 1967.)

ANTIBODY FORMATION

General Characteristics of the Latent/Induction Period

We have now followed an antigen from its injection into an experimental animal, where it is eliminated and triggers the differentiation of lymphocytes and plasma cells prior to antibody synthesis. Antigen is first eliminated from the system by phagocytosis and normal metabolic catabolism, mediated by appropriate enzymes. The first effects of antigen elimination are detectable in the serum and next in macrophages of various tissues and organs such as the liver, lymph nodes, and spleen. Each of these organs is equipped morphologically for antigen trapping, because of the substantial development of its phagocytic RES system. Approximately one week after the disappearance of antigen, antibody appears in the serum, followed by a second burst of antigen elimination.

After the first injection of antigen, there is a lag of several days prior to the appearance of detectable amounts of antibody in the serum. This is the *latent* or *induction* period. Certainly the length of the latent period is very much affected by the kind, dosage, and route of antigen administration, as well as the age, species, and general physical condition of the host. The latent period occurs prior to the appearance of antibody in the serum. However, it reflects nothing of what happens at the cellular level, when antibody synthesis is demonstrable within one hour after antigen administration. Often the first antibody appears in the blood prior to the complete elimination of antigen from the circulation. If this happens and antigen and antibody combine, such antigen-antibody complexes are then rapidly excreted, prior to the appearance of easily measurable free antibody some days later. Presumably this rapid elimination of antigen-antibody complexes is due to their preferential attachment to phagocytic cells.

The Primary Response

Catabolic elimination of antigen must precede immune elimination. Immune elimination is of course the result of the combination of antigen with antibody. The latent phase is that period when there is no identifiable antibody in the serum, but antibody secreted by single cells can easily be detected. As the latent period ends, the primary antibody response is now demonstrable throughout the entire animal. Antibody gradually increases during the next few days, but it does not reach a high level. It persists for a few weeks at the most; it plateaus and then begins to drop. The general shape of the primary response curve is the typical sigmoid curve with an extended decay period.

The Secondary or Memory Response
Introduction

If a second dose of antigen is given, any remaining antibody is rapidly removed by combination with the antigen; this results in a fall in the detectable antibody in the blood (Fig. 12-15). Almost immediately thereafter, within one to three days, there

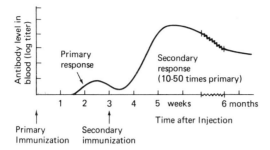

Fig. 12-15 The antibody response. (*From*: Weir, 1971, *Immunology for Undergraduates.*)

is a spectacular rise in the level of antibody, which reaches a peak. Actually, this antibody far surpasses that of the primary response and can be ten to fifty times higher than the primary response. This accelerated response to antigen during the secondary response is the *memory response* or the *anamnestic response*. In other words, the host's immune system "remembers" that it has been confronted with antigen previously and it remains primed for a second encounter. All the conditions that govern the primary response also pertain to the secondary response, except that the latent period is greatly abbreviated, the titer is heightened significantly, and the amount of antibody that is detectable is much extended when compared to the primary response.

Specific Characteristics

Because the anamnestic response is crucial to the very essence of the adaptive immune response, this phase of vertebrate immunity merits further discussion. One can induce memory at any time after the primary response. In fact, even after several years, when the primary response titer has dropped to zero, the anamnestic response can still be induced. However, after a considerably longer time, such a secondary response will not be as spectacular as one induced by an earlier secondary challenge, where the interval between the primary response and the second injection of antigen is shorter. There is, however, a physiologic limit to the number of times the memory response can be elicited; the animal usually reaches its limit after some three to five booster injections that are spaced rather closely. It should be obvious now that this remarkable capacity for memory is advantageous for certain natural infections, and of course it is demonstrable under controlled laboratory conditions. That certain antigens may be closely related can exert a profound effect on the outcome of a secondary response. The more closely related are the antigens, the greater likelihood there is of inducing a secondary response to a second antigen that is not precisely the same as the first antigen that induced the primary response.

There are certain generalities regarding the antibody that is produced during both responses. The antibody of the primary response is rich in IgM (immunoglobulin M), which has a half-life of only eight to ten days. The secondary response contains more IgG that has a half-life of twenty-five to thirty-five days. The contributions of

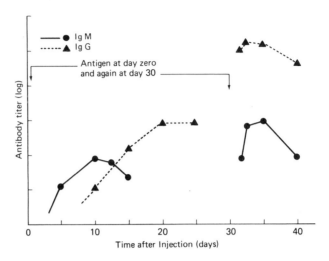

Fig. 12-16 The primary and secondary immune response of IgG and IgM. The IgG response is delayed after the primary injection but comes to be the dominant immunoglobulin after a few days and especially after the anamnestic response. The IgM primary response precedes the IgG response but the anamnestic response is very feeble. (*From*: Barrett, 1970, *Textbook of Immunology*.)

both IgM and IgG are illustrated in Fig. 12-16. Here it is obvious that a secondary IgM response is only one-tenth that of IgG. Although IgG is referred to as the memory component, IgM is also synthesized during a secondary response. In fact, secondary IgM is somewhat higher than that of the primary response. There is one possible danger in uncontrolled secondary administration of antigen, particularly concerning soluble antigens. Following primary antigen administration, some of the antibody that is formed is capable of fixing to tissue cells. Such cell-bound antibody may be anaphylactic antibody, mast cell degranulating antibody, cytotoxic antibody, or homocytotropic antibody. These can be attached to the injected antigen while still attached to the tissue cells. In certain cases, this *in vivo* cell-bound antigen-antibody reaction can trigger a set of reactions that may actually be lethal to the animal. Such a response is often referred to as *anaphylactic shock* and is often fatal; it can be easily demonstrated experimentally in the guinea pig, but it can occur in humans too; therefore, this kind of immune response is of much clinical interest.

Changes in Amphibian Lymphoid Organs After Immunization
Rana

Antigen elimination and localization in cells and organs precedes or probably even occurs simultaneously with the differentiation of lymphocytes and plasma cells. Haptens play a role in provoking the lymphocyte differentiation, whereas particulate antigens such as SRBC induce changes in responding tissues. This can be seen in bullfrog tadpoles after SRBC immunization (Figs. 12-17, 12-18), where the number of mitotic figures and plasma cells even in the thymus increase, and mitotic figures are obvious in the lymph gland (Fig. 12-19). Blast cells apparently increase in number and are usually located in pairs (Fig. 12-20), an arrangement suggesting cell division

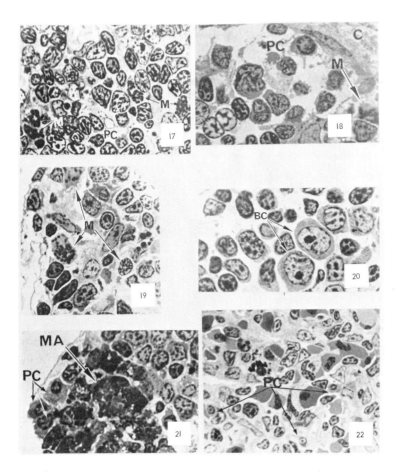

Figs. 12-17–12-22   (*From*: Moticka, et al. *J. Immunol.* **110**: 855, 1973.)

(Fig. 12-21). Some plasma cells have highly vacuolated cytoplasm, a possible processing artifact, and are mobile; they regularly pass through vascular channels by diapedesis and end up within sinusoids (Fig. 12-22).

The spleen's appearance is different: The number of blast cells within the parenchyma does not increase; thus mitoses are rare. The frequency of mitotic figures is, in fact, less than it is in the lymph gland. However, as Fig. 12-22 illustrates, plasma cells are more prominent after antigen stimulation. This first observation of antibody synthesis by the thymus is important, since the thymus is usually believed to be a depository of *T* cells that mediate cell immunity in mammals, without any importance attributable to antibody.

Xenopus Laevis

As Manning and Turner (1972) demonstrated, adult *Xenopus* can be immunized with human gamma globulin (HGG) antigens that can be easily emulsified in an equal volume of complete (CFA) and incomplete Freund's adjuvant. Strong precipitating antibody develops and is measurable thereafter for several months. During antibody synthesis the white pulp of the spleen is occupied by numerous large pyroninophilic cells. Injections of both antigen and CFA always lead to greater pyroninophilia and a peculiar vacuolation phenomenon that does not occur after injections of only CFA. Turner (1969) found vacuoles in the white and red pulp of the spleen that appear to phagocytose colloidal carbon for as long as one year after immunization. These vacuoles are not peculiar to *Xenopus* or to immunization with soluble antigens; Moticka et al. (1973) saw vacuoles beginning at eight weeks in *Rana catesbeiana* after immunization with SRBC. Intracellular melanin accompained by vacuolation appears in association with the phagocytes of larval bullfrog spleens. The weight of the toad's spleen increases considerably after immunization with HGG in adjuvant before and during serum antibody production. Cell proliferation and differentiation of pyroninophilic cells occurs in the splenic white pulp, but to a lesser extent in the red pulp, suggesting differential sensitivities of splenic cells to antigens. For example, spleens from toads immunized with SRBC exhibit greater cell proliferation in the white pulp, especially toward the periphery of the follicles, than spleens from toads immunized with HGG.

The spleen may not be vital to antibody synthesis, since good responses occur after splenectomy. In fact, antibody activity may not result from splenic regeneration, since splenectomy can be complete in most situations. Cells in other sites contribute to antibody synthesis. Kidney lymphoid cells increase after HGG injection in adjuvant, but not after SRBC injections. After booster injections good antibody production is stimulated, but splenic histology changes little. For example, large pyroninophilic cells characteristic of the primary response do not reappear. In the white pulp, follicles are compact and often exhibit central melanin deposits. In the liver there is no evidence of lymphocyte responses or pyroninophilia following antigenic stimulation. Essentially there are no pyroninophilic cells or vacuolation in the gut or in the kidney. In *Xenopus* the important effect of adjuvant seems more marked. According to Manning and Turner,

> it may be that [this species] is at an evolutionary stage where it is well equipped for efficient antibody production against . . . antigens, [such as bacteria], which occur in particulate form, . . . but when dealing with circulating soluble materials, its somewhat primitive antigen-trapping mechanisms may perhaps be a major limitation.

Further analysis of toad spleen cells by light and electron microscopy reveals a basic similarity of toad small lymphocytes and large pyroninophilic cells to those of mammals. Plasma cells are notably absent in both control and immunized toads, suggesting that proliferation alone occurs in the spleen and that later, migration, differentiation, and antibody secretion can be measured in other sites. There is controversy on the question of memory and its correlation with lymphoid organ structure. Anamnestic responses have been demonstrated in amphibians lacking germinal centers, (e.g., in *Bufo* by Lin et al. 1971, and Manning and Turner 1972). Thus, apparent morphologic features are not always common to, or essential for, an anamnestic response. Clustering of large numbers of lymphocytes capable of making contact with antigen seems to be the prime requisite for antibody synthesis.

THE INFLUENCE OF ENVIRONMENTAL TEMPERATURE
ON ANTIBODY PRODUCTION

Introduction

In order to compare the effects of temperature on the synthesis of antibodies, it
is necessary to utilize a poikilothermic vertebrate (fish, amphibian, or reptile) or a
hibernating mammal. Although mammals are homiotherms, with more or less
constant temperatures that are regulated internally, the hibernating mammal
approaches the condition of the poikilotherms; yet little is known about this aspect
of mammalian physiology. Some believe that as long as mammals are in hibernation,
even after immunization, antibodies are not formed. Such a contention is based on
an analysis of the primary response to only a few antigens using relatively insensitive
methods for detecting antibodies. In fact, there is not much known about the state
of the immune machinery, with the possible exception of phagocytosis, during hibernation. We can now compare what happens in poikilothermic vertebrates, where
temperature can be controlled, with the hibernating mammal. There is no information
on antibody synthesis in any bird species in a state of torpor.

Adult Teleost Fishes

Fish have been exceedingly important to the analysis of the temperature-regulating
events during antibody synthesis. In fact the first accounts related to more recent
efforts in comparative immunology were devoted to studies of temperature and
antibody synthesis (Cushing 1942, Bisset 1948, Hildemann and Cooper 1963). Recently, two investigators (Avtalion 1969, and Trump and Hildemann 1970) have
consistently used bovine serum albumin (BSA) as antigen. Avtalion's first experiments were designed to test the hypothesis that production of antibodies at low
temperature is possible if the fish have previously been in natural contact with antigens
or exposed experimentally to these antigens at high ambient temperatures. To this
end fish were initially immunized by injections into the caudal muscle of BSA in an
emulsion of Freund's complete adjuvant. The fish were grouped in the following
way. One group was kept continually at 25°C; a second group at 12°C; the third and
fourth groups at 25°C when injected with antigen and then transferred to 12°C. The
third group was transferred at the eighth day after immunization and before appearance of detectable antibodies, and the fourth group was transferred at the fifteenth
day, when antibody synthesis had already begun. At 254 days, three fish from the
first group showed no antibodies to BSA and were then given a secondary injection
with 5mg BSA in complete Freund's adjuvant.

Antibody synthesis during the secondary response began immediately after the
injection and the maximal antibody titer was higher than in the primary response
(Fig. 12-23). The second group, kept continually at 12°C, served as controls. In this
group, no antibodies to BSA were detected. The third group, kept at 25°C for eight
days and then at 12°C, showed a rising antibody titer at this relatively low temperature.
An interesting result was obtained after the 104th day in three fish that survived.
After a secondary immunization there was, instead of an increase, a decrease in

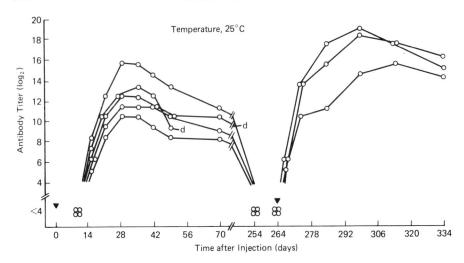

Fig. 12-23 Primary and secondary responses to bovine serum albumin in carp continually kept at 25°. d, Dead; ▼, antigenic stimulation; ○, antibody titer of individual carp as detected by the passive hemagglutination method. (*From*: Avtalion, *Immunol.* **17**: 927, 1969)

antibody titer, which Avtalion attributes to the formation *in vivo* of antigen-antibody complexes. Later there was a typical anamnestic response characterized by rising antibody titers (Fig. 12-24, Avtalion 1969). The last group, kept at 25°C for fifteen days and then placed at 12°C after the first appearance of circulating antibodies, showed a rising titer of antibody despite the low temperature (Fig. 12-25). Thus, antibody production can occur at a low ambient temperature in fish that have been previously exposed to antigens at a higher temperature. The implications of this work are twofold: fish are able under certain conditions to respond immunologically at low temperature, and fish possess immunological memory.

Trump's adult goldfish, *Carassius auratus*, were immunized with BSA by intracardiac, intraperitoneal, and intramuscular routes. Bleedings were performed at

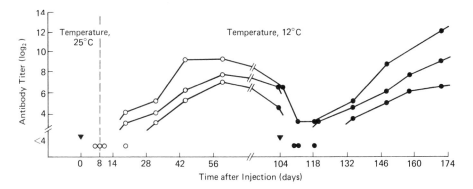

Fig. 12-24 Carp kept at 25° for 8 days and then transferred, before appearance of first circulating antibodies, to 12°. ▼, Antigenic stimulation; ○, antibody titer of pooled sera of four fish as detected by the passive hemagglutination method; ●, antibody titer of the individual surviving carp. (*From*: Avtalion, *Immunol.* **17**: 927, 1969.)

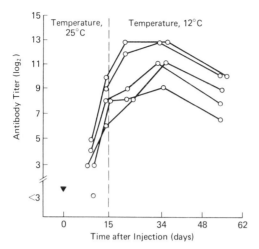

Fig. 12-25 Carp transferred from 25° to 12° after beginning of antibody synthesis. ▼, Antigenic stimulation; ○, antibody titer of individual carp as detected by hemagglutination method. (*From*: Avtalion, *Immunol.* **17**: 927, 1969.)

three-to-four-day intervals until peak antibody was noted. For the primary response, no antibody was detected before the seventeenth day after cardiac immunization in fish maintained at 20°C (Fig. 12-26); by the thirty-eighth day, 80% of the fish had responded, and a mean peak titer of 5 was reached at fifty days. All fish produced anti-BSA by day 10 at 25°C, but no antibody was detected at seven days. By twenty days, in most animals there were peak titers that persisted as long as 245 days after immunization (Fig. 12-27). At 30°C, the anti-BSA response was extremely different in many respects. Although the induction or latent period was apparently seven days, peak titers were reached by thirteen days. It was interesting that the mean highest titer was only 3, and antibody production was sustained for a significantly shorter time period at 30°C than at other temperatures.

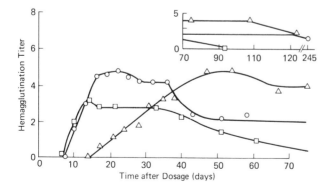

Fig. 12-26 The mean anti-BSA primary response at 20° (△), 25° (○), and 30° (□). The responses of goldfish maintained at three different temperatures to weight-adjusted doses of BSA are indicated as hemagglutination titers. The different groups of fish are indicated by the temperature of their environment. (*From*: Trump & Hildemann, *Immunol.* **19**: 927, 1970.)

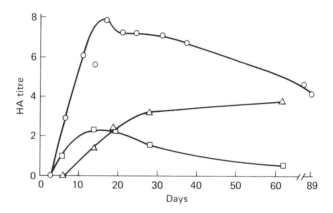

Fig. 12-27 The mean anti-BSA secondary responses at 20° (△), 25° (○), 30°(□). The responses of goldfish maintained at three different temperatures to a secondary dose of BSA are indicated as Hemagglutination titres. The different groups of fish are indicated by the temperature of their environment. (*From:* Trump & Hildemann, *Immunology,* **19**: 621, 1970).

For the secondary response, the mean induction period at 20°C following secondary stimulation occupies seven days. Most peak titers were reached by thirty days, but the rate of secondary antibody production at this temperature was still notably slower than the rates of primary responses at higher temperatures. The titers never exceeded those of the primary response at this temperature, but contrary to the findings of the primary response, antibody production remained stable up to sixty days after secondary stimulation. At 25°C, accelerated production of anti-BSA began three days post secondary immunization. The rate was one-and-a-half times faster than it was during the primary response. Peak titers at this temperature exceeded primary responses at any temperature. Antibody production began to decline at approximately twenty days after its peak, although antibody remained detectable for more than ninety days.

The secondary response at 30°C, the highest temperature, was interesting because it was so feeble in comparison to titers at other temperatures. Despite the half-time necessary to induce secondary responses, the rate and magnitude of antibody production was less than it was during the primary response at this temperature. Actually, by extrapolation, there probably would not have been antibody at seventy-five days. According to Trump and Hildemann the magnitude of goldfish anti-BSA responses after secondary immunization decreases at temperatures of 25°, 20°, and 30°C. This may reflect the number of memory cells available for stimulation. At all the temperatures, the induction or latent period of the secondary responses was shorter than during the primary response. In the 30° group only the rates of antibody appearance increase following secondary immunization. Thus, peak titers are reached in a comparatively shorter time.

Low temperatures do depress the immune responses of poikilothermic vertebrates. However, there can be a rise in antibody titer, as revealed by Avtalion's carp, which were kept at low temperature after short initial period at a high temperature, following the first antigenic challenge. This occurs regardless of whether the fish are removed to low temperature before or after the first appearance of circulating antibodies. Similarly, it also occurs if carp are immunized against bacteria and held at 20°–23°C for seven weeks after first immunization. They continue to produce rising titers of specific antibodies even after a transfer to 10°C.

Adult Anuran Amphibians

Fully developed anuran amphibians have been excellent sources of information on antibody formation. Except for minimal work on urodeles (and nothing on the apodans), anurans have formed the core for understanding antibody synthesis in amphibians. Their antibodies have specific molecular characteristics of extreme importance to the evolution of antibody synthesis in terrestrial vertebrates.

Toads kept at room temperature or even higher produce varying antibodies to injections of particulate antigens (Elek et al. 1962). Beginning at nine days, agglutinins appear in the blood stream, peak at thirty-six days, and then decline. However, similar immunization schedules using particulate antigens at 8°C result in a lack of circulating antibody synthesis. If toads are immunized in the cold and brought to 27°C for sixty hours, they will produce circulating antibody between the forty-fifth and seventy-ninth day post-immunization. Raising the temperature before or after this period is not effective. Agglutinins, thus, seem to be formed by the toad at two stages: antibody production itself is slightly affected by lowering the temperature to 8°C but the release of antibody into the circulation is affected by higher temperatures.

In the frog *Rana temporaria*, Alcock (1965) found specific agglutinating antibody synthesized to phenolized *Brucella abortus*, *Salmonella pullorum*, or live cultures of *Azotobacter agilis* at 19°C. Similarly, those receiving *Azotobacter agilis* cultures produce precipitating antibody against the polysaccharide coat of these bacteria. Frogs injected with either plain or alum-precipitated bovine serum albumin (BSA) produced no specific antibody. Another antigen, killed *Brucella abortus*, is ineffective if injected as suspensions into frogs kept at 10°C. Antibodies of two distinct molecular sizes are produced against *Brucella abortus*. *Salmonella pullorum* induces frog antibodies of diverse molecular sizes throughout the immune response. The heavy, macromolecular antibodies appear first and are followed by the appearance of antibodies of lighter molecular weight. Other serum protein components also increase during antibody production.

Lin and Rowlands (1973) recently studied thermal regulation of the immune response in toads after single injections of bacteriophage f2. Toads kept at 15°C had a markedly inhibited immune response as compared to controls kept at 25°C. The appearance of serum antibodies was delayed in toads at 15°C during the first post-immunization week, but their peak antibody levels were similar to those in toads maintained at 25°C throughout. In another experiment, transfer of toads from 25°C to 15°C at two weeks after immunization only temporarily depressed serum antibody levels, but causes a marked delay in conversion from heavy to light antibodies.

Adult Reptiles

After studying antibody synthesis in the California desert lizard, *Dipsosaurus dorsalis*, Evans (1963) concluded that the response is regulated by varying the ambient temperature. Using a typhoid vaccine as antigen, he found that the antibody response was poor or nonexistent at 25°C, good at 35°C and moderately good at 40°C. This is approximately 10° warmer than similar conditions in carp. If lizards are immunized at 35°C and transferred to 25°C, the antibody response is inhibited; in the reverse situation, the response is enhanced. Actually, an analysis of the cellular events would be profitable, since we can view those cells involved in antibody synthesis prior to their release of antibodies into the serum.

Wetherall and Turner (1972) used the lizard *Tiliqua rugosa*, a member of the reptilian family Scincidae, which probably originated during the Triassic period from

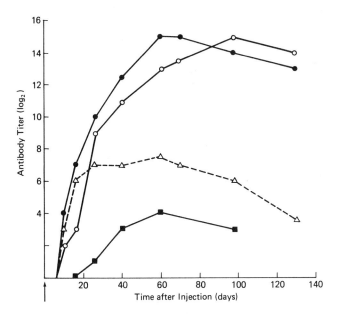

Fig. 12-28 Kinetics of antibody production by lizards immunized i.p. with 30 mg BSA and maintained at different temperatures.

●———● Response of 10 lizards maintained at 30° to BSA plus CFA.
○———○ Response of 5 lizards maintained at 25° to BSA plus CFA.
△-----△ Response of 7 lizards maintained at 30° to BSA without CFA.
■———■ Response of 5 lizards maintained at 20° to BSA plus CFA.

Each point on the curves represents the arithmetic mean of the $\log_2$ titers of the lizards within that group. (*From*: Wetherall & Turner, AJEBAK, **50**: 79, 1972.)

a group of extinct forms, the Eosuchia. These gave rise earlier to the Rhynchocephalia, of which the tuatara is the sole surviving member. *Tiliqua* is a diapsid reptile bearing live young, and it occurs in certain dry, sandy locations throughout Australia, where it is known as the sleepy, or bobtailed, lizard. For studies of antibody synthesis the lizards were immunized and maintained at 20°, 25°, and 30°C (Fig. 12-28). Maximum titers attained at 30°C and 25°C were identical and were reached at seventy-seven and ninety-eight days respectively, but at 20°C, the maximum titer was obtained at sixty days and was much slower than at 30° and 25°C. After immunizing lizards with BSA and maintaining them at 30°C for twenty to twenty-five days, when the rate of antibody production was maximal, if they were moved to 20°C antibody levels peaked, remained steady for two to three weeks and then slowly decreased. As shown in Fig. 12-29 similar results are obtained with lizards immunized with *Salmonella typhimurium* at 30°C and 20°C.

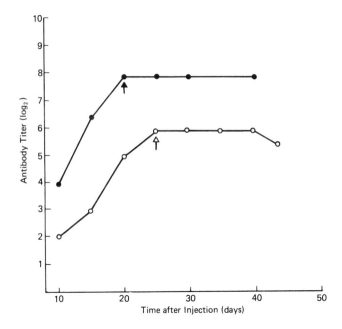

Fig. 12-29 The effect of a decrease in environmental temperature on antibody production in the lizard. The environmental temperature of the lizards was decreased from 30° to 20° at the times indicated by the arrows.

●———● Lizard response to BSA + CFA.
○———○ Lizard response to *S. Typhimurium* + CFA.

(*From*: Wetherall & Turner, AJEBAK, **50**: 79, 1972.)

Mammals—The Hibernating Ground Squirrel

McKenna and Musacchia (1968) studied antibody synthesis in the ground squirrel, *Citellus tridecemlineatus*. Their work is particularly interesting and merits a detailed coverage of their techniques, since the squirrel's antibody response was studied during hibernation. The hibernaculum temperature was 5–7°C; nonhibernating control squirrels were kept at 22°C ± 1°C during the winter months. The antigen was influenza A virus vaccine (strain PR$_8$), an antigen known to be effective even in bullfrog larvae. To study the primary response, ground squirrels previously in hibernation for at least two to four days were each given a single intraperitoneal injection of 1 ml of vaccine diluted with 0.85% NaCl to contain 5×10^3 chick-cell agglutinating (CCA) units, an indicator of the virus's potency. The animals were not awakened during the immunization. For secondary responses, they were given 5×10^2 CCA intraperitoneally one month after the initial injection and sacrificed five days later.

After primary immunization, hibernating ground squirrels can produce circulating antibody; in fact, even a secondary response may be obtained. Hibernating squirrels show a greater range in titers than controls. The time courses of both primary and secondary responses in all squirrels are shown in Fig. 12-30. Active animals show responses to primary and secondary antigen stimulation typical of most mammals.

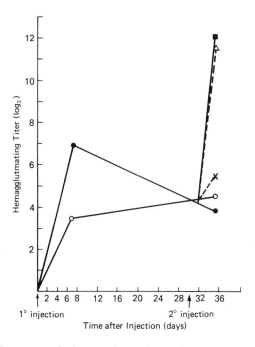

Fig. 12-30 Time course of primary and secondary antibody responses in all animals studied. Group 1. ●———● 1° active; 2. ■———■ 2° active; 3. ○———○ 1° hibernating; 4. x———x 2° hibernating; 5. △———△ 2 hibernating—then active. (*From:* McKenna & Musacchia, *Proc. Soc. Exp. Biol. Med.,* **129**: 120, 1968.)

By contrast, squirrels kept in hibernation for the full thirty-five days after primary stimulation show an increasing antibody titer from seven to thirty-five days. It is unknown whether the antibody formed by the hibernating squirrels is immunoglobulin *M* or *G*. These data are important to clarify some early conflicts in information on the capacity of hibernating animals to synthesize antibody. It is probably immune clearance, one of the earlist events of the latent period that can occur during hibernation. If the animals remain in hibernation the ability to synthesize antibody is lost, since the steps leading to antibody formation, i.e., induction, maturation, and proliferation, must be initiated. Actually the comparison here may be somewhat unwarranted, for none of the poikilotherms so far have been maintained at such low temperatures. Still this information on temperature regulation of antibody synthesis is important.

BIBLIOGRAPHY

Ada, G. L., Parish, C. R., Nossal, G. J. V., and Abbott, A. 1967. The tissue localization, immunogenic, and tolerance-inducing properties of antigens and antigen-fragments. Cold Spring Harbor Symposia on Quantitative Biology, V, **32**: 381–393. Cold Spring Harbar New York: The Cold Spring Harbor Laboratory of Quantitative Biology.

Alcock, D. M. 1965. Antibody production in the common frog, *Rana temporaria*. J. Pathol. and Bact. **40**: 31.

Avtalion, R. R. 1969. Temperature effect on antibody production and immunological memory, in carp (*Cyprinus carpio*) immunized against bovine serum albumin. Immunology **17**: 927.

Bissett, K. A. 1948. The effect of temperature upon antibody production in cold-blooded vertebrates. J. Path. Bact. **60**: 87.

Cooper, E. L. 1967. Lymphomyeloid organs in amphibia. I. Appearance during larval and adult stages of *Rana catesbeiana*. J. Morph. **122**: 381.

Cushing, J. E. 1942. An effect of temperature upon antibody production in fish. J. Immunol. **45**: 123.

Diener, E., and Nossal, G. J. V. 1966. Phylogenetic studies on the immune response. Localization of antigens and immune response in the toad, *Bufo marinus*. J. Immunol. **10**: 535.

Dixon, F. J. 1957. Characterization of the antibody response. J. Cell. Comp. Physiol. **50**: 27.

Elek, S. D., Rees, T. A., and Gowing, N. F. C. 1962. Studies on the immune response in a poikilothermic species, *Xenopus laevis daudin*. Comp. Biochem. Physiol. **7**: 255.

Evans, E. E. 1963. Comparative immunology. Antibody responses in *Dipsosaurus dorsalis* at different temperatures. Proc. Exp. Soc. Biol. Med. **112**: 531.

Hildemann, W. H., and Cooper, E. L. 1963. Immunogenesis of homograft reactions in fishes and amphibians. Fed. Proc. **22**: 1145.

Kent, S. P., Evans, E. E., and Attleberger, M. H. 1964. Comparative immunology. Lymph nodes in the amphibian, *Bufo marinus*. Proc. Soc. Exptl. Biol. Med. **116**: 456.

Lin, H. H., and Rowlands, D. T. Jr. 1973. Thermal regulation of the immune response in South American toads (*Bufo marinus*). Immunology **24**: 129.

Lin, H. H., Caywood, B. E., and Rowlands, D. T. 1971. Primary and secondary immune response of the marine toad (*Bufo marinus*) to bacteriophage f2. Immunol. **20**: 373.

Manning, M. J., and Turner, R. J. 1972. Some responses of the clawed toad, *Xenopus laevis*, to soluble antigens administered in adjuvant. Comp. Biochem. Physiol. **42**: 735.

Marchalonis, J. J. 1971. Immunoglobulins and antibody production in amphibians. Am. Zool. **11**: 171.

McKenna, J. M., and Musacchia, X. J. 1968. Antibody formation in hibernating ground squirrels (*Citellus tridecemlineatus*). Proc. Soc. Exptl. Biol. Med. **129**: 720.

Moticka, E. J., Brown, B. A., and Cooper, E. L. 1973. Immunoglobulin synthesis in bullfrog larvae. J. Immunol. **110**: 855.

Sigel, M. M., Acton, R. T., Evans, E. E., Russell, W. J., Wells, T. G., Pinter, B., and Lucas, A. H. 1968. T_2 bacteriophage clearance in the lemon shark. Proc. Soc. Exptl. Biol. Med. **128**: 977.

Trump, G. N., and Hildemann, W. H., 1970. Antibody responses of goldfish to bovine serum albumin: primary and secondary responses. Immunology **19**: 621.

Turner, R. J. 1969. The functional development of the reticuloendothelial system in the toad, *Xenopus laevis* (Daudin). J. Exp. Zool. **170**: 467.

Wetherall, J. D., and Turner, K. J. 1972. Immune response of the lizard, *Tiliqua rugosa*. Aust. J. Exp. Biol. Med. Sci. **50**: 79.

Chapter 13

The Immunoglobulins

INTRODUCTION

The most unique feature of vertebrate immunity is the ability to synthesize antibodies in response to antigenic stimulation. This uniqueness is particularly noteworthy from two points of view: whereas invertebrates occur in larger numbers than vertebrates that occupy the same environmental niches, the antibody-synthesizing capacity appears to be strictly limited to vertebrates. Secondly the exquisite specificity that governs each antibody produced in response to countless numbers of antigens is phenomenal.

Antibodies or immunoglobulins are a group of structually related proteins produced by plasma cells, secreted into the serum or tissue fluids, and characterized by certain physicochemical and biological properties. Most immunoglobulins are associated with the gamma globulin fraction of serum. They are called *gamma globulins*

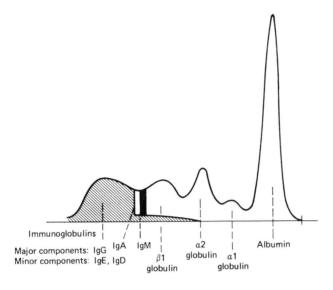

Fig. 13-1 Electropherogram obtained by UV scanning of paper electrophoresis strip and showing diagrammatically the main components of human serum and the immunoglobulin classes. (*From*: Weir, 1971, *Immunology for Undergraduates.*)

because they migrate more slowly toward the anode in an electric field at pH 8.6; this was different from the groups of faster proteins termed the *alpha* and *beta globulins* that migrated toward the cathode (Fig. 13-1).

Immunoglobulins of mammals can be divided into five major classes, usually called IgM, IgG, IgA, IgD, and IgE, which differ physicochemically and immunologically (Table 13-1). All vertebrates synthesize immunoglobulins resembling the IgM class. Concentrated studies of crossoptygerian fishes, ancestors of the urodele amphibians and a species more primitive than the anurans, suggest that IgG immunoglobulins probably first evolved in anuran amphibians. Those vertebrates considered more phylogenetically advanced than amphibians possess multiple classes of immunoglobulins that resemble IgM, IgG, and possibly other classes of antibodies of mammals. As in other fundamental aspects of immunity, the structural properties of mammalian immunoglobulin molecules serve as the convenient model for comparative studies. The information in this chapter has been derived from numerous sources, but summarized primarily from the recent and complete work of Marchalonis and Cone (1973).

METHODS OF CHARACTERIZING IMMUNOGLOBULINS

Antibodies from all vertebrate groups have been isolated and characterized by physicochemical methods. Since a detailed description of these methods is beyond the scope of this book, they will not be considered in detail. Instead, several examples will

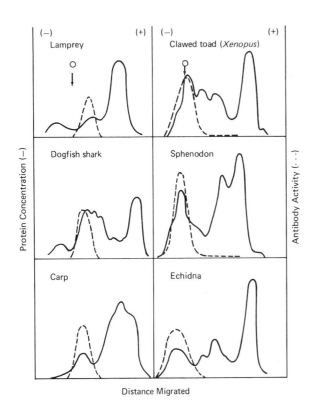

Fig. 13-2 Analysis of antisera from diverse vertebrate species by zone electrophoresis on starch. The species investigated are as follows: lamprey *Petromyzon marinus*, a cyclostome; dogfish shark, *Mustelus canis*, an elasmobranch; carp, *Cyprinus carpio*, a teleost fish; *Xenopus laevis*, an anuran amphibian; the tuatara, *Sphenodon punctatum*, a reptile, and the echidna, *Tachyglossus aculeatus*, a monotreme mammal. ○, indicates the position of the origin. ——, total protein. ——, antibody activity. (+) anode. (−) cathode. (*From*: Marchalonis & Cone, AJEBAK, **51**: 461, 1973.)

Table 13-1

Some properties of the immunoglobulin classes of man.

	γG	γA	γM	γD	γE
Serum concentration mg/100 ml	800-1,680	140-420	50-190	3-40	0·01-0·14
Molecular weight	150,000	150,000 to 400,000	950,000	180,000	190,000
Sedimentation co-efficient	6·7S	7S to 11S	18-20S	6·2-6·8S	8·2S
Cross the placenta?	Yes	No	No	No	No
Light chains	κ,λ	κ,λ	κ,λ	κ,λ	κ,λ
Heavy chains	γ	α	μ	δ	ϵ
Heavy chain Molecular weight	53,000	64,000 (52,000)	70,000	60,000-70,000	72,500
Sub-classes known	4	2	2	?	?
Molecular formula	$\gamma_2\kappa_2$ $\gamma_2\kappa_2$	$(\alpha_2\kappa_2)m$ $(\alpha_2\kappa_2)m$	$(\mu_2\kappa_2)_5$ $(\mu_2\lambda_2)_5$	$\delta_2\kappa_2$ $\delta_2\lambda_2$	$\epsilon_2\kappa_2$ $\epsilon_2\lambda_2$
Carbohydrate content (%)	2	6-10	9-12	12·7	11·7
Antibody activity?	Yes	Yes	Yes	Yes	Yes
Complement Fixation?	Yes	No	Yes	?	?

(*From*: Marchalonis & Cone, AJEBAK, 51 : 461. 1973.)

be presented to illustrate the type of information that can be derived and used for comparative studies.

Zone electrophoresis on starch separates proteins on the basis of their electric charges and molecular weights and allows antibody activity to be localized. Figure 13-2 summarizes and compares those characteristics of antibody activity from various vertebrates that are demonstrable by zone electrophoresis. Antibody activity is always localized in the more slowly migrating components, the γ and β globulins.

Fractionation by ultracentrifugation on linear sucrose gradients allows estimation of the molecular size of proteins (Fig. 13-3). For example, mammalian antibodies are resolvable into two major components on the basis of size. IgM molecules are characterized by a sedimentation coefficient of approximately 19S, and the IgG molecules have a coefficient of approximately 6.7S. When compared to the mammalian pattern, differences in the sedimentation patterns for antibody molecules from other vertebrate classes are quite evident. The dogfish shark, carp, and tuatara (*Sphenodon*) possess only 19S-type molecules, while the clawed toad has both 19S and 7S molecules. The lamprey is unique as the size distribution of it's antibody activity correlated with a

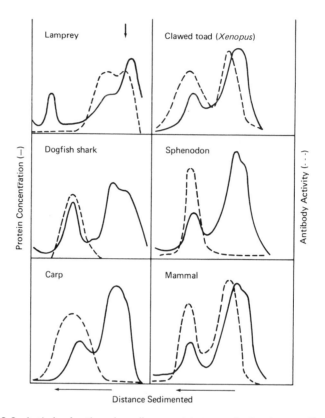

Fig. 13-3 Analysis of antisera from diverse vertebrate species by ultra-centrifugation on linear gradients of sucrose. Sedimentation proceeded from right to left. The species studied here are those listed in Fig. 14-3 except a typical mammalian pattern is given. ———, total protein. ----, antibody activity. (*From*: Marchalonis & Cone, AJEBAK, **51**: 461, 1973.)

diffuse area ranging from molecules that have sedimentation coefficients of approximately 7S to 16S.

Gel filtration in dissociating solvents separates the two types of polypeptide chains common to all immunoglobulins on the basis of size. This facilitates determination of properties such as molecular weight, amino acid composition, and primary sequence data. Table 13-2 shows that light and heavy chains are characteristic of all vertebrate immunoglobulins and that they possess a wide range of molecular weights.

STRUCTURE OF MAMMALIAN IgM AND IgG

The pioneer work of Porter (1967) is important in understanding the chemistry of immunoglobulins. He used the proteolytic enzyme papain and the reducing agent cysteine and succeeded in splitting the rabbit IgG molecule into three fragments. Two fragments contain an antigen-binding site and a third crystallizable fragment. These fragments were called *fragment antigen-binding* (*Fab*) and *fragment crystallizable* (*Fc*)

Table 13-2

Polypeptide chain structure of vertebrate immunoglobulins.

Animal	Immuno-globulin	Molecular weight	Carbohy-drate content	Light	Heavy	Molecular formula
Lamprey (a)	6·8S	(188,000)	ND	24,000	69,000	$L_2\mu_2$
	15 S	ND	ND			$(L_2\mu_2)_n$
Dogfish	7 S	198,000	7·6	20,500	73,400	$L_2\mu_2$
Shark (b)	17 S	982,000	8·7	20,100	71,600	$(L_2\mu_2)_5$
Carp (c,d)	13 S	720,000		24,000	71,400	$(L_2\mu_2)_4$
Lungfish (e)	19 S	(950,000)	?	23,100	70,300	$(L_2\mu_2)_5$
(Australian)	5·9 S	(122,000)	?	23,000	38,000	$L_2\nu_2$
Bullfrog (f)	18·0 S	(920,000)	10·8	20,000	72,100	$(L_2\mu_2)_5$
	6·7 S	(150,000)	2·1	22,000	53,600	$L_2\gamma_2$
Turtle (g)	18·8 S	900,000	ND	22,500	70,000	$(L_2\mu_2)_5$
	5·7 S	120,000	0·9	22,500	38,000	$L_2\nu_2$
Chicken (h)	15-16 S	890,000	2·6	22,000	70,000	$(L_2\mu_2)_5$
	7·1-7·4 S	170,000	2·2	22,000	67,000	L_2Y_2
Echidna (i)	19 S	950,000	6·4	22,500	69,000	$(L_2\mu_2)_5$
	7 S	150,000	1·5	22,500	49,000	$L_2\gamma_2$

(*From*: Marchalonis & Cone, AJEBAK, 51 : 461. 1973.)

respectively. The two noncrystallizable Fab fragments, with a molecular weight of 52,000, retained antibody activity. However, the Fc fragment, with a molecular weight of 48,000, was devoid of antibody activity and was crystallizable in the cold.

From Edelman's laboratory (1967) came equally important information on the structure of the IgG molecule. The molecule, treated with reducing agents in the presence of urea, is split into single peptide chains by reduction with thiol compounds. From this information we now know that the IgG molecule is composed of four polypeptide chains of two types. One type, a long chain, is referred to as the *heavy* (*H*) *chain* and a second, short chain, is called the *light chain* (*L*). Each Fab fragment is composed of one *L* chain and a portion of an *H* chain. The *Fc* fragment is composed of the remaining portions of two *H* chains. Each *L* chain contains 210–230 amino acids, and each *H* chain has 420–440 amino acids. The chains are paired in such a way that the molecule consists of two identical halves. Each half contains one *H* chain and one *L* chain. One disulfide bond links two symmetric *H* chains together, and another disulfide bond links each of the symmetric *L* chains to one of the *H* chains. Figure 13-4 is a widely accepted model of the IgG molecule, that details the physical relations of the molecule's polypeptide chains (Gally and Edelman 1972). (For earlier accounts see: Fougereau and Edelman 1965; Edelman and Gally 1969).

The presence of specific heavy chains (γ, μ, α, δ, and ϵ) defines the class of immunoglobulin. Two types of light chain have been defined (κ and λ), and each class of heavy chain may combine with either light chain. Figure 13-5 is a diagrammatic representation of human γG (a) and γM (b). γM immunoglobulin usually occurs as a polymer containing five units, each of which is, in general, similar to the basic γG

GENETIC CONTROL OF IMMUNOGLOBULIN SYNTHESIS

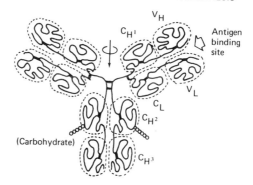

Fig. 13-4 A model of the structure of a human IgG molecule. The variable regions of heavy and light chains (VH and VL), the constant region of the light chain (Cl), and the homology regions in the constant region of heavy chain (CH1, CH2, and CH3) are thought to fold into compact domains (delineated by dotted lines), but the exact conformation of the polypeptide chains has not been determined. The vertical arrow represents the two-fold rotation axis through the two disulfide bonds linking the heavy chains. A single interchain disulfide bond links CL and CH, and a single intrachain disulfide bond is present in each domain. Carbohydrate prosthetic groups are attached to the CH2 regions. (*From*: Gally, J. A. & Edelman, G. M. *Ann. Rev. Genetics,* **6** : 1, 1972.)

molecule. The striped portions of the molecules represent variable (V) regions, a unique property of immunoglobulins characterized by marked heterogeneity in amino acid sequence in a normal individual. Furthermore, the V-regions represent approximately the first 110 residues from the terminal amino acids in both the heavy and light chains. One set of V-regions is apparently shared by all heavy chains but the κ and λ

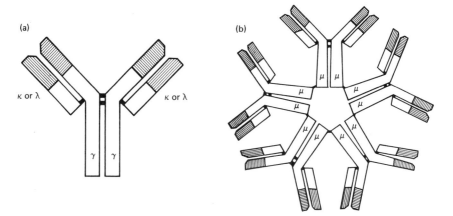

Fig. 13-5 Schematic representations of the structures of human γG and γM immunoglobulins. (a) Human γG immunoglobulin. (b) Human γM immunoglobulin. Striped portions of the molecules represent variable (V) regions; the constant (c) regions are unmarked. γ, γ heavy chain; μ, μ heavy chain; or light chains. (b) is reduced relative to (a). Disulfide bonds are represented by heavy bars. (*From*: Marchalonis & Cone, AJEBAK, **51** : 461, 1973.)

light chains each possess distinct sets of V-regions. Apparently the amino acid sequence observed in the V-region of any given antibody can be correlated with the binding specificity of that antibody.

IMMUNOGLOBULINS OF DIVERSE VERTEBRATES

Ostracoderm-Derived Vertebrates: the Agnathans

Hagfish and lampreys occupy a critical position in the phylogenetic development of immunity. They are considered to be the only surviving examples of the oldest vertebrate line. According to recent fossil evidence, these jawless vertebrates may even have a separate ancestry and may have evolved from two distinct groups of ostra-coderms or preostracoderm fishes (Bardack and Zangerl, 1968).

Fresh normal hagfish serum regularly contains saline agglutinins for sheep erythrocytes at a 1 : 4 or 1 : 8 titer. These agglutinins reside in the macroglobulin (IgM) fraction and are heat-labile inasmuch as the sera, after heating at 56°C for thirty minutes, loses all antibody activity. Specific agglutinins can be induced against sheep erythrocytes. Hagfish that received weight-adjusted dosages every fourteen days over a seventy-day period at 18°C show 2^3–2^5-fold rises in specific hemagglutination titers. In contrast to naturally occurring agglutinins, induced agglutinins are heat stable and display a high degree of specificity for the antigens of sheep erythrocytes. Like the natural agglutinin, the induced agglutinin has been shown to be, by means of chro-matographic and immunoelectrophoretic analyses, limited to a major macroglobulin fraction similar to, but distinguishable from, the IgM of higher vertebrates.

Hagfish produce antibody detectable by a variety of methods to keyhold limpet hemocyanin (KLH). When hagfish anti-KLH serum is fractionated and assayed for antibody activity, it shows an unusual profile on Sephadex G200 columns in compari-son to shark and rabbit serum fractionated on the same column (Fig. 13-6). Most of the antibody activity is concentrated in two fractions (IA and IB) from the first peak; very little antibody activity is associated with fraction II, which may reflect slight contamination from fraction I. Fraction II is free of antibody activity even from hyperimmune serum, but it does contain a protein closely resembling gamma globulin as revealed by immunoelectrophoresis. This protein is eluted first from DEAE-cellulose as the most positively charged protein (Figs. 13-7 and 13-8). It shows a distinct pink color like the third G200 fraction when highly concentrated. Naturally occurring sheep erythrocyte hemagglutinins are consistently located in the first G200 peak or, after ion-exchange fractionation, in the last two peaks. Ion-exchange chro-matography of the third Sephadex-G200 fraction results in a good separation of the main component, which has the mobility of a mammalian gamma globulin, although no antibody activity is associated with it (Fig. 13-9). When serum is analyzed by ultracentrifugation, two major, distinct components of $S_{20,w} = 9$ and 20, appear in addition to several minor ones. The macroglobulin fraction, in relatively pure form at a concentration of 4.7 mg/ml, shows a sedimentation coefficient $S_{20,w}$ of about 28 (Fig. 13-10).

Lampreys immunized with bacteriophage f_2 (Marchalonis and Edelman, 1968) produce specific 6.6S and 14S antibodies. Antigenic analysis of the 6.6S antibody shows it to be similar or identical to the 14S antibody. They consist of diffusely

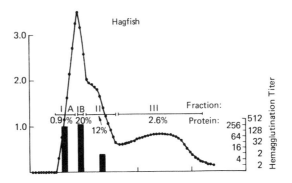

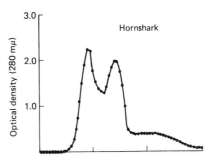

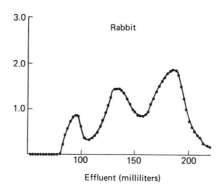

Fig. 13-6 Sephadex-G 200-gel filtration: Elution pattern of hagfish-anti-KJH serum in comparison to normal shark—and rabbit serum. Fractions I, II, III represent the major, reconcentrated peaks. The bars demonstrate the location of specific KLH antibody activity in the first two peaks. Note the protein concentration of the fractions. (*From*: Thoenes & Hildemann, 1970.) In *Developmental Aspects of Antibody Formation and Structure* (Prague: Publishing House Czechoslovakia Academy of Sciences)

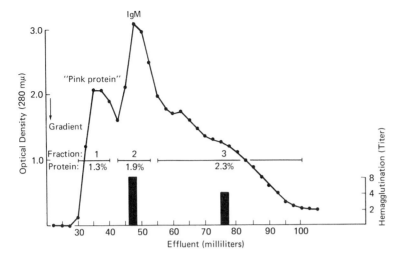

Fig. 13-7 DEAE-cellulose chromatography of normal hagfish serum and demonstration of naturally occurring hemagglutinins, mainly in fraction 2, also 3, but not in 1, where the "pink protein" is eluted. (*From*: Thoenes & Hildemann, 1970.) In *Developmental Aspects of Antibody Formation and Structure* (Prague: Publishing House Czechoslovakia Academy of Sciences)

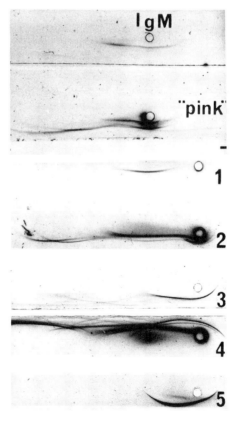

Fig. 13-8 Immunoelectrophoresis of the G 200-fractions I and III of Fig. 13-6 illustrating IgM and "pink protein." (*From*: Thoenes & Hildemann, 1970.) In *Developmental Aspects of Antibody Formation and Structure* (Prague: Publishing House Czechoslovakia Academy of Sciences)

Fig. 13-9 Immunoelectrophoresis of purified hagfish serum proteins. 1. G 200 fraction I, after DEAE-cellulose chromatography (IgM); 2. G 200 fraction II, after DEAE-cellulose chromatography (7S IgM?); 3. G 200 fraction III, after DEAE-cellulose chromatography ("pink protein"); 4. Hagfish-whole serum; 5. Purified mouse IgM as reference. The concentration of the fractions were about 10 mg hagfish serum was undiluted, and mouse IgM was 20 mg/ml. Rabbit-anti-hagfish serum undiluted. (*From*: Thoenes & Hildemann.) In *Developmental Aspects of Antibody Formation and Structure* (Prague: Publishing House Czechoslovakia Academy of Sciences)

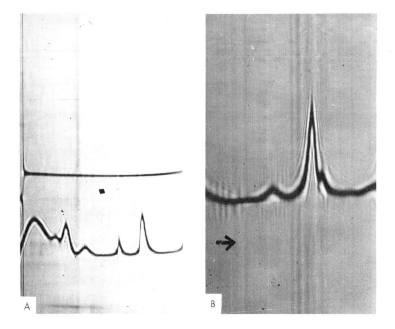

Fig. 13-10 Analytical ultracentrifugation. Schlieren patterns of hagfish serum proteins. (a) While serum, diluted with 1 2% NaCl (10 mg protein/ml). The two major, distinct peaks have S_{20},w-values of 9.2 and 20.6 respectively. 59,780 RPM, analyzer angle 75°. (b) Purified high-molecular protein (IgM), 5 mg/ml, solvent 0 14M Na(a. 0.01M sodium-phosphate, pH 7.0. S_{20},w is 28.0; 59,780 RPM, analyzer angle 49°. (*From*: Thoenes & Hildemann, 1970.) In *Developmental Aspects of Antibody Fomation and Structure* (Prague: Publishing House Czechoslovakia Academy of Sciences)

heterogeneous light and heavy chains that appear to be linked via noncovalent bonds rather than interchain disulfide bonds.

On the basis of this data, it appears that representatives of the oldest living vertebrates are capable of forming antibodies consisting of light chains and heavy chains comparable to the μ chain of mammalian γM macroglobulins. It is imperative however to have additional information, to determine the possible relationship between hagfish and lamprey immunoglobulins and the immunoglobulins of other vertebrates.

Cartilaginous Fish

Immunoglobulins from several species of sharks have been studied in considerable detail. Two types of immunoglobulins have been distinguished on the basis of size, a 17–19S and a 7S antibody. Structural studies on these molecules are summarized in Table 13-3. Characterization of isolated light and heavy chains suggest they are indistinguishable from each other except for size. Thus, they do not represent separate immunoglobulin classes but closely related proteins.

Sting rays (Marchalonis and Schonfeld, 1970) possess a major immunoglobulin component with a molecular weight of approximately 360,000 (11S). The molecule can be resolved into light and heavy chains similar to the light chains of other vertebrates and the μ heavy chains of the IgM immunoglobulin class.

Table 13-3

Structural characteristics of elasmobranch antibody.

Species	s rate	Molecular weight			Carbohydrate content (%)
		Intact protein	Heavy chain	Light chain	
Dogfish shark	17	982,000	71,600	20,100	8.7 (anthrone)
	7	198,000	73,400	20,500	7.6
Nurse shark	19		70,000	22,000	3.5 (orcinol)
	7				3.6
Lemon shark	19	800–900,000	71,000	22–23,000	3.7 (orcinol)
	7	160,000	71,000	22–23,000	3.5

(*From*: Grey, Adv. Immunol. **10**: 51, 1969.)

Bony Fish

The gar, *Lepisosteus platyrhincus* (Bradshaw et al., 1971), is a holostean fish whose immunoglobulin characteristics place it at a point where evolutionary lineages diverged leading to the more advanced fishes. When purified gar 14S immunoglobulin obtained by DEAE-cellulose chromatography is followed by Sephadex G-200 gel filtration, it has a molecular weight of $\sim 650,000$ and a relatively high hexose content. It is composed of disulfide-linked H (MW $\sim 70,000$) and L (MW $\sim 22,000$) polypeptide chains present in equimolar amounts. This 14S protein is a tetrameric form of IgM. Immunoelectrophoretic analysis of fractions from Sephadex G-200 with rabbit anti-gar H- and L-chain antisera show that this is the only class of immunoglobulin present in gar serum.

Data on the more advanced fishes, the teleosts, is fragmentary. Immunoglobulins of the giant grouper, *Epinephelus itaira* (Clem, 1971), have sedimentation coefficients of 16S and 6.4S. The 16S has a molecular weight of $\sim 700,000$, is composed of H and L chains, and resembles IgM on the basis of chain properties. The 6.4S molecule appears to be a fragment of the 16S molecule.

Dipnoi

The Australian lungfish, *Neoceratodus forsteri*, shows anatomical and embryological similarities to amphibians and is regarded as an "uncle" of the tetrapods rather than a direct ancestor (Romer, 1967). The lungfish has two types of antigenically related proteins, characterized by sedimentation coefficients of 19.4S and 5.9S. Both proteins possess light polypeptide chains which resemble typical immunoglobulin light chains in molecular weight (23,000) and behavior in gel electrophoresis. The 19.4S proteins are similar to γM immunoglobulins of other vertebrates in size and chain structure. Heavy polypeptide chains from these molecules are comparable to the μ-chain in molecular weight (70,000) and gel electrophoretic properties. The heavy chain of the 5.9S immunoglobulin-like protein differs from those of the major classes of vertebrates in possessing a molecular weight of approximately 40,000. In both proteins, the light and heavy chains are linked through disulfide bonds. Marchalonis once believed that this protein might be unique to lungfish and proposed the term *IgN*. However, antibodies with similar properties have been found in ducks, turtles, and rabbits.

Amphibians

The urodeles constitute a major group of amphibians more primitive than the anurans. The recent examination of the mudpuppy, *Necturus maculosus* (Marchalonis and Cohen 1973), is of importance. *Necturus* has a serum immunoglobulin with a molecular weight of 900,000. After reduction of disulfide bonds and analysis under dissociating conditions, the molecule resolves into polypeptide chains resembling light chains and μ-type heavy chains, MW 22,000 and 70,000. This immunoglobulin is related antigenically to the IgM like immunoglobulins of the toad, *Bufo marinus*, and the clawed toad, *Xenopus laevis*. Unlike the anurans, *Necturus* does not possess detectable amounts of low molecular weight immunoglobulins.

Xenopus laevis is one of the most primitive anuran amphibians. Hadjii-Azimi (1971) found antibodies in *Xenopus* resembling the mammalian γM and γG immunoglobulins. *Xenopus*' γM class of immunoglobulin is similar to human IgM, but γG differs from human IgG. Immunization with HGG, BSA, and *Octopus vulgaris* haemocyanin (Hc), causes antibody activity that is similar to 19S and 7S synthesis. The 19S protein has heavy chains with a molecular weight of 74,500, similar to human μ-chains of 73,900. The 7S protein differs from the human IgG with a heavy chain molecular weight of 64,500. The light chains of both immunoglobulins of *Xenopus* have a molecular weight of 26,700, similar to human immunoglobulin light chains at 25,000.

The 19S and 7S immunoglobulins of *Xenopus* represent two distinct immunoglobulin classes that are characteristic of anuran amphibians. The proteins are antigenically related, as their light chains are identical in molecular weight (23,000), and both exhibit electrophoretic behavior on acrylamide gel. However, the heavy chains differ. The 19S heavy chain resembles the μ-chain of γM immunoglobulins of other vertebrates with a molecular weight of 71,300, whereas the heavy chain of the light 7S immunoglobulin is comparable to the μ-chain of γG in electrophoretic behavior and molecular weight of 52,700.

Antibodies to bacteriophage f2 occur in the serum of the toad *Bufo marinus* two weeks after primary immunization and reach peak levels at six weeks. Although both IgM and IgG antibodies are present, most of the antibody activity persists in the IgM fraction until eight weeks after immunization. After a second injection of antigen, four weeks after primary immunization, total serum-antibody activity increases markedly, and IgG antibodies occur as early as four weeks after the second antigen injection (Lin et al. 1971). A good immune response to bovine γ-globulin can also be induced in the toad (Lykakis, 1969). Two classes of immunoglobulins, homologous with mammalian γM (19S) and γG (7S) antibody, are produced during the course of immunization. The conversion from 19S to 7S antibody activity occurs approximately one month after primary immunization.

Rana catesbeiana immunoglobulins have the same chain structures as those of mammals (Marchalonis and Edelman, 1966). The molecular weights of light chains of both immunoglobulins is 20,000. Heavy chains of the γM-class have molecular weights of 72,100, and those of the γG-class have a molecular weight of 53,600. The carbohydrate content of the γG-immunoglobulin is 2.1% and that of the γM-protein is 10.8%. The amino acid compositions of both classes is also similar to those of mammals.

Reptiles

Among the living reptiles, the tuatara (*Sphenodon punctatum*) of New Zealand is the most primitive. Its ancestors were progenitors of the major group of reptiles, which includes dinosaurs, lizards, snakes, and the branch giving rise to birds. The tautara possesses 19S, γM, and 7S immunoglobulins of a distinct class. The behavior of the heavy chain of the tuatara 7S immunoglobulin is distinct from that of the lungfish "nu" chain and resembles more closely that of the γ chain. The turtles represent a line distinct from that of the tuatara, as do the therapsids, which were ancestral to mammals. The turtles possess immunoglobulins resembling those of the lungfish in general characteristics. Undoubtedly turtles possess two immunoglobulin types (Grey, 1963). Ambrosius (1966) and Ambrosius et al. (1969) have found two types in the tortoise corresponding to the $\gamma_{ss}(\gamma)$ globulin and one corresponding to the $\gamma_{M^1}(\beta_{2_M})$ globulin of mammals. Although it awaits confirmation, Coe (1972) suggests the presence of a "surprisingly complex IgG system involving four different serum proteins" in the painted turtle, *Chrysemys picta*. If this is true it means that the reptiles possess greater diversity in immunoglobulin structure than all the vertebrates except the mammals.

At least three immunoglobulin classes have been found in the sea turtle *Chelonia mydas* (Benedict and Pollard 1972) and in the common turtle *Pseudamys scripta* (Leslie and Clem 1972). Three different sizes of immunoglobulins containing anti-dinitrophenyl activity were isolated by Leslie and Clem (1972) from turtles immunized with dinitrophenyl bovine γ globulin. Their sedimentation coefficients were ~17S, 7.5S, and 5.7S. Their molecular weights were 850,000, 180,000, and 120,000. The 17S immunoglobulin was similar to IgM; it was composed of five subunits each with a molecular weight of ~170,000. The heavy and light chain molecular weights were 70,000 and 22,500, respectively. The 7.5S molecule had *H* chains of ~67,500 and *L* chains. The 5.7S molecule had *H* chains of ~35,000 and *L* chains. Partial reduction of the 5.7S molecule results in the formation of half molecules of ~61,000. Antigenic analysis suggests that the 5.7S molecule may be a fragment of the 7.5S molecule. Neither the 7.5S *H* chains nor the 5.7S *H* chains cross-reacted with the 17S *H* chains.

In another group of reptiles, Saluk et al. (1970) found two antigenically distinct types of *L*-chains in the Florida alligator, *Alligator mississippiensis*. They suggest that these are under the control of independently segregating genes comparable to κ and λ in man.

Birds

Among avian species, the chicken and the duck have been studied in greatest depth. Chickens possess a low molecular weight immunoglobulin, which Leslie and Clem (1969) call IgY because its heavy chain fits into none of the standard categories.

It possesses a molecular weight of 67,000 and is generally referred to as chicken IgG. Ducks possess IgM and two low molecular weight classes, one of which probably resembles the IgY of chickens and the other is similar to the IgN of the lungfish. Birds may represent variants of the reptilian pattern of immunoglobulin structure. Ducks possess a mercaptoethanol-sensitive, slowly sedimenting anti-BSA antibody, which by gel filtration and radioimmunoelectrophoresis does not behave like a mammalian $7S\gamma$ globulin (Grey, 1963). This antibody is larger in size than the $7S\gamma$ protein, migrates separately from the $7S\gamma$ globulin line, and/or bears a striking resemblance in some of its characteristics to the $\beta_2 A$ (1A) immunoglobulin described in the mammal. Mercaptoethanol-sensitive, slowly sedimenting antibody occurs in nonmammalian vertebrates such as the chicken, frog, goldfish, and turtle. The presence of this class of antibody in inframammalian species, to the apparent exclusion in the cold-blooded vertebrates at least of the mercaptoethanol-resistant antibody, suggests that this class of antibody represents a stage in the evolution of the immune response that in the mammal has become largely superceded by mercaptoethanol-resistant $7S\gamma$ globulin.

The H chain of chicken IgG and IgM possesses a common antigenic determinant revealed by the use of rabbit antisera absorbed with L chains. Sera of rabbits immunized with γ chains cross-react with IgM, but not if the intact IgG molecule is used for immunization. Sera of rabbits immunized with IgM cross-react with γ chains but not with IgG. Thus, there is a common determinant on the H chains, "hidden" in the IgG molecule, but accessible on the IgM molecule.

One of the parameters needed for a detailed analysis of the behavior of avian IgG both with respect to the aggregation of the molecule and with respect to the structure is the molecular weight of the monomeric species (Hersh et al. 1969). To date, the following three molecular weights have been reported for chicken IgG: 1.74×10^5, 2.06×10^5, and 1.65×10^5 daltons (D). As background information, it was necessary to determine again the molecular weight of chicken IgG and to include the values for two closely related IgG immunoglobulins: namely, the Japanese quail (*Coturnix coturnix*) and the ring-necked pheasant (*Phasianus colchicus*). Chicken IgG has a molecular weight near 1.70×10^5 D, which is lower than the previously reported value of 2×10^5 D and is more in agreement with the value of 1.74×10^5 D obtained by light scattering, it is also closer to the value of 1.65×10^5 D. The molecular weights of pheasant and quail IgG were close to the value obtained for chicken IgG; thus, at least for these three avian species, the molecular weights of the IgG are somewhat higher than the values for most mammalian species.

The pigeon is unrelated to the chicken or duck, is readily available, and is frequently used in other biologic studies (Guttman et al. 1971). After pigeons were immunized with bovine serum albumin, the antibody responses were delayed in onset, and six of seventeen pigeons failed to produce detectable hemagglutinating antibody until after a second or third injection. Only four of seventeen birds produced precipitating antibody. Mercaptoethanol-sensitive antibody persists after the primary stimulus, since the hemagglutination titers of some sera collected after the third injection could still be reduced by treatment. Immunoelectrophoresis and autoradiography revealed the presence of antibodies with mobilities similar to human IgG and IgM. A heat-labile, skin-sensitizing antibody is detected and has a minimum latent period of twenty-four hours and other characteristics similar to human homocytotropic antibody.

Monotreme and Marsupial Mammals

Monotreme mammals, or the prototheria, include the duckbill platypus and spiny anteaters from Australia. They are quite different from other mammals and for this reason it is believed that they must have diverged from the ancestors of other members of the class at the very beginning of mammalian history. It is further suggested by Romer that they may have evolved as a separate stock from the therapsids, ancestral mammal-like reptiles from which all mammals arose. Still, their immunoglobulin characteristics are not unlike other mammals. According to Marchalonis and Cone (1973), the echidna possesses two major classes of immunoglobulin that are similar in general properties to the IgM and IgG antibodies of man.

With regard to marsupials, Thomas et al. (1972) reported that the quokka, *Setonix brackyurus*, possesses immunoglobulins similar to the IgM, IgG, and IgN classes described for other species. The American opossum, another marsupial, may be different (Rowlands and Dudley 1968). When the serum proteins of the opossum are compared with a eutherian mammal, the rabbit, the electrophoretic distribution of proteins appears qualitatively similar, with five separate peaks in each. However, significant quantitative differences are obvious (Fig. 13-11, a and b). In opossums, the

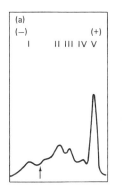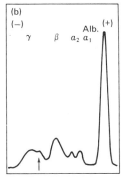

Fig. 13-11   Electrophoretic comparison of the serum proteins of the opossum and rabbit. (a) Electrophoresis of whole adult oppossum serum. The arrow indicates the origin. (b) Electrophoresis of whole adult rabbit serum. The arrow indicates the origin. (*From*: Rowlands & Dudley, *J. Immunol.*, **100**: 736, 1968.)

albumin peak represents an appreciably smaller portion of the total protein than it does in the rabbit. In addition, in the opossum, peaks II and III (β and α_2) were in excess of those in the rabbit. Two major classes of immunoglobulins have been isolated; these appear to be similar to those of eutherian mammals. The rate of conversion from macromolecular antibodies to smaller molecular weight antibodies among opossums is much more nearly like that seen in lower vertebrates than in other mammals.

IMMUNOGLOBULIN EVOLUTION

There is a remarkable similarity among immunoglobulin chains of diverse vertebrate species, based upon electrophoretic properties, molecular weight, and carbohydrate content. Heavy chains seem to be related, since the heavy chains of the lamprey, the dogfish shark, and the catfish resemble the human μ chain more closely than the other chains. Based on computer information and comparisons with other well-studied proteins such as cytochrome C and haemoglobulin, there is a tentative conclusion that IgM immunoglobulins evolved in a highly conservative fashion among vertebrate species.

The information derived from the structure of heavy chains is given a molecular interpretation in Fig. 13-12. The lengths of the chains are proportional to their molecular weights. The basic unit in the diagram corresponds to a polypeptide segment of molecular weight 12,000. Light γ and μ chain representation is based upon

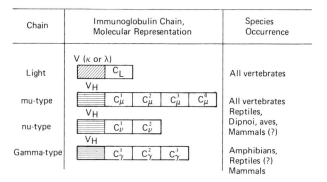

Fig. 13-12 Molecular representation of immunoglobulin polypeptide chains. The lengths of the chains are proportional to the carbohydrate-free molecular weight. The basic unit is a homology region of approx. 110 amino acids. The variable region (VL or VH) is placed at the amino terminal end of the molecule. C, constant regions. The particular class of the C region homology units is given by the subscript. The superscript numeral gives the position. CL can be either CK or C_λ. (*From*: Marchalonis & Cone, AJEBAK, **51**: 461, 1973.)

new sequence data; the diagram of the "nu" chain is hypothetical. In the figure there is an emphasis on the high degree of duplication characteristic of vertebrate immunoglobulins. Because of a lack of primary sequence information, it is not completely clear if the γ-like heavy chain of amphibians is homologous to the γ chain of mammals; there is, however, suggestive physicochemical evidence. Furthermore, similar data are required for avian immunoglobulins; it is conceivable that the low molecular weight heavy chains of birds represent an independent gene duplication from the one that produced the γ chain gene in mammals. This would support convergent evolution rather than any ancestral relationship.

The previous information was concerned with the evolution of the constant (C) region. Within any given species, four-fifths of the μ chain is composed of a constant sequence. Table 13-4 summarizes the partial sequences of amino acids from the N-terminal ends of light and heavy chains of a variety of lower species, thus providing information on the phylogenetic patterns of variation within the V regions. There are strong homologies between the K chain of man and the light chains of paddlefish, leopard shark, and the African lungfish. There are also obvious homologies among the V_H regions of diverse vertebrate species. Human V_H regions can be broken down into three subclasses on the basis of amino acid sequence, regions shared among heavy chains of all classes. In fact, V-region subclasses are present even in the leopard shark; thus the genetic events underlying V-region evolution must have occurred early in vertebrate phylogeny. Immunoglobulins of primitive vertebrates do resemble those of man in amino acid sequence diversity. Furthermore, there is a high degree of homology among immunoglobulins from species that diverged over 200 million years ago.

Gene control of immunoglobulin structure began early in the evolution of vertebrates. The emergence of vertebrate immunoglobulins is revealed in the hypothetical scheme in Fig. 13-13. We may begin with the ancestral gene, which probably coded

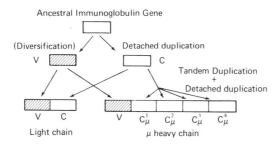

Fig. 13-13 Genetic scheme for the origin of vertebrate immunologlobulins. The events depicted here occurred by the phylogenetic level of cyclostomes. (*From*: Marchalonis & Cone, AJEBAK, **51**: 461, 1973.)

for a polypeptide of 110 amino acids. It later underwent a detached duplication to form the V gene and the C gene. These two genes now formed separate genetic compartments, which continued to duplicate. At the level of the elasmobranchs, V-region subgroups emerged. C-region duplications to form classes occurred within the ancestors of the Dipnoi and Amphibia. Marchalonis and Cone believe that the mechanism of V-region diversification occurred early in evolution, such that the ancestral polypeptide may have resembled a V region. Such a polypeptide probably paired with another to form a specific combining site on the outer surfaces of "protolymphoid" cells. There it served as a recognition unit or receptor for the detection of foreign antigen. Those detached duplications that formed C-region genes may have been a means of removing recognition units from the cell surface, freeing them into a fluid (e.g., serum). It is necessary to study deuterostomate invertebrates and protochordates, the nearest relatives to chordates, in order to estimate the time of primary divergence. According to this model, it is possible for V and C genes to fuse, so that an intact polypeptide can be synthesized at the time of the first duplication. The creation of light chains and μ heavy chains by fusion of V and C genes and the tandem duplication of constant homology regions probably occurred over 300 million years ago, preceding the divergence of the ancestors of elasmobranchs and mammals.

Litman et al. (1971) believe that the evolution of immunoglobulins has occurred along three distinct lines: 1) immunoglobulins of ostracoderm-derived vertebrates possess certain structural characteristics making their relationships to other immunoglobulins questionable; 2) immunoglobulins of modern vertebrates that evolved from placoderms, e.g., osteichthyes, (paddlefish) and some of the chondrichthyes (sharks), are of both high and low molecular weight classes. The heavy chains of these classes are indistinguishable on the basis of amino acid composition, carbohydrate composition, antigenic relationship, and molecular weight; 3) immunoglobulins represented by

Table 13-4

N-terminal amino acid sequences of vertebrate immunoglobulins.

| Species | Chain | Residue number | | | | | |
		1	2	3	4	5	6
Lamprey	light	Asp					
Leopard shark	light	Asp	Ile	Val	Leu	Thr	Glx
			Pro	Ile	Met		
					Val		
Paddlefish	light	Asp	Ile	Val	Ile	Thr	
					Leu		
Lungfish	light	Asp	—	—	Leu	Thr	Glx
Man	K	Asp	Ile	Val	Met	Thr	Gln
		Glu	Val	Gln	Leu		
			Met	Leu			
Man	λ	PCA	Ser	Val	Leu	Thr	Gln
			Tyr	Ala		Ala	
				Glu			
Man	V$_H$I	PCA	Val	Gln	Leu	Val	Gln
				His			
	V$_H$II	PCA	Val	Thr	Leu	Lys	Glu
						Thr	
						Arg	
	V$_H$III	Glu	Val	Gln	Leu	Leu	Glu
			Ile			Val	
Leopard shark	HS 1	PCA	Val	Pro	Gly	—	Gln
	HS 2	PCA	Asp	Leu	Pro	Thr	Pro
	V$_H$(ub)	Glu	Ile	Val	Leu	Thr	Gln
			Val				
Lamprey	mu	Asp					
Paddlefish	mu	Asp	Ile	Val	Ile	Thr	

(*From*: Marchalonis and Cone, AJEBAK, 51 : 461, 1973)

other osteichthyes (lung fishes), Amphibia, Reptilia, Aves, and Mammalia that also possess both high and low molecular weight immunoglobulin classes.

Litman et al. adhere to the last argument; they offer further physicochemical evidence supporting this evolutionary scheme and, at the same time, give insight into the genetic mechanisms governing immunoglobulin synthesis (Table 13-5). The molecular weight is consistent: approximately 70,000 for the heavy chains of the high molecular weight immunoglobulins. Heavy chains of low molecular weight immuno- globulins possess identical molecular weights in all elasmobranch (shark) and a chondrostean (paddlefish) species. In the holostean *Amia calva* there is a reduction in molecular weight of these heavy chain classes. The low molecular weight immuno- globulins of all other species uniformly possess heavy chains that bear partial (lung- fishes, bullfrog, turtle, chicken) or nonidentical (rabbit, human) antigenic relationships to heavy chains of the corresponding high molecular weight immunoglobulin class. A distinct class of heavy chains in the low molecular weight immunoglobulins of the Amphibia and Aves is established in the dipnoid fishes (lungfish), Reptilia, and other avian forms. In the future, more information will help to resolve controversies on the evolution of immunoglobulins.

Table 13-5

Molecular weight values of heavy chains from phylogenetically critical
species of vertebrata.

Class		High molecular weight (HMW)	Low molecular weight (LMW)	Complete antigenic relationship between HMW and LMW
Chondrichthyes	Horned shark			
	Heterodontus francisci	70,000	70,000	+
	Nurse shark			
	Ginglymostoma cirratum	70,000	70,000	+
	Leopard shark	77,000	76,500	
	Triakis semifasciata	70,000	70,000	+
	Lemon shark			
	Negaprion brevirostris	71,000	71,000	+
	Dogfish shark			
	Mustelus canis	71,600	73,400	+
Osteichtyes	African lungfish			
	Protopterus aethiophicus	70,000	38,000	−
	Australian lungfish			
	Neoceratodus forsteri	70,280	37,950	−
	Paddlefish	75,300		
	Polyodon spathula	70,000	70,000	+
	Bowfin			
	Amia calva	70,000	52,000	+
Amphibia	Bullfrog			
	Rana catesbiana	72,100	53,600	−
Reptilia	Turtle			
	Chelydra serpentina	70,000	38,000	−
Aves	Chicken			
	Gallus domesticus	70,000	66,000	−
	Duck			
	Anas sp.		36,000	−
Mammalia	Rabbit			
	Oryctolagus cuniculus	70,000	53,000	−
	Human			
	Homo sapiens	70,000	50,000	−

(*From* Litman et al., Immunochem. 8 : 345, 1971)

BIBLIOGRAPHY

Ambrosius, H. 1966. Beiträge zur immunobiologie poikilothermer wirbeltiere. IV. Weitere immunologische und immunchemische untersuchungen an schildkröten. Zeit. für Imm. forschung. Allerg. und Klnis. Immunol. **130**: 41.

Bardack, D., and Zangerl, R. 1968. First fossil lamprey: a record from the Pennsylvanian of Illinois. Science **162**: 1265.

Benedict, A. A., and Pollard, L. W. 1972. Three classes of immunoglobulins found in the sea turtle, *Chelonia mydas.* Folia. Microb. **17**: 75.

Bradshaw, C. M., Clem, L. W., and Sigel, M. M. 1971. Immunologic and immunochemical studies on the gar, *Lepisosteus platyrhincus.* II. Purification and characterization of immunoglobulin. J. Immunol. **106**: 1480.

Clem, L. W. 1971. Phylogeny of immunoglobulin structure and function. IV. Immunoglobulins of the giant grouper, *Epinephelus itaira.* J. Biol. Chem. **246**: 9.

Coe, J. E. 1972. Immune response in the turtle (*Chrysemys picta*). Immunology **23**: 45.

Edelman, G. M. 1967. Studies on the primary and tertiary structure of γG immunoglobulin. Nobel Symposium **3**: 89.

Edelman, G. M., and Gally, W. E. 1969. The antibody problem. Ann. Rev. Biochem. **38**: 415.

Fogereau, M., and Edelman, G. M. 1965. Corroboration of recent models of the γG immunoglobulin molecule. J. Exp. Med. **121**: 373.

Gally, J. A. and Edelman, G. M. 1972. Genetic control of immunoglobulin synthesis. Ann. Rev. Genetics **6**: 1.

Grey, H. M. 1963. Phylogeny of the immune response: studies on some physical chemical and serologic characteristics of antibody produced in the turtle. J. Immunol. **91**: 819.

Guttman, R. M., Tebo, T., Edwards, J., Barboriak, J. J., and Fink, J. N. 1971. The immune response of the pigeon (*Columba livia*). J. Immunol. **106**: 392.

Hadjii-Azimi, I. 1971. Studies on *Xenopus laevis* immunoglobulins. Immunology **21**: 463.

Hersh, R. T., Kubo, R. T., Leslie, G. A., and Benedict, A. A. 1969. Molecular weights of chicken, pheasant, and quail IgG immunoglobulins. Immunochem. **6**: 762.

Leslie, G. A., and Clem, L. W. 1972. Phylogeny of immunoglobulin structure and function. VI. 17S, 7.5S and 5.7S anti-DNP of the turtle, *Pseudamys scripta.* J. Immunol. **108**: 1656.

Lin, H. H., Caywood, B. E., and Rowlands, D. T. Jr. 1971. Primary and secondary immune responses of the marine toad, *Bufo marinus*, to Bacteriophage f2. Immunology **20**: 373.

Litman, G. W., Frommel, D., Chartrand, S. L., Finstad, J., and Good, R. A. 1971. Significance of heavy chain mass and antigenic relationship in immunoglobulin evolution. Immunochem. **8**: 345.

Lykakis, J. J. 1969. The production of two molecular classes of antibody in the toad, *Xenopus laevis*, homologous with mammalian γG (7s) immunoglobulins. Immunology **16**: 91.

Marchalonis, J. J., and Edelman, G. M. 1966. Phylogenetic origins of antibody structure. II. Immunoglobulins in the primary response of the bullfrog *Rana catesbeiana.* J. Exp. Med. **124**: 901.

Marchalonis, J. J., and Schonfeld, S. A. 1970. Polypeptide chain structure of sting ray immunoglobulin. Biochem. Biophys. Acta **221**: 604.

Marchalonis, J. J., and Cohen, N. 1973. Isolation and partial characterization of immunoglobulin from a urodele amphibian (*Necturus maculosus*). Immunol. **24**: 395.

Marchalonis, J. J., and Cone, R. E. 1973. The phylogenetic emergence of vertebrate immunity. AJEBAK **51**: 461.

Porter, R. R. 1967. The chemical structure of the heavy chain of immunoglobulins. Nobel Symposium **3**: 81.

Romer, A. S. 1967. Major steps in vertebrate evolution. Science **158**: 1629.

Rowlands, D. T. Jr. and Dudley, M. A. 1968. The isolation of immunoglobulins of the adult opossum. (*Didelphys virginiana*). J. Immunol. **100**: 736.

Saluk, P. H., Krauss, J., and Clem, L. W. 1970. The presence of two antigenically distinct light chains (K and λ?) in alligator immunoglobulins. Proc. Soc. Exp. Biol. Med. **133**: 365.

Thomas, W. R., Turner, K. J., Eadie, M. E., and Yadav, M. 1972. The immune response of the quokka (*Setonix brachyurus*). The production of a low molecular weight antibody. Immunol. **22**: 401.

Chapter 14

Activities of Immune Cells

INTRODUCTION

Although advanced invertebrates have discrete organs that generate leukocytes, only vertebrates possess a thymus, spleen, and subsidiary lymphoid accumulations. During the development of reptiles, birds, and mammals, the yolk sac or its equivalent, and later, the bone marrow or a comparable organ, serve as sources of stem cells. Such potential immunologically competent cells receive further instructions in the thymus or bursa of Fabricius of birds (or its analogue in other vertebrates) and differentiate into two immunocytes, the T cell and B cell. T cells effect cellular immune responses (e.g., graft rejection) and B cells synthesize antibody. It should be stressed that the T and B concept of the two-component immune system is based on the discrete dual lymphoid organ system of birds (the thymus and the bursa of Fabricius). Whether this strict delineation exists in other vertebrates including mammals is problematic. The bird information supports the need for still more valuable contributions that can be gained by the comparative approach to immunology.

The thymus is derived from endoderm in ontogeny from evaginations of the developing pharynx, and in phylogeny it persists in all vertebrates. For cell mediated immunity, the most primitive immune response phylogenetically, the appropriate (thymus) environment for T cell maturation is constant. However, where those stem cells that are destined to become the B variety receive final instructions is controversial, since the location for B-cell differentiation in most vertebrates is unclear. The T and B lymphocyte concept is worthy of intense investigation since its analysis in poikilothermic vertebrates has hardly been studied at all. Yet the thymus occupies a central role in the immune response of the poikilotherms (Fig. 14-1).

Because the study of antibody-mediated immunity began with vertebrates, a definition of the immune response has always implied that antibody synthesis must occur. However, studies of adoptive transfer and the graft-vs.-host response (GVH), two specific immunologic reactions, were instrumental in focusing on the importance of cells in immunity. In addition to lymphocytes and plasma cells, other leukocytes, such as granulocytes, monocytes, and the ubiquitous macrophage, are also important and necessary in effecting immunologic responses.

Immune cells can be demonstrated within organs in response to antigen. The whole organ-organism approach is valuable, yet a study of component cells is also desirable. With the development of cell culture procedures, *in vitro* approaches to immunological problems are increasingly useful in poikilothermic vertebrates, since

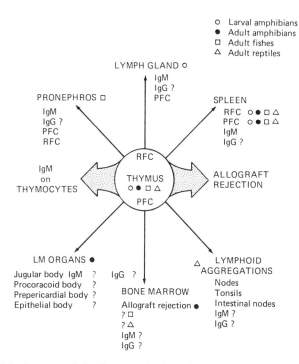

Fig. 14-1 Summary of the thymus and other principal lymphoid organs in fishes, amphibians, and reptiles. The two horizontal arrows represent the principal role of the thymus in all lower vertebrates. Complementary organs or possible precursors of other organs in these three groups are joined by unidirectional diagonal arrows. (*From*: Cooper, *Cont. Topics in Immunobiol.*, **2**: 13, 1973.)

they often involve organs not ordinarily encountered in mammals. One such example is the pronephros of fish, a developmental precursor of the kidney of advanced vertebrates, and a part of the immune system (see Chap. 7). Immunologic specificity and memory occur in animals where immunocytes possess the capacity to divide. Lymphocytes incorporate tritiated thymidine, indicating DNA synthesis, an event in cell division. It is by means of mitosis that primed lymphocytes, initially immunized with a particular antigen, can pass such immunity on to daughter cells.

Until recently, the usual method for demonstrating antibody from an immune animal was to obtain its serum after empirical immunization periods. Putatively, immune serum is then reacted with the antigen and various tests are employed. For example, if antigens such as erythrocytes or bacteria are used, tests for the presence of antibody often involve the demonstration of agglutinations. Soluble antigens usually lead to antibody, demonstrable by precipitin methods, although there are other approaches. To determine what cells or organ regions are involved in antibody synthesis, histologic sections can be prepared and certain immunohistologic techniques employed, notably the use of fluorescent dyes; contact of antigen and antibody leads to recognizable fluorescence.

Such analyses were and still are valuable, yet procedures allowing at the same time quantitative analyses and the identification of viable immune cells, actively producing antibody, are equally desirable. With the advent of Jerne's approach and some later modifications, modern cellular immunology became more evident. According to Jerne's technique, antibody-forming cells derived from animals previously immunized with sheep erythrocytes (SRBC) can be readily identified. Such cells, in the presence of SRBC and complement (a heat-labile component of serum), will lyse the surrounding SRBC. This mixture, usually layered onto agar, becomes riddled with plaques and clear sites. These represent single cells secreting antibody (plaque-forming cells: PFC) that lyse the erythrocytes.

A second *in vitro* technique searches for antibody still attached to the surfaces of viable immune cells (immunocytoadherence). Recognition and enumeration of these cells is important, as they represent antigen-sensitive cells revealed as rosette-forming cells (RFC) that are equipped with antibody receptors for recognizing or sensing antigens. Cells involved in antibody synthesis can be enumerated and classified after mixing them with an antigen, usually erythrocytes. These readily adhere to the surface of active cells, creating rosettes. Single rows of erythrocytes adhering to lymphocyte surfaces indicate cytophilic antibody, but multiple rows identify cells actively secreting antibody. Thus, the rosette test can enable a study not only of the specific cell types, but also the antibody synthesizing capabilities of the cell.

A third test involves measuring the incorporation of radioactively labelled precursors into lymphocytes. Actively dividing lymphocytes will incorporate tritiated thymidine and those that synthesize RNA or protein with other precursors such as proline or leucine. One can readily characterize whether a lymphocyte is of the T or B variety by its response to mitogens, agents that cause lymphocytes to enlarge (blast transformation) and divide. In all vertebrates studied to date phytohemagglutinin (PHA) stimulates T cells and lipopolysaccharide (LPS) stimulates B cells. When lymphocytes from different animals of the same species are mixed together in allogeneic combinations, the histocompatibility differences existing between the cell types cause mutual stimulation (MLC). Small lymphocytes become large, take on characteristics of primitive blast cells, transform, and divide. These more recent facts, coupled with information gained from the whole organ and organism, are responsible for newer insights into immune response mechanisms.

INVERTEBRATE COELOMOCYTES *IN VITRO* AND *IN VIVO*

Introduction

If we assume that the various types of vertebrate immunocytes originated from a common cell precursor found in invertebrates, we must be able to trace known characteristics of vertebrate cells to analogous ones in invertebrates. Just as biologists recognize a universality of cells, tissues, and functional organ systems (e.g., digestion, reproduction), undoubtedly an equivalent universality exists for the immune system. We can conclude firmly that the phagocytic cell or macrophage is readily identifiable throughout the phylogenetic scale. It is the T and B cells whose precise phylogenetic origin still remains unclear.

Annelids

A substantial amount of *in vivo* evidence favors cell-mediated immunity as the primitive immune response. In annelids, coelomocytes migrate and effect transplant rejection, measurable by coelomocyte enumeration. Coelomocytes from worms previously grafted can adoptively transfer this response to nongrafted hosts, conferring on them the ability to show memory by accelerated rejection of a test graft. Earthworm coelomocytes can respond *in vivo* and *in vitro* to PHA, showing increased H[3] thymidine incorporation. Coelomocytes also respond by increased uptake of H[3] uridine *in vitro*, also a characteristic of vertebrate *T* cells; however uridine incorporation is a necessary indicator of any cell's viability. Finally, earthworm coelomocytes readily form RFC when mixed with SRBC. Whether this represents a specific reaction implicating the presence of coelomocyte receptors for SRBC is unknown. Earthworms and other coelomate invertebrates possess antigen-sensitive (receptor) cell(s) and effector cell(s), which are capable of destroying foreign tissue antigens. Perhaps the coelomocyte receptor, surface-bound like vertebrate antibody, is demonstrable in the coelomic fluid, as antibodies are in vertebrate serum. Thus, at least in the annelids there are responses that strongly suggest cell-mediated reactions by a primitive T cell type.

Tunicates

It is among this group of protochordates that we see the capacity to exhibit cell responses reminiscent of those found in vertebrates. Protochordates are close to the vertebrates phylogenetically, and for this reason leukocyte responses could be more meaningful from the viewpoint of evolutionary origins. Circulating leukocytes will form rosettes to SRBC and readily respond *in vivo* and *in vitro* to PHA by increased incorporation of H[3] thymidine. *In vivo*, leukocytes resembling the vertebrate small lymphocyte actively invade tunic allografts but not autografts. Thus, a primitive *T*-cell response also appears to be present in the tunicates.

LYMPHOCYTES AND PLASMA CELLS *IN VITRO*

Agnatha

The first and only study devoted to *in vitro* characterizations of immune cells of Agnatha, cyclostomes or jawless fishes, is that of A. J. Cooper (1971). Ammocoetes, or juvenile lampreys, live burrowed in mud and obtain their food by an ancestral mode of filter feeding. They possess typical blood lymphocytes and localized lymphoid aggregations, as well as the haemapoietic typhlosole, a spiral invagination of the midgut wall. The thymus is an unimpressive "patch" of pharyngeal gill pouch tissue. Peripheral blood leukocytes are easily separated from erythrocytes by differential centrifugation and can be maintained in culture satisfactorily for four days, but thereafter viability falls sharply. What is essential to cellular immunologists is the response of cultured lymphocytes to PHA. When ammocoete lymphocytes are mixed in culture with PHA, typical transformations into blast cells occur. They show increased incorporation of H[3] thymidine, and, to further support the evidence for cell division, mitotic figures are readily demonstrable. In addition to this PHA response, lymphocytes derived from at least two different donors and mixed in culture also interact together and show morphological transformation (MLC response). That lymphocytes do divide by mitosis seems fundamental to the evolution of immunologic competence.

The phylogenetic development from cyclostomes to mammals remains constant with regard to specificity; however, the anatomical and physiological necessities (e.g.

kinds of lymphoid organs) for recognizing and reacting to antigens have required various modifications throughout the phylogenetic scale. According to Cooper (1971),

> As mitosis is phylogenetically as old as the nucleus, and proliferative response as old as regeneration, the only initial physiological innovation required of evolution is adaptive specificity which itself might easily be considered a logical extension of the inter-cellular co-ordination and recognition processes fundamental to metazoan organization. Non-specialized effector processes such as allogeneic inhibition or phagocytosis (apparently reaching back to echinoderms [or even earlier in phylogeny], around which level of larval organization vertebrate origins most likely lie) would be pre-adaptive to the evolution of an adaptive, specific, proliferative response in a suitable, probably amoebocytic, cell line, giving at once a functional immunological system of sorts for selection to work on. A crude memory would follow readily if some of the cells involved had a reasonably long life, and if recognition involved a degree of irreversible differentiation. The relationships of humoral and cell-bound adaptively synthesized antibodies and recognition receptors might also depend on whether immunoglobulins were fundamental in proto-immunological responsiveness—which would tend to make them physically similar—or whether the two advanced effector systems developed in parallel, necessitating only the common features dictated by the nature of recognition and the sites responsible for it.

Teleosts

The pronephros of fish is intriguing, since it is a phylogenetic precursor of the excretory system and at the same time is involved with antibody synthesis. It would be difficult, however, to examine this structure for antibody-producing cells (APC) phylogenetically, since, beginning with the reptiles, it may be only an embryonic organ persisting *in ovo* or *in utero*. Although the physicochemical properties of antibodies in fish have been studied by Clem (see Chap. 13), the location of antibody-forming cells in particular organs has only begun to receive attention.

According to Avtalion (personal communication) antibody-producing cells occur in the kidney, spleen, and pronephros of goldfish after a primary intraperitoneal injection of the antigen *Salmonella typhi* 0-901. PFC are demonstrable *in vitro* eighteen days after antigen injection, attain peak numbers, and return to background levels before those in the kidney and pronephros. Ortiz-Muniz and Sigel (1971) have investigated antibody formation in the thymus, spleen, and pronephros from two species of marine teleosts, the gray snapper, *Lutjanus griseus*, and the grouper, *Mycteroperca bonaci*, after immunization with bovine serum albumin (BSA) or bovine gamma globulin (BGG). Fragments of tissue were grown *in vitro*, and afterwards the culture fluids and sera were assayed for antibodies. All three tissues synthesize γM macroglobulin antibody *in vitro* for up to thirty days. Antibody is detectable as early as three days after beginning the cultures and titers are maximum at six days. Pronephros and spleen produce antibody that remains at peak levels for twelve days, but then it falls. Thymic antibody, rare in most vertebrates, begins to decline after fifteen days and is undetectable on day 30. Antibody production by all tissues can be depressed by adding puromycin to the cultures; this inhibits amino acid incorporation into protein.

Lymphoid cell activities from the pronephros of the blue gill, *Lepomis macrochirus*, are interesting. Smith et al. (1967) immunized blue gills with SRBC, and found that in the pronephros or spleen (or both), PFC are detectable in most fish six days after immunization. Maximum numbers of active cells appear after a secondary booster injection of antigen on days 13 and 14. It is surprising that more PFC occur in the pronephros than in the spleen. PFC also occur in the pronephros of immunized rainbow trout, *Salmo gairdneri* (Chiller et al. 1969a). Kinetic studies reveal plaques initially, two to six days after SRBC injection, and peaks at about day 14. Both small and large plaques can be obtained from spleen and anterior kidney cells of rainbow trout.

Sera from all vertebrates contain complement, a heat-labile component absolutely necessary for lysis of RBC and gram-negative bacteria. Complement is a complex group of serum proteins, which, in low concentration, can bring about RBC lysis of areas of the erythrocyte membrane. To study immune hemolysis in mammals, complement is usually obtained from the guinea pig. However, the source of complement among poikilothermic vertebrates is crucial; it seems to act effectively only if derived from closely related species. For example, combined spleen and kidney tests for PFC reveal that complement is most effective in the salmon if obtained from three different species of salmon or rainbow trout (Table 14-1). In searching for PFC in amphibians and reptiles, it is likewise necessary to employ complement from closely related species.

Table 14-1

Influence of complement source on development of Jerne plaques and tube hemolysis by immune trout cells and sera respectively.

Complement Source	Plaques		Hemolysis Test
	Spleen	A. kidney	
Human	−	−	−
Rabbit	−	−	−
Guinea pig	−	−	−
Mouse	−	−	−
Rat	−	−	NT*
Chicken	−	−	NT
Frog (*Rana pipiens*)	−	−	NT
Axolotl (*Siredon mexicanum*)	−	−	−
Rainbow trout (*Salmo gairdneri*)	+	+	+
Coho salmon (*Oncorhynchus kisutch*)	+	+	+
Sockeye salmon (*Oncorhynchus nerka*)	+	+	+
Chinook salmon (*Oncorhynchus tshawytscha*)	+	+	+
Sole (species unknown)	−	−	−
Carp (*Cyprinus carpio*)	−	−	−
Pacific hake (*Merluccius productus*)	−	−	−
Flounder (species unknown)	−	−	NT
Dogfish (*Squalus acanthias*)	−	−	−
Cod (species unknown)	−	−	−
Herring (*Clupea harengus pallasi*)	−	−	NT
Tilapia (*Tilapia macrocephala*)	−	−	NT
Catfish (*Ictalurus nebulosus*)	−	−	NT
Ratfish (*Hydrolagus colliei*)	−	−	NT
Rockfish (*Sebastodes sp*)	−	−	−
Whiting (*Theragra chaleogrammus*)	−	−	−

*NT = Not tested.
(*From*: Chiller et al., *J. Immunol.*, **102**: 1202, 1969.)

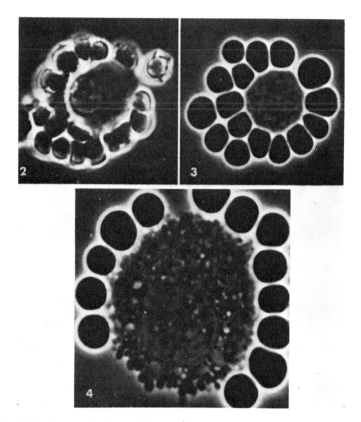

Fig. 14-2 A rosette-forming cell from the anterior kidney of an immunized rainbow trout showing characteristics of a plama cell, including an eccentric nucleus and a cartwheel arrangement of the nuclear chromatin. (Phase contrast ×2000.)

Fig. 14-3 A rosette-forming cell from the anterior kidney of an immunized rainbow trout showing blast-like characteristics. Note the large, pale nucleus and the high nuclear-cytoplasmic ratio. (Phase contrast ×2000.)

Fig. 14-4 A rosette-forming cell from the anterior kidney of an immunized rainbow trout showing characteristics of a macrophage. Note the numerous cytoplasmic vacuoles and the surface microvilli. The single layer of adhering sheep erythrocytes is in contrast with the multiple layering of erythrocytes seen with other cell types. (Phase contrast ×2500.) (From: Chiller, et al., J. Immunol., 102: 1193, 1969.)

Chiller et al. (1969b) have used cells from the pronephros in tests for RFC from the rainbow trout, *Salmo gairdneri*, immunized with SRBC. Naturally occurring RFC are found in tissues from unimmunized trout, and several diverse cell types can form rosettes (Figs. 14-2 to 14-4). With the electron microscope it is easy to visualize typical lymphocytes and macrophages (Figs. 14-5, 14-6). After immunization, the percentage of RFC in the spleen ranges from 0.3–3.0 and in the pronephros from 0.14–0.18. Most splenic RFC appear to be small, medium, or large lymphocytes, but those from the pronephros are more varied and comprise plasma cells, macrophages, and blast-like cells. Although there is no known quantitative relationship between serum agglutinins and number of RFC, hemagglutinin titers of at least 1:64 are required before rosettes are obvious in trout.

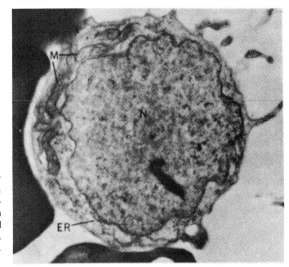

Fig. 14-5 A rosette-forming cell of the anterior kidney of an immunized rainbow trout with morpho-characteristics of a lymphocyte, including a large nucleus, *N*, surrounded by a thin rim of cytoplasm, large mitochondria, *M*, and a small amount of endoplasmic reticulum, *ER* (×*14,000*). (*From*: Chiller, et al., *J. Immunol.*, **102**: 1193, 1969.)

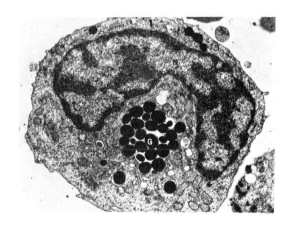

Fig. 14-6 A rosette-forming cell from the anterior kidney of an immunized trout. The crescent-shaped nucleus, *N*, and the osmiophilic granules, *G*, are characteristic features of a macrophage (×*6900*). (*From*: Chiller, et al., *J. Immunol.*, **102**: 1193, 1969.)

Amphibians
  RFC and PFC in Alytes obstetricans

The midwife toad tadpole, *Alytes obstetricans*, has been used to study the ontogenetic development of antigen receptor cells, RFC and PFC (Du Pasquier 1965a, b; 1968; 1970a, b). Antigen receptor cells develop first and are easily demonstrable as RFC. Most RFC resemble lymphocytes and are thymus dependent, as indicated by their reduction after thymectomy. Despite the presence of background levels of RFC in normal immunized tadpoles, the number of RFC increase after immunization with heterologous erythrocytes. Young tadpoles synthesize no antibodies if spleens contain less than 6×10^3 cells. PFC begin to appear in tadpoles with 9×10^4 spleen cells. Thus, the onset of PFC appearance can be determined in relation to spleen size.

The specificity of the response can be easily tested by using HRBC and SRBC. After injections with one RBC, RFC corresponding to the other erythrocyte are absent. PFC apparently synthesize mercaptoethanol sensitive macroglobulin (IgM), since plaque formation can be inhibited by incubating the spleen cells and erythrocyte mixture with mercaptoethanol.

Several speculations stem from Du Pasquier's work regarding the existence of natural RFC in *Alytes* larvae. Natural RFC originate as thymic cells with surface antibody that could emigrate to and reproduce in the spleen or in other lymphoid foci during larval development. They may represent a primitive, but necessary, cadre of cells inherently capable of recognizing antigen. With regard to lymphocyte surface antibody, at least some preformed IgM may pass from mother toads, remain viable in the yolk, and protect larvae until their natural capacity for independent synthesis develops.

RFC and PFC in Xenopus laevis

In *Xenopus* and other anurans, larval maturation is determined on the basis of external morphological criteria (stages). At stage 49 the thymus acquires its mature lymphoid structure, and at stage 50 the spleen completes its lymphocyte differentiation. Larvae beyond stage 50 show substantial increases in spleen RFC six to ten days after the injection of SRBC (Table 14-2). Thymic RFC also show low but increased frequencies at stage 50. Thus, the timing and magnitude of the RFC response in *Xenopus* depends on the maturation stage of the spleen and thymus.

Table 14-2

Summary of immuno-cytoadherence assays with Xenopus larvae

Series	Group	Stage at injection	Days after injection	No. larvae	RFC/10⁶ cells*	
					Spleens	Thymi
I	A	Late-50	(Background)	34	168 ± 21	10 ± 1
			6–10†	12	308 ± 20	30 ± 4
	B	51	(Background)	34	168 ± 21	10 ± 1
			6–10†	11	725 ± 77	46 ± 13
	C	53	(Background)	4	32	7
			6–8‡	10	130 ± 170	58 ± 10
II	D	49/50	(Background)	20	94 ± 5	8 ± 1
			6–10§	28	1240 ± 400	45 ± 22
	E	48/49	(Background)	20	94 ± 5	8 ± 1
			6–8	16	1840 ± 370	13 ± 1
III	F	48	(Background)	15	257	11
			13–22‡	17	281 ± 48	9 ± 1
	G	48	(Background)	22	214 ± 24	30 ± 4
			10–11	16	171 ± 21	10 ± 1

*Except for background determinations in groups C and F, numbers indicate means of multiple assays of each group of larvae carried out during the designated time intervals. Variation is expressed in terms of standard error of the mean.

†Since larvae of groups A and B were siblings of approximately the same chronological age, a single set of background determinations was taken for both groups.

‡A single background determination was carried out for this group of larvae.

§A single set of background determinations was taken for groups D and E as explained in footnote†.

From: Kidder et al., J. E. E. M., 29: 73, 1973.

Bufo Marinus
  Immunocytoadherence (ICA) using bacteria as antigens

Immunocytoadherence can also be demonstrated using bacteria. To assay for anti-body-forming cells (AFC), Diener and Marchalonis (1970) immunized marine toads, *Bufo marinus*, with the antigen *Salmonella adelaide flagella*. Afterwards, the spleen cells are washed and mixed with motile bacteria of *Salmonella adelaide*. AFC can be recognized by the adherence of bacteria to the surfaces of cells secreting antibody. As might be predicted, a significant number of AFC first appear at three days following immunization, with a peak at seven days (Fig. 14-7). Serum antibody measured by bacterial immobilization lags behind, but antibody titer peaks by fourteen days.

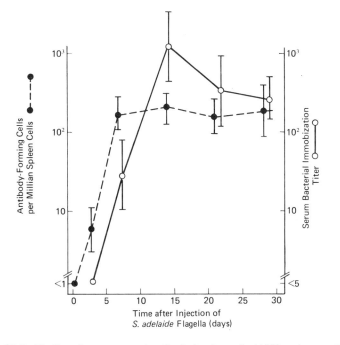

Fig. 14-7 Kinetics of appearance of antibody-forming cells (AFC) and serum titers in the primary response of *B. marinus* to *S. adelaide* flagella.
          ●———● AFC per million spleen cells
          ○———○ serum bacterial immobilization titer
Each point represents the geometric mean of data obtained from six animals. Vertical bars indicate $\log_{10}$ of the standard deviation. (*From*: Marchalonis, *Am. Zool.*, **11** : 171, 1971.)

The AFC population consists of lymphocytes, immunoblasts, and plasma cells. During the early phases of antibody synthesis, the most active cells are small and medium lymphocytes. Incorporation of H^3 thymidine reveals that the majority of AFC found during the logarithmic phase of the response result from mitosis (Fig. 14-8). The titers and numbers of AFC in fishes and toads are comparable in magnitude to those obtained in mice or rats following primary stimulation with antigen. Thus, the toad's primary response to the same antigen is basically similar to mammals.

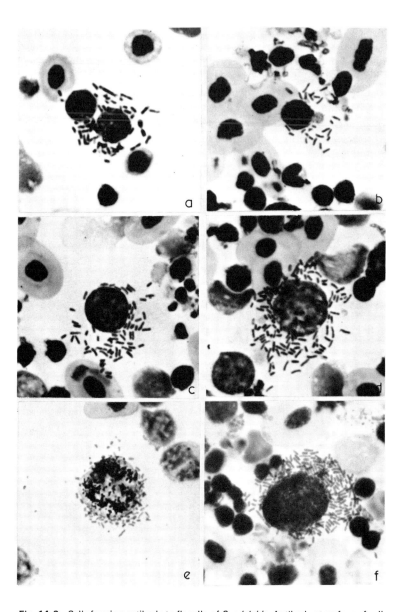

Fig. 14-8 Cells forming antibody to flagella of *S. adelaide*. Antibody at surface of cells causes adherence of *Salmonella* bacteria (×*1320*). (a) Teleost; *Perca fluviatilis*; lymphocyte, diameter 7μ. (b–f) Amphibian: *Bufo marinus*. (b) lymphocyte, diameter 6.5μ. (c) lymphocyte, diameter 9μ. (d) lymphocyte, diameter 12μ. (e) dividing cell labeled with tritiated thymidine autoradiography, diameter 16μ. (f) immunoblast, diameter 16.5μ. (*From*: Diener, *Transpl.*, **2**: 309, 1970.)

With the electron microscope it is possible to detect radioactive-labelled antigen in the toad's jugular body, an arrangement similar to localization in the follicles of mammalian lymph nodes. Antigen is detectable on the surfaces of cells but not within the cell. Diener and Marchalonis (1970) conclude that

> the major patterns of differentiation and proliferation of immunologically competent cells, antigen retention, and immunoglobulin structure emerged at the phylogenetic level of amphibians.

Blastogenesis

Transformation of small lymphocytes, in response to nonspecific mitogens, to larger blast cells followed by mitosis are characteristics of vertebrate lymphocytes. In *Bufo marinus*, untreated spleen and peripheral blood lymphocytes can be cultured and compared to cells treated with PHA (Fig. 14-9). According to Goldshein and

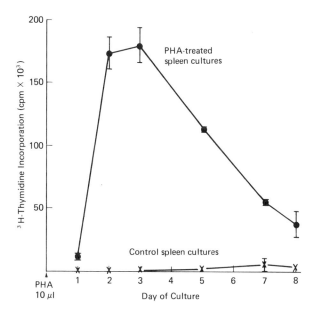

Fig. 14-9   Kinetics of the PHA response. 1.5×10^6 splenic leukocytes were incubated with and without $10\mu 1$ of PHA in ACM supplemented with toad serum. Cultures were pulsed at various intervals with 1.5μ Ci of tritiated thymidine for 16 hr. The points plotted are means ±S.D. of counts from duplicate tubes. (*From*: Goldshein & Cohen, *J. Immunol.*, **108**: 1025, 1972.)

Cohen (1972), 70% of the spleen cells and 30% of the peripheral blood leukocytes are viable after seven days of culture. Decrease in peripheral blood leukocytes occurs during the first forty-eight hours in culture, a feature common also to the leukocytes of guinea pigs, rats, mice, hamsters, and cats. After addition of PHA, high incorporation levels occur at forty-eight to sixty-four hours and are maximum at seventy-two to eighty-eight hours afterwards (Fig. 14-10).

Autoradiographic analysis of lymphocyte cultures reveals three major categories of responding cells, occasionally organized into clusters: unlabeled small lymphocytes, unlabeled blast cells, and labeled blast cells. Each cluster contains ten to twenty

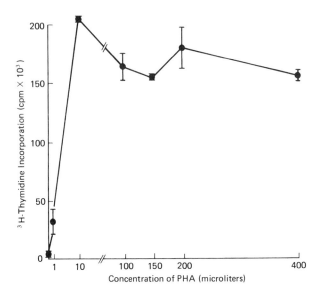

Fig. 14-10 Effect of PHA concentration on tritiated thymidine incorporation. 1.5×10^6 splenic leukocytes were incubated with varying amounts of PHA in ACM supplemented with toad serum. After 3 days, cultures were pulsed with 1.5 Ci of tritiated thymidine for 16 hr. The points plotted represent means S.D. of counts from duplicate tubes. (*From*: Goldshein & Cohen, *J. Immunol.*, **108**: 1025, 1972.)

cells with an approximate 1:1:2 ratio of unlabeled blasts to labeled blasts to unlabeled small lymphocytes. According to Goldshein and Cohen (1970):

> [*as all lymphocytes from vertebrates respond to PHA*], *it would seem that during the evolution of immunologic competence and regardless of the complexity and diversity of lymphoid tissue, the proliferative ability of the small lymphocyte appears early. Since mammalian lymphocyte transformation in the MLC probably involves the interaction of histocompatibility antigens with appropriate receptor sites, such sites probably evolved at least as early as anuran amphibians.*

Density Profiles of AFC

It is common to classify populations of lymphocytes by conventional morphological and functional methods. However, a finer delineation is possible by subdividing lymphocytes with respect to their distribution according to density. In one such attempt, Kraft et al. (1971) gave adult toads (*Bufo marinus*) a single, intraperitoneal injection of polymerized flagellin protein (POL). Cells from spleens were dissociated and counted with a Coulter counter equipped with a particle distribution analyser or were dispersed in plasma albumin density gradients. The results obtained are expressed as a density distribution fraction that relates total cells (or total AFC) per density increment to fraction density. The number of AFC in the early response stages are relatively homogeneous and confined to light density regions. Later, AFC are found in more dense regions (Figs. 14-11 and 14-12).

This gradual increase in toad lymphocyte complexity, from a light, single density region to a progressively more dense one, suggests a correlation between cell density

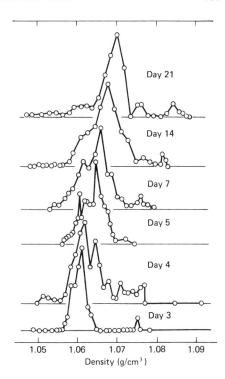

Fig. 14-11 Changes in toad spleen AFC density distribution during the course of the response to POL. Cells from six spleens, comprising approximately 6×10^6 lymphoid cells, were used for each experiment. Each point was repeated 2-6 times, with little variation in the basic patter. Typical profiles are presented. All curves are normalized to the same peak height, regardless of absolute AFC numbers in fractions. (*From*: Kraft & Shortman, *J. Cell. Biol.*, **52**: 438, 1972.)

Day 21
Day 14
Day 7
Day 5
Day 4
Day 3

1.05   1.06   1.07   1.08   1.09
Density (g/cm³)

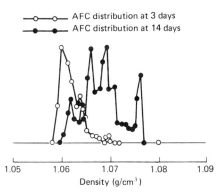

——○——○—— AFC distribution at 3 days
——●——●—— AFC distribution at 14 days

Fig. 14-12 Higher resolution comparison of toad spleen AFC density distribution profiles 3 and 14 days post-POL stimulation. Conditions are as in Fig. 14-11, except that the analysis involved more points in gradients encompassing a narrower density range. (*From*: Kraft & Shortman, *J. Cell. Biol.*, **52**: 438, 1972.)

1.05   1.06   1.07   1.08   1.09
Density (g/cm³)

and stage of immunocyte maturation. Thus separation of toad cells by density is an excellent model for investigating AFC differentiation. If density heterogeneity reflects a complex differentiation sequence in the toad, the latter may in part be simpler than it is in mammals such as the rat, since toad cells only produce IgM AFC. In the toad there is a trend for AFC to settle out toward the dense end as the response develops. The toad response may be more synchronized, since most of the AFC at day 5 are progeny of cells observed at day 3.

A second physical parameter for showing AFC differentiation is cell size. Cell size is demonstrable by using sedimentation velocity separation (Kraft and Shortman 1972). In *Bufo marinus*, AFC found early in the response (10–14μ diameter) are usually much larger than typical spleen small lymphocytes (6–8μ diameter). Differences in size distribution are broad in contrast to the narrower differences in density distribution. During the response, the AFC population exhibits a continuous shift towards a smaller size. Finally many AFC are equal to spleen small lymphocytes (6–8μ diameter) in size.

There are several advantages in using cell size measurements to monitor AFC development. First, it is possible to obtain pure preparations of immature AFC, which differ more in size than in density from most spleen lymphocytes. Second, size yields a higher degree of selection between dividing and nondividing AFC, since early in the response there is a broad range in size. This extends from large to small cell, suggesting that stages in the differentiation pathway involve a series of halving divisions without intermediate growth. This important information approaches the source and mechanism of differentiation of immune cells from preexistent blast cells capable of division or from nondividing small lymphocytes.

Cell Cooperation in the Newt

At least two cell types cooperate in mammals and birds to effect immunity: the thymus-derived *T* cell and the bursa, or bone marrow-derived, *B* cell. Ruben et al.

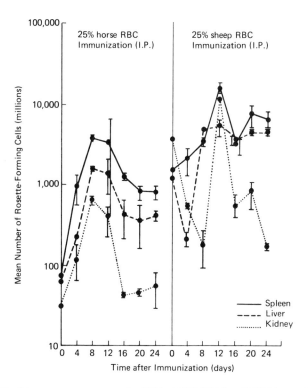

Fig. 14-13 Primary response curves after 0.25 ml, 25% HRBC and SRBC immunization (ip). Each point represents the average number of rosette-forming cells/10[6] in 2-4 aliquots of cells pooled from spleen, liver and kidney of 4-6 adult newts. (*From*: Ruben, et al., *Cell. Immunol.*, **6**: 300, 1973.)

(1973) recently tried to determine whether two or more cooperating cell populations in the newt respond to haptens when heterologous erthrocytes are used as carriers (Fig. 14-13). Cellular cooperation is determined in the newt by its response to the hapten trinitrophenol (TNP) coupled to chicken (CRBC) or toad (TRBC) erythrocytes, using the rosette assay test.

Enhancement of the hapten response occurs by carrier preimmunization. Newts injected with TNP-CRBC and assayed eight days later exhibit no TNP-specific RFC. When CRBC are injected four days prior to the TNP-CRBC injection, however, 1000 RFC/10^6 specific for the hapten are generated in the spleen; 350 TNP-RFC /10^6 in the liver; and 250 TNP-RFC /10^6 in the kidney. Similar results are obtained after preimmunization with toad cells, followed by TNP-TRBC. Apparently no hapten-specific RFC are produced when the immunogen used to preimmunize differs from that used as the TNP-carrier in the second challenge. Ruben et al. believe that two cell populations must interact in the newt: one specific for the carrier, which in turn assists the other in generating the antihapten response. These findings suggest that cellular cooperation probably exists at the evolutionary level of the amphibians.

Reptiles
The turtle

Maturation of immune competence in the turtle occurs several months after hatching. The immunological competence of spleens from the snapping turtle, *Chelydra serpentina*, has been studied successfully *in vitro*. Spleen fragments exposed to sheep (SRBC) and mouse (MRBC) produce agglutinins. Cultures stimulated with SRBC are always negative to MRBC, and those that are positive to MRBC are unable to agglutinate. Thus the response is specific. In addition, adult turtle spleen cells can elicit splenomegaly or hepatomegaly *in vitro*, suggesting a graft-vs.-host reaction (Sidky and Auerbach 1968).

The Lizard

There is relatively much information on the pattern of immunological maturation in mammals and birds, but the facts are not clearly defined for poikilothermic vertebrates, particularly reptiles. Kanakambika and Muthukkaruppan (1972a,b) provide an important glimpse into the immune capacity of the lizard *Calotes versicolor*. This is a garden lizard whose eggs can be readily obtained and incubated in the laboratory. The hatchlings are easily immunized by a single intraperitoneal injection of 25% SRBC; PFC are analyzed using modification of the original Jerne technique. The spleen of one-day-old lizards is oval and reddish and about 0.5 mm in length; it contains approximately 8×10^5 leukocytes. Lymphocytes are arranged uniformly but not into definite follicles. Leukocyte suspensions from immunized lizards of all ages mixed with SRBC and complement derived from *Calotes* serum contain significant numbers of PFC at all ages, ranging from 25–2186 PFC/10^6 leukocytes. The response is specific, since no anti-SRBC activity is demonstrable to rat erythrocytes.

Using essentially the same approach as in the hatchling, the PFC response is easily demonstrated in adults. After immunization, splenic vascularity increases, and dense lymphocyte accumulations characteristic of the darkly stained areas are reduced.

Mitotic figures become more frequent, especially in lightly stained areas. The most striking feature is the profuse development of blood spaces after antigenic stimulation, which may represent a reaction peculiar to lizards. Background counts range from 0–8.0 PFC/10^6 leukocytes/spleen from unimmunized lizards. Thus, all adults with 10 PFC/10^6 leukocytes are considered positive responders. Prior to testing, it is necessary to heat-inactivate the thermolabile lysin to SRBC found in fresh serum at titers up to 1:16. By the seventh day, PFC are readily obvious in most spleens; they peak at fourteen days and are followed by a slow decline. Antibody is detectable in the serum after fourteen days, reaching a maximum level of 1:1600 for hemolysins and 1:80 for hemagglutinins at twenty-one days, followed by a decline. At forty days after a primary immunization, the secondary antibody is 2-ME sensitive, indicating that it is the universal vertebrate IgM type. At fourteen days there are no plaques in the thymus, bone marrow, cloacal complex, lung, liver, or kidney. However, blood leukocytes from immunized lizards produce clear plaques like those in spleens. Obviously the information gained from studying antibody-forming cells in reptiles is highly relevant to phylogeny because of their taxonomic position.

Birds
  Diverse approaches

Apparently all animal immunocytes, including those from invertebrates, possess the capacity to respond to mitogens. In representative mammals, lymphocytes derived from the peripheral blood or thoracic duct show rapid increases in RNA and protein synthesis during the first hours after exposure to PHA. By contrast, increase in DNA synthesis occurs, but with a delay of twenty-four hours or more. The work of Alm (in press) with birds has been important. Using conventional procedures he isolated lymphocytes from spleens of unoperated but irradiated chickens (Cx) and bursectomized, irradiated (Bx) chickens whose bursa of Fabricius was surgically removed at hatching. At various times after the addition of PHA from 0–48 hours, incorporation of H^3 thymidine, H^3 uridine, and H^3 leucine in each culture is determined.

In general the rate of incorporation of H^3 uridine into RNA and H^3 leucine into protein accelerates during the first four hours after the addition of PHA, with a linear increase in twenty-four to thirty-six hours. The rate of increase of PHA-induced RNA synthesis is significantly higher for Bx chickens, suggesting that among the lymphoid cells there are proportionally more PHA reactive cells. Increases in H^3 thymidine incorporation into DNA begin at sixteen hours. Apparently the bursa does not significantly affect those cells that are sensitive to PHA.

As in other vertebrates, the periarteriolar lymphoid sheaths in the spleen are termed thymus-dependent regions, since lymphoid cells are depleted after thymectomy and antigen induces hyperplastic changes. Large pyroninophilic lymphoid cells appear and proliferate in the periarteriolar lymphoid sheaths within twenty-four hours after immunization with SRBC. During the ensuing three to four days, cell proliferation extends into the red pulp. Antibody-forming plasmablasts and mature plasma cells appear. On day 4, germinal center formation becomes prominent. Therefore, germinal center and plasma cell development in chickens seems to be independent of the bursa of Fabricius.

In chickens, antigen-stimulation of both thymus- (T) and bursa- (B) dependent cells leads to the concomitant production of a lymphocyte mitogenic factor. Thymectomy abolishes lymphocyte stimulation by both the antigen PPD (purified protein derivative) and the phytomitogen PHA. Bursectomy significantly reduces lymphocyte responses to PPD, but lymphocyte stimulation to both PPD and PHA remains significantly higher than in thymectomized birds. Thus, the lymphocyte mitogenic factor can be generated in the complete absence of the bursal system but is abolished by total thymectomy. Mitogenic factors may mediate lymphocyte transformations in birds and may regulate and facilitate interactions between T cells and B cells during immunological responses.

Surface-bound antibody on lymphoid cells renders them capable of binding antigen such as SRBC to form rosettes. RFC can be inhibited by reaction with anti-θ antiserum; theta (θ), an antigen in mice peculiar to thymocytes, is thymus-dependent and may be restricted to RFC. In birds, because antibody-producing cells are bursaldependent and are thought to be the sole carriers of surface immunoglobulin, the precise origin of so-called thymus-derived RFC is questionable. To study such a problem in birds is less complicated than it is in mammals, since the organs of the immune system are structurally and functionally divisible. After bursectomy of 17-day-old chick embryos (Hemmingsson and Alm, 1972) found that a significant proportion of RFC and PFC are absent suggesting, in chickens, that RFC are bursadependent. Despite several other interpretations, RFC may differentiate in the bursa microenvironment under the influence of a thymic hormone; alternatively RFC or their precursors may differentiate thymic characteristics.

The spleen and accessory spleen of chickens readily form PFC after intravenous injections of SRBC. In previously splenectomized birds, PFC are demonstrable in small regenerated splenules. Keily and Abramoff (1969) found that the chicken spleen, like the spleens of other vertebrates, is highly vascular and, in fact, difficult to remove without invariably spilling some of the spleen cells during dissection. Such cells form splenules of varying sizes that are fully capable of showing immune responses. These same splenectomized birds do not have an impaired capacity to reject skin allografts, suggesting an absence of T cells that participate in cell-mediated immune responses. By contrast, the caecal tonsil, the lacrimal gland, and the gland of Harder are negative for PFC. Because of the location of the latter two organs, topical inoculation of antigen into the eye orbit by dropping SRBC onto the eyeball stimulates the production of PFC in the Harderian gland and the spleen. These avian lymphoid foci in the oculonasal region are important components of the chicken's immune system.

Examination of the Bursa of Fabricius by Fluorescein

In addition to these diverse approaches utilizing cells, there is an excellent technique developed by Coons (1956), which easily localizes the presence of antibodyproducing cells within an organ. The fluorescent antibody technique detects specific antibodies in tissues by means of a fluorescent dye conjugated to a soluble protein antigen. Tissue sections thought to contain antibody-producing cells treated with the antigen-dye conjugate, when examined with a fluorescent microscope, will fluoresce and therefore reveal the presence of specific antibodies. After immunizing the ringnecked pheasant *Phasianus colchicus* with bovine gamma globulin and the fluorescent dye 5-dimethylamino-10 naphthalene sulfonyl chloride, the bursa of Fabricius is removed, frozen in isopentane, and stored in a deep freeze at $-45°C$. Examination of tissue sections shows fluorescing cell groups or clones in triple inoculated birds; the response is more intense in twice-inoculated birds. This observation, made early in the 1960s, was important in defining a function of the avian bursa of Fabricius.

MAMMALS

Marsupials
Opossum

The opossum is a primitive metatherian mammal that bears extrauterine embryos. Because of its position in the mammalian taxonomic scheme, it is useful in determining immune response events, especially from the developmental viewpoint. Its immune response is considered more primitive than that of higher eutherian mammals; e.g., it apparently has only two immunoglobulin classes analogous to IgM and IgG and also weaker effector ends for delayed hypersensitivity. Antigen clearance rates (*Serratia marcescens*) by pouch young up to ten weeks of age is significantly lower than those of the adults. The adult condition is reached by twelve weeks. Phagocytosis is confined primarily to macrophages in the liver, lungs, and spleen.

Peak PFC in adult opossum spleens occur on the seventh day. In younger seventy-day-old opossums, PFC to SRBC are absent, nor are their antibody-producing cells to BSA demonstrable from spleens by a standard immunofluorescent sandwich technique. When compared to mice, such low numbers of PFC may reflect the lower cell density of the opossum spleen producing a proportionally lower percentage of immunocompetent cells capable of responding to SRBC stimulation. The opossum seems to react more slowly immunologically apparently because of deficient central and efferent limbs of the immune response; the afferent limb seems comparable to higher mammals.

Quokka

The quokka (*Setonix brachyurus*) is a marsupial mammal from Western Australia, interesting because it has a superficial and a thoracic thymus. Blood leukocytes from the normal quokka, thymectomized quokka, and thymectomized quokka replanted with superficial thymus grafts from another marsupial, the tammar (*Macropus eugenii*) provide interesting and comparable *in vitro* information to that of other vertebrates relative to cytotoxicity, PHA stimulation and mixed leukocyte reactions (Ashman et al. 1972). When mixed together with immune serum, leukocytes in the presence of complement will lyse, die, and take up eosin, a red stain. After an appropriate incubation period, it is possible to determine the extent of cytotoxic antibodies directed against the cells. Sera from thymectomized quokkas previously grafted with xenogeneic tammar thymus grafts, or from intact or thymectomized controls tested against both allogeneic tammar leukocytes and leukocytes from the donor animal, show no cytotoxic antibodies. PHA stimulates T lymphocytes, resulting in increased incorporation of H^3 thymidine. Quokka leukocytes produce a dose response curve to PHA similar to that of man and the mouse. In neonatally thymectomized quokkas, PHA-sensitive cells in the peripheral blood circulation are found to be reduced somewhat in numbers when the quokkas are tested after permanently emerging from the pouch. With regard to mixed lymphocyte cultures, assuming antigenic differences, quokka and tammar cells will stimulate each other and cause increased incorporation of H^3-thymidine into DNA. Thymectomy causes a 50% reduction in lymphocyte reactivity in the "one-way" leukocyte stimulation test; this is reduced still further by 20% in thymectomized quokkas that receive tammar thymus; a xenogeneic implant does not reconstitute the loss created by the absent thymus.

Apparently quokka immune responses share characteristics with equally primitive marsupials as well as with more advanced, eutherian mammals. Effective sensitization to produce a skin response to 2, 4-dinitrofluorobenzene (DNFB) compares very favorably with the dose employed for rabbits, but it is considerably more vigorous than that required to sensitize guinea pigs, marmosets, and monkeys. Quokkas do respond by giving delayed-type hypersensitivity, but because a vigorous regime is necessary, this suggests a weaker immune response; it usually requires intradermal injection of DNFB emulsified in olive oil, just as in the North American opossum, *Didelphys virginiana*. That removal of both the superficial and the thoracic thymus fails to induce an early "wasting syndrome," and the normal rejection of skin allografts in juvenile quokkas (Ashman and his colleagues) is at variance with findings in murine systems and indeed all other vertebrates. It supports, however, the interpretation of Morris (1973), who used fetal lambs, that thymectomy does not affect cellular responses. Such responses are not without precedent, for fetal human thymocytes can show mixed lymphocyte reaction evidenced by increased uptake of thymidine. Thus, fetal thymocytes as young as thirteen weeks can initiate certain cellular immune reactions. Essentially, then, newborn quokkas are like fetuses from advanced eutherian mammals. The precise nature of the response to allografts in thymectomized quokkas must therefore remain controversial. Although marsupial responses by comparison are weaker, they do undoubtedly possess respectable immune systems.

Nude Mice

The thymus remained an enigmatic organ despite the facts attributed to it by the prescience of early comparative immunologists like Beard. Its function, so crucial to the immune response of vertebrates, only began to be appreciated in the early 1960s with Miller's pioneering works (Miller, 1961). Recently, though, another advantageous approach to deciphering thymus physiology besides removing it is its natural condition in the nude mouse. Mice homozygous for the mutation *nude* (nu/nu) lack recognizable thymus tissue and seem depleted of thymus-derived T lymphocytes by both functional and histological criteria (Kindred 1971, Mitchell et al. 1972). Nude mice are unable to show various *T*-cell dependent immune responses such as allograft rejection, reactivity to phytohemagglutinin (PHA), and the proliferative response to *Hemophilus pertussis*. Furthermore, antibody production to a thymus-dependent antigen such as SRBC is reduced. B cells are independent and provide an interesting approach to another parameter of the nude mouse. Feldman et al. (1972) finds a normal antibody response to dinitrophenylated polymeric flagellin, an antigen that elicits normal responses in the absence of T lymphocytes; in other words, it is a T-independent antigen. By contrast, a T-dependent antigen, SRBC, elicits no response; this could be restored, however, by introducing a population of pure T lymphocytes. *In vitro* cell-mediated immune responses, i.e., spleen cells from nude mice, yield no cytotoxic response, a T cell reaction. Spleens from nude mice are thought to be devoid of T lymphocytes but possess B cells capable of producing normal IgM antibody.

Placental Mammals—Antibody Producing Cells in Diffusion Chambers

Several phases of the antibody synthetic response are easily demonstrable by growing lymphoid cells in cell-tight diffusion chambers. These chambers are constructed of filter membranes on either side of a donut-shaped disc that allows easy entrance and egress of molecules, but not cells. Using diffusion chambers, Urso and Makinodan (1964) found a linear $\log_2$ relation between antibody titer and nucleated cell number.

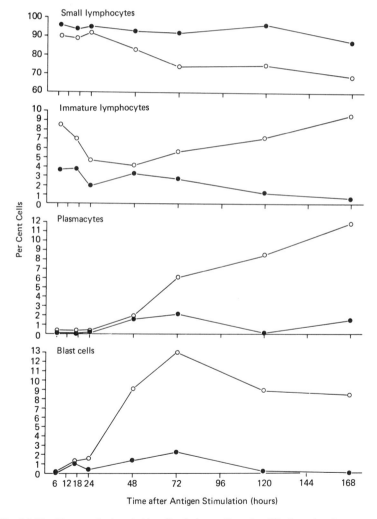

Fig. 14-14 Changes in lymphoid cells during culture in diffusion chambers. ○, experimental; ●, control. Each point represents the mean of two to five determinations from 6 to 120 hr. One determination was made at 168 hr. (*From*: Urso & Makinodan, *J. Immunol.*, **90**: 897, 1963.)

Lymphoid cells are monitored beginning six hours after antigenic stimulation with BSA (Fig. 14-14). Blast cells begin to increase shortly after the first day, reach a peak on the third day, and then decrease slightly. The number of plasma cells begins to rise one day later and continues to rise up to the seventh day. Immature lymphocytes resembling plasmatocytes increase from the second to the seventh days, and small lymphocytes decrease after the first twenty-four hours through the third day and remain low through the seventh day.

Cell changes correlate with antibody synthesis. Antibody is first detectable in the chamber fluid on the third day after antigenic stimulation (Fig. 14-15). Later the antibody titer rises logarithmically to a peak on about the seventh day. A similar curve is obtained when the percentage of antibody-containing cells is determined.

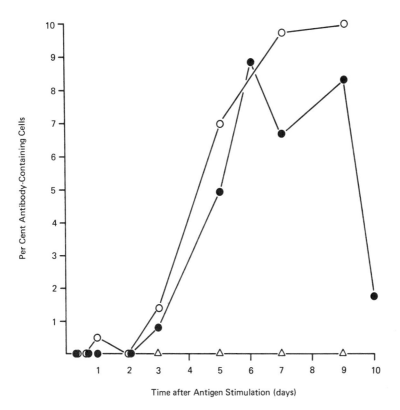

Fig. 14-15 Antibody production by lymphoid cells cultured in diffusion chambers. ○, experimental titer; △, control titer; ●, antibody containing cells. Each point after the first day represents the mean of 4 to 13 determinations. First-day points based on 1 to 2 determinations. (*From*: Urso & Makinodan, *J. Immunol.*, **90**: 897, 1963.)

Antibody-containing cells are first detected on the third day, and their numbers rise logarithmically to a peak about a week after antigenic stimulation. At this time there is a corresponding increase in the number of competent cells containing diffusely distributed antibodies in the cytoplasm. The relative number increases from a low of about 50% on day 3 to a high of 100% on day 6. Using methyl-green pyronin

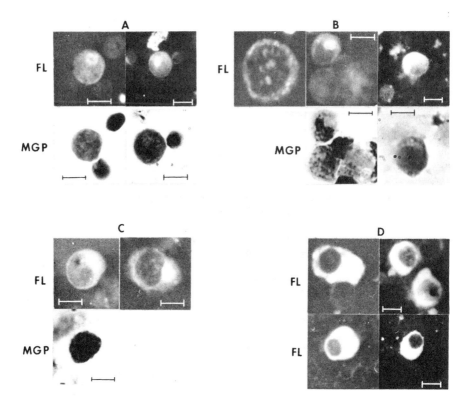

Fig. 14-16 Changes in antibody containing cells found in diffusion chambers at various intervals after antigenic (bovine albumin (BSA) stimulation (×550). FL refers to cells stained for antibody by fluorescent anti-BSA. MGP refers to the same fluorescent cells subsequently stained with methyl green-pyronin. The bright areas in the cell indicate antibody. (A) 3 days after antigen; note the island in the nucleus containing antibody and the same island after MGP staining; (B) 3 to 5 days after antigen; note the island containing antibody partly in the nucleus and cytoplasm, and the antibody as nuclear rods (or dots); (C) 3 to 7 days after antigen: note the island containing antibody in the cytoplasm; (D) 7 to 9 days after antigen; note the antibody in islands or diffused throughout the cytoplasm, and also as nuclear rods (or dots). Scale marker, 5μ. Identical numbers indicate identical cells. (*From*: Urso & Makinodan, *J. Immunol.*, **90**: 897, 1963.)

stain, it has been found that discrete antibody-positive islands are clear and the position of a nuclear island coincides with that of the nucleolus (Fig. 14-16).

Cell division is crucial to antibody synthesis, as can be revealed by the uptake of H^3 thymidine (H^3T), the mitotic index, and mean dividing time during the log and stationary phases following antigenic stimulation. In Fig. 14-17, when preimmunized cells are cultured with BSA antigen and exposed to H^3T on day 2, the percentage of labelled cells increases about four-fold within a day. By contrast, when cells of the control group, preimmunized cells cultured without BSA, are exposed to H^3T on day 2, a four-fold increase in percentage of labelled cells requires about two days. Thus, the dividing time of cells stimulated with a soluble antigen in the log phase of activity is about twelve hours, and twenty-four hours in the absence of antigenic stimulation. However, if cells are exposed to H^3T at the onset of the stationary phase (day 5 after

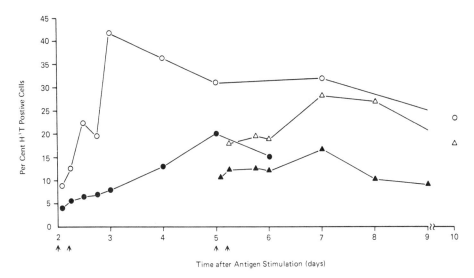

Fig. 14-17 H³T uptake by lymphoid cells as a function of time after culturing in diffusion chambers. ○, △, preimmunized cells cultured with bovine serum albumin antigen (BSA); ●, ▲, preimmunized cells cultured without BSA. Arrows pointing to the abscissa indicate the times cells were exposed to H³T (10 c/exposure). Each point represents one to two determinations. (*From*: Urso & Makinodan, *J. Immunol.*, **90**: 897, 1963.)

antigenic stimulation), the division time is estimated at approximately twenty-four hours. Thus competent cells divide at a high rate with a characteristically shorter division time during the latent and log phases.

Most, if not all, of the antibody-containing cells in the stationary phase of activity are descendants of immature cells that arise by somatic division. To test this, both the experimental and control groups are exposed to H³T four times at fifteen- to twenty-four-hour intervals beginning on day 3 after antigenic stimulation (Fig. 14-18). The frequency of cellular division among competent cells is about twice as high than that of the total cell population in the experimental group and about four times higher than that of controls. Some of these cells are shown in Fig. 14-19 after staining with the immunofluorescent reagent, followed by autoradiographic treatment and giemsa stain.

To verify that cells are dividing it is necessary to treat them with colchicine, which arrests them in the metaphase stage of mitosis. Colchicine treatment on days 5, 6, and 7 reveals that the mitotic index is always higher (three to five times) in both experimental and control groups than among cells without colchicine. Figure 14-20 shows some representative cells in mitosis. The first two cells received no colchicine, but the latter four did. The chromosomes that are clearly visible in the fluorescent cytoplasmic background stain green after application of methyl green, a stain specific for DNA.

Before the advent of *in vitro* procedures, it was known that antigens stimulated lymphoid cells to divide *in vivo*. From this information we knew that division is necessary if lymphocytes are to show memory. The ability to culture cells has made available valuable quantitative information pertinent to various stages of the immune response.

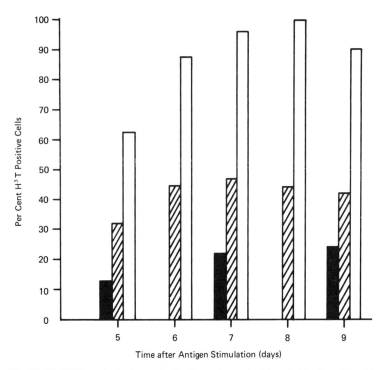

Fig. 14-18 H³T uptake by immunized and non-immunized lymphoid cells cultured in diffusion chambers. □ antibody-containing cells; ▨, experimental (immunized) cells; ■, control (non-immunized) cells. (*From*: Urso & Makinodan, *J. Immunol.*, **90**: 897, 1963.)

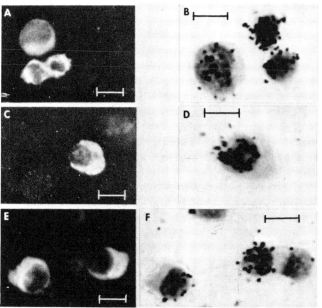

Fig. 14-19 Antibody-containing cells labeled with H³T in diffusion chambers (×*750*). A, C, E show cells stained for antibody in the cytoplasm, and B, D, F the same cells after autoradiography and staining with Giemsa. Note the grains of H³T in the nuclei. A, B, 6 days; C, D, 7 days; E, F, 8 days after antigen stimulation. Scale marker, 5μ. Identical numbers indicate identical cells. (*From*: Urso & Makinodan, *J. Immunol.*, **90**: 897, 1963.)

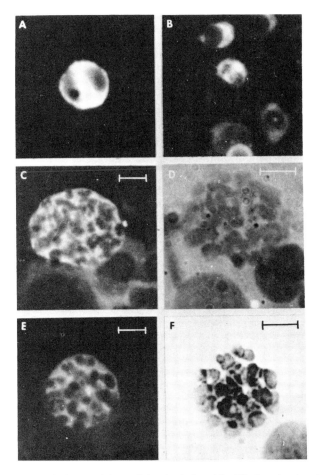

Fig. 14-20 Antibody-containing cells in mitosis found in diffusion chambers (×770). A, B, Antibody-containing cells without colchicine treatment in anaphase or telophase; C, E, Antibody-containing cells after colchicine treatment. Note the typical chromosomes in a fluorescent cytoplasmic background. D, F, the same cells shown in C and E after staining with methyl green. Scale marker, 5μ. (*From*: Urso & Makinodan, *J. Immunol.*, **90**: 897, 1963.)

Immunologically competent cells duplicate vigorously by somatic division at the onset of immunologic activity. The latent phase occurs during the first forty-eight hours and the log phase commences on the third day, reaching a stationary phase a week after antigenic stimulation. There is a direct relationship between antibody titer of the chamber fluid and the percentage of antibody-containing cells during the first week after antigenic stimulation. The mitotic index begins to rise one day after antigenic stimulation and reaches a peak on day 3. Before the stationary phase, competent cells divide at a frequency significantly higher than that of incompetent cells. Thus, all competent cells in the stationary phase are descendants of immature cells that have arisen by somatic division, a necessary feature of immune reactivity.

SUMMARY

Among the bony fishes, the thymus, the pronephros, and the spleen are major sites for the generation of plaque-forming and rosette-forming cells (PFC, RFC) that synthesize IgM immunoglobulin. Thymocytes of fishes and larval amphibians show IgM antibodies first, prior to their appearance in the spleen. In addition to the previously-mentioned tests, which demonstrate antibody synthesis and cells bearing surface antibody, lymphocytes can be maintained in culture for other tests. If challenged with mitogens such as PHA and LPS, T and B lymphocytes are stimulated much as they would be after antigenic challenge during normal immune responses. Similarly, when allogeneic lymphocytes are mixed in culture, they transform to blast cells capable of division, a necessary attribute if lymphocytes are to generate others capable of memory. The *in vitro* situation is extremely useful and the results are proving to be remarkably consistent throughout the phylogenetic scale. From what happens to immune cells *in vitro*, we can predict what may occur in the whole organism.

BIBLIOGRAPHY

Alm, G. V. *In vitro* studies of chicken lymphoid cells. I. Phytohemagglutinin-induced DNA, RNA and protein synthesis in spleen cells from control-irradiated and bursecto-mized-irradiated chickens. Acta Path. Microbiol. Scand. (in press).

———. The *in vivo* spleen response to sheep erythrocytes in bursectomized irradiated chickens. Acta Path. Microbiol. Scand. (in press).

Ashman, R., Keast, D., Stanley, N. F., and Waring, H. 1972. The *in vitro* response to phytohemagglutinin (PHA) of leucocytes from intact and thymectomized quokkas. Aus. J. Exp. Biol. Med. Sci. **50**: 337.

Chiller, J. M., Hodgins, H. O., Chambers, V. C., and Weiser, R. S. 1969a. Antibody response in rainbow trout (*Salmo gairdneri*). I. Immunocompetent cells in the spleen and anterior kidney. J. Immunol. **102**: 1193.

Chiller, J. M., Hodgins, H. O., and Weiser, R. S. 1969b. Antibody response in rainbow trout (*Salmo gairdneri*). II. Studies on the kinetics of development of antibody-producing cells and on complement and natural hemolysin. J. Immunol. **102**: 1202.

Coons, A. H. 1956. Histochemistry with labeled antibody. Inter. Rev. Cytology **5**: 1.

Cooper, A. J. 1971. Ammocoete lymphoid cell populations *in vitro*. In *Fourth Leukocyte Culture Conference*, ed. O. R. McIntyre, pp. 137–146. New York: Appleton-Century-Crofts.

Diener, E., and Marchalonis, J. 1970. Cellular and humoral aspects of the primary immune response of the toad, *Bufo marinus*. Immunol. **18**: 279.

Du Pasquier, L. 1965a. Recherches sur les aspects cellulaires et humoraux de l'intolérance aux homogreffes chez le têtard d'*Alytes obstetricans*. Thèses 3-éme Cycle Enseigne-ment supérieur, No 336 Bordeaux.

———. 1965b. Aspects cellulaires et humoraux de l'intolérance aux homogreffes chez le tetard d'*Alytes obstetricans*. Role du thymus. C. R. Acad. Sci. (Paris) D 261 1144.

———. 1968. Les protéines sériques et le complexe lymphomyèloïde chez le tetard d'*Alytes obstetricans* normal et thymectomisé. Ann. Inst. Pasteur **114**: 490.

———. 1970a. L'acquisition de la compétence immunologique chez les vertébrés. Etude chez la larve du crapaud accoucheur *Alytes obstetricans*. Thèses Doctorat ès Sciences, Université de Bordeaux No 290.

————. 1970b. Immunologic competence of lymphoid cells in young amphibian larvae. Transplant. Proc. **2**: 293.

Feldman, M., Wagner, H., Basten, A., and Holmes, M. 1972. Humoral and cell-mediated responses *in vitro* of spleen cells from mice with thymic aplasia (nude mice). AJEBAK **50**: 651.

Goldshein, S. J., and Cohen, N. 1972. Phylogeny of immunocompetent cells. I. *In vitro* blastogenesis and mitosis of toad (*Bufo marinus*) splenic lymphocyte in response to phytohemagglutinin and in mixed lymphocyte culture. J. Immunol. **108**: 1025.

Hemmingsson, E. J., and Alm, G. V. 1972. The effect of embryonic bursectomy on the rosette-forming cell in the chicken. Eu. J. Immunol. **2**: 380.

Kanakambika, P., and Muthukkaruppan, V. R. 1972a. The immune response to sheep erythrocytes in the lizard, *Calotes versicolor*. J. Immunol. **109**: 415.

————. 1972b. Immunological competence in the newly hatched lizard, *Calotes versicolor*. Proc. Soc. Exptl. Biol. Med. **140**: 21.

Keily, D., and Abramoff, P. 1969. Studies of the chicken immune response. III. Cellular and humoral antibody production in the splenectomized chicken. J. Immunol. **102**: 1058.

Kindred, B. 1971. Immunological unresponsiveness of genetically thymusless (nude) mice. Europ. J. Immunol. **1**: 59.

Kraft, N., and Shortman, K. 1972. Differentiation of antibody-forming cells in toad spleen. A study using density and sedimentation velocity cell separation. J. Cell Biol. **52**: 438.

Kraft, N., Shortman, K., and Marchalonis, J., 1971. Density distribution analysis of a primary antibody-forming cell response. Immunology **20**: 919.

Miller, J. F. A.P. 1961. Immunological function of the thymus. Lancet **2**: 748.

Mitchell, J., Pye, J., Holmes, M. C., and Nossal, G. J. V. 1972. Antigens in immunity. The localization of antigen by congenitally athymic (nude) mice. Aust. J. Exp. Biol. Med. Sci., **50**: 637.

Morris, B. 1973. Effect of thymectomy on immunological responses in the sheep. In *Contemporary Topics in Immunobiology*, eds. A. J. S. Davies and R. L. Carter, II, 39–62.

Ortiz-Muniz, G. and Sigel, M. M. 1971. Antibody synthesis in lymphoid organs of two marine teleosts. J. Ret. Soc. **9**: 42.

Ruben, L. N., van der Hoven, A., and Dutton, R. W. 1973. Cellular cooperation in hapten-carrier responses in the newt, *Triturus viridescens*. Cell. Immunol. **6**: 300.

Sidky, Y. A., and Auerbach, R. 1968. Tissue culture analysis of immunological capacity of snapping turtles. J. Exptl. Zool. **167**: 187.

Smith, A. Mason, Potter, M., and Merchant, E. Bruce. 1967. Antibody-forming cells in the pronephros of the teleost, *Lepomis macrochirus*. J. Immun. **99**: 876.

Urso, P., and Makinodan, T. 1963. The roles of cellular division and maturation in the formation of precipitating antibody. J. Immunol. **90**: 897.

Chapter 15

Immunosuppression

IMMUNOSUPPRESSION

The process of suppressing the immune response is of interest for several reasons. By suppressing immunity one effectively abrogates the response. In clinical situations that involve transplants, it is advantageous to abrogate partially or even permanently the host's reaction to a foreign graft. Until an appropriate matching system for host-donor incompatibilities is discovered, the only tool remaining is to suppress the host's natural response, rendering it incapable of rejecting or reacting against an antigen. Unfortunately, at the same time this cripples the host, making it vulnerable to infection. Suppression by chemicals or irradiation is possible, but potentially dangerous. It is readily apparent how difficult it is to regulate and balance doses of the immunosuppressant with the host's immune system. Suppression is not to be confused with tolerance, a state of nonreactivity to an antigen that is induced by and is specific for a particular antigen. Suppression, by contrast, involves the use of some outside agent that bears no relationship to the antigen in order to inactivate the immune system.

Ways of suppressing the immune response may be divided into several categories: chemical, physical, and biologic, all of which act at certain strategic points in the immune response. The immune response can be suppressed by the use of a number of chemicals often used in cancer chemotherapy. Usually these compounds are grouped into several classes: corticosteroids, purine analogs, folic acid antagonists, and alkylating agents. Regardless of the chemical class, they all act by interrupting cell division and/or inhibition of RNA or DNA synthesis. Both RNA and DNA synthesis are essential to the immune response. A second major method of suppression is produced by the effects of ionizing irradiation. When experimenting, it is necessary to remember that various species respond differently to irradiation. In general, mammals and birds require relatively low doses of irradiation to significantly depress the immune system. Invertebrates, fishes, amphibians, and reptiles require higher doses of irradiation. A third way to suppress the immune response is by removing organs that generate immunologically competent cells. Such ablations involve thymectomy and bursectomy in birds, and thymectomy and splenectomy that can be performed in all vertebrates. The absence of each of these organs leads to predictable deficiencies in the immune response whose cause is ultimately referable to the ablated organ.

EFFECTS OF DRUGS, TEMPERATURE AND IRRADIATION IN POIKILOTHERMS

Metabolic Drug Antagonists in Fundulus Heteroclitus

Allograft rejection is one end result of immune cells having divided and synthesized nucleic acids and/or proteins. Drugs can be used to interfere with the production of these two important cell products, thereby altering the immune response capacity. If protein or nucleic acid synthesis is restricted antibody production is also inhibited, and the result is prolonged survival of tissue allografts. Scale transplantation in any teleost fish is especially useful in screening those compounds that delay allograft rejection. Fish are readily available, inexpensive, and the technique of grafting is simple, requiring only moderate skill, physical equipment, and facilities. As sterile conditions are not essential and protective dressings are unnecessary, fish are good subjects for laboratory experiments. Furthermore, numerous transplants, including autograft controls, may be performed on a single fish. The use of multiple donors minimizes the opportunities for weak reactions among genetically similar fish. Fish are thus useful in evaluating the effect of drugs on the allograft reaction.

Response to a foreign antigen in the adult fish, *Fundulus heteroclitus* cannot occur if antibody synthesis is selectively inactivated by drugs. Much evidence supports the efficacy of cortisone in suppressing allograft reactions. Without suppression, *Fundulus* rejects scale allografts maximally at three days. Daily intraperitoneal injections of a 1-mg suspension of cortisone acetate to grafted fish, beginning on the day of transplantation, has no effect on the survival of scale allografts. However, more potent preparations of cortical hormones are suppressive. Injections of 2 mg of 6-fluorohydrocortisone acetate on the day of transplantation and two days later result in longer allograft survival. About half of all the pigment cells then undergo fragmentation, the signal of graft rejection.

Likewise, 2 mg of delta-1-hydrocortisone sodium succinate has a distinct protective effect. Though no pigment cell breakdown occurs until the third day, incipient destruction begins on the fourth day, but disintegration is still not complete by the fifth day. Daily injections of 1 mg chloramphenicol sodium succinate have no detectable effect; however, 10 mg chloramphenicol results in survival of allograft pigment cells beyond the third day; all are usually destroyed by the sixth day. Finally, too, 0.1 mg injections of tetracycline hydrochloride have no protective effect, but larger doses such as 1 mg prolong survival of allografts. Thus, if the dose is large enough, antibiotics can interfere with the immunological response of host fish against foreign grafts.

The injection of substances that inhibit nucleic acid synthesis are successful in protecting scale allografts from the immune response of the host, but the doses are often toxic. When 1 mg of 5-fluorouracil is given daily, beginning on the day of operation, scale allografts show no signs of pigment cell breakdown, but many fish die after two to six days. Similarly, injections of 2 mg of 5-fluorodeoxyuridine (FUDR) result in protection of allografts up to eight days, but the fatality rate accompanying use of this drug is high.

Although near lethal doses of such drugs effectively prolong the survival time of allografts, no protection is given when the doses are reduced to 1/100 of the above

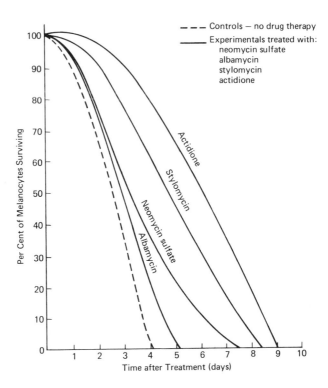

Fig. 15-1   The antibiotics albamycin and neomycin sulfate hardly affected the survival of allografts, but stylomycin and actidione prolonged the survival until the 8th and 9th days. (*Redrawn* from Cooper, *Transpl.*, **2**: 2, 1964.)

levels. Neomycin sulfate is toxic at 5 mg and slightly effective at 1 mg. Some melanocytes are still intact through the seventh day, while in control groups they are intact only until the fifth day. One mg of stylomycin is effective in prolonging graft survival. The survival end-point of control groups is four days, while for experimental groups it is eight days. The antibiotic actidione also prolongs allograft survival. At 0.001 mg it is not toxic, and grafts survive until the seventh day. At 0.01 mg, graft survival is prolonged until the ninth day, but there are a greater number of deaths. As is summarized in Fig. 15-1, each of these drugs can effectively be used to prolong allograft survival.

Temperature

Information regarding the effects of temperature on the immune response has been derived from experiments with poikilothermic vertebrates. All of their metabolic processes are strictly temperature-dependent, as their body temperatures at any given time are equivalent to that of their particular ambient environment. The mean survival time of scale transplants on the goldfish *Carassius auratus* changes as body temperature either decreases or increases. Hence, the lower the temperature, the longer the time required for the end-point of immune reactions to be reached. For example, at 28°C, the response is relatively abrupt. Incipient breakdown of melanocytes or other pigment cells is detectable two days after operation, and all are destroyed by the third day. By contrast allografts made at 21°C undergo no pigment cell disintegration until the fifth or sixth day after grafting. Those maintained at 14°C require fourteen to sixteen days to become disrupted, while those at 7°C remain intact for twenty-six days or more.

Effects of Drugs and Temperature on Immune Suppression in Goldfish

As in the killifish, *Fundulus heteroclitus*, allograft rejection in the goldfish *Carrasius auratus* is dependent on drug dosage (Levy 1963). For example, 5 mg/kg of mercaptopurine (MP) has practically no effect on the scale chromatophores; 10 mg/kg has a slight effect. Doses of 25 and 50 mg/kg delay allograft rejection significantly. Although blood flow occurs in 10% to 20% of the scales of fish treated with 25 or 50 mg/kg of 6-MP on the fifth day after transplantation, it does not occur in the scales of control fish beyond the second or third day after transplantation. Doses of 50 mg/kg or less of 6-MP are nontoxic and produce similar results, but higher doses usually kill the fish after seven days or more.

A dose-dependent response is also observed when fish are injected with hydrocortisone acetate. Though less than 25 mg/kg does not markedly affect allografts, larger doses delay rejection. It is interesting that pretreatment one or two days prior to transplantation does not alter the normal rejection pattern. Rejection is delayed only if the drugs are injected on the day of and on the days following transplantation. This suggests that the action of the drug is immediate, perhaps on those cells that recognize antigens.

When either 6-MP or hydrocortisone acetate is administered in 50 mg/kg doses on the day of transplantation, and 5 mg/kg of 6-MP or hydrocortisone acetate is given daily for fourteen days afterwards, allograft reaction is delayed. Clearly, goldfish, too, exhibit the behavior in which nearly lethal doses of certain drugs delay the allograft rejection response (Figs. 15-2 to 15-4).

Stutzman's work (1967) using imuran has shown that the median survival time (MST) of allografts at 16°C at a level of 50 mg/kg is about 17.4 days, but at 100 mg/kg, it is about 18.3 days. As the MST of grafts in control fish at this temperature is about 17.3 days, there is no significant difference between these results. At 26°C however, moderate but significant prolongation of graft survival can be seen; the MST of grafts in groups given 100 mg/kg is about 7.2 days, but only 5.1 days for control groups.

When 3.0 mg/kg methotrexate is administered at 3.0 mg/kg, the MST is about 16.9 days. At 26°C the MST is about 6.2 days. Comparison with control MSTs suggests that substantial prolongation of graft survival is not induced by this drug, but that there is a significant difference in the rate of allograft rejection as a consequence of temperature. Perhaps the most significant result of the methotrexate therapy is suppression of the inflammatory response without concomitant prolongation of graft survival. Consequently, it can be inferred from the immunosuppression data that is already known, that allograft rejection is mediated by multiple processes, one or more of which occurs independently.

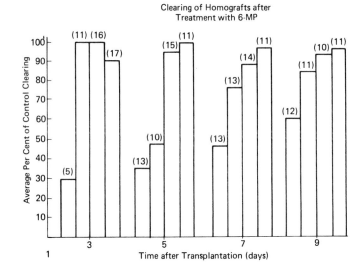

Clearing of Homografts after
Treatment with 6-MP

Average Per Cent of Control Clearing

Time after Transplantation (days)

1

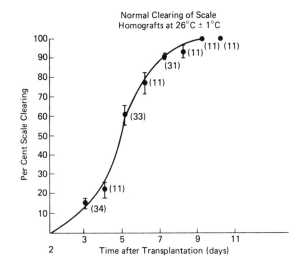

Normal Clearing of Scale
Homografts at 26°C ± 1°C

Per Cent Scale Clearing

Time after Transplantation (days)

2

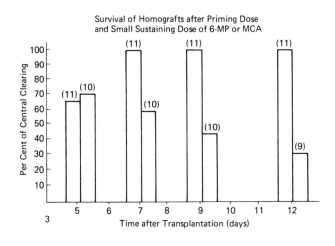

Survival of Homografts after Priming Dose
and Small Sustaining Dose of 6-MP or MCA

Per Cent of Central Clearing

Time after Transplantation (days)

3

Immunosuppression by Irradiation
  Fundulus heteroclitus

X-irradiation has been used to analyze the problem of allograft survival, the origin of cells responsible for allograft survival, the origin of cells responsible for allograft rejection, and the nature of the lymphomyeloid complex among poikilotherms. Irradiation dosage is an important factor (Fig. 15-5). When *x*-rays are admin-

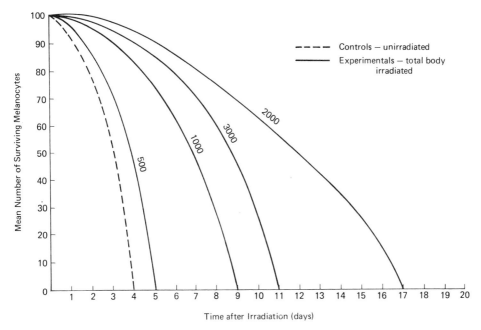

Fig. 15-5 Irradiation at 500r prolonged graft survival one day past controls; at 1000r grafts survived until the 9th day. At 2000–3000r the number of deaths increased, but at 2000r deaths were less and therefore graft survival was longer at 17 days. (*Redrawn* from Cooper, *Transpl.*, **2**: 2, 1964.)

istered at 500r six hours prior to scale grafting, allograft survival is extended by only one day. At 1000r allograft survival is prolonged only two days. Higher doses of 2000r to 3000r produce longer graft survival concomitant with an increase in the number of deaths. As can be seen, at 3000r most animals die before complete allograft rejection.

  Oryzias latipes

Irradiation has proven successful in studying transplantation immunity in *Oryzias latipes*, a small teleost fish native to Japan. Ugami and Kukita (1969) exchanged fin,

Fig. 15-2 Fish were injected i.p. with 6-MP dissolved in 0.05 N NaOH on day of transplant and on 3 successive days. Numbers in parentheses represent number of scales used for the average value.
Fig. 15-3 Dots and bars represent mean s.e.m. and parentheses the number of scales observed. Fish were injected on day of transplantation and on 3 successive days with 0.6% saline.
Fig. 15-4 Fish given 50 mg/kg of drug on day of transplant and 5 mg/kg every day during experiment. Numbers in parentheses indicate number of drug treated scales used for average. (*From*: Levy, *Proc. Soc. Exp. Biol. Med.*, **114**: 47, 1963.)

rather than scale, allografts between adult *Oryzias* and maintained them at several temperatures. Their findings suggest that allograft rejection is clearly inhibited if hosts are irradiated with 1000r immediately before transplantation. Moreover, the median survival time of fin allografts decreases as the interval between irradiation and transplantation is increased. By contrast, after transplantation, once the immunologic machinery is set into motion it is not easily disrupted by destructive irradiation. Irradiation at colder temperatures has fewer effects than it does at warmer temperatures. Though temperature is the ultimate influence on the immune response, irradiation interferes with the proliferative activities of lymphocytes in the spleen, thymus, and pronephros.

Anuran Amphibians

Total body irradiation halts the immune response in anuran amphibians. Bone marrow is capable of restoring transplantation immunity in frogs exposed to damaging irradiation, for it is a source of lymphocytes capable of reacting to tissue alloantigens. A source of autogeneic marrow is obtained by shielding the right hind limb in the center of a block of lead to allow negligible exposure to the irradiation treatment. The immunologic capacity can subsequently be tested by exchanging skin allografts five days post-irradiation. Normal frogs reject allografts at approximately fourteen days at 25°C. Frogs given total body irradiation begin to die seven days post-irradiation. The mean survival time is fifteen days, but grafts are intact at the last death. By contrast, graft survival in frogs given total body irradiation with one limb shielded is delayed by two days, and the death rate is lower than in the total body irradiated group (Cooper and Schaefer 1970).

The importance of bone marrow in transplantation immunity is further revealed by the effect of irradiation on the neutrophil level. The neutrophil level of control groups rises about two days post-irradiation from 15% to 70%, indicating the animal's susceptibility to infection. In a partially shielded group, the neutrophil levels rise only to an approximate 35%. In addition, the lymphocyte level in partially shielded frogs falls from 70% or 80% to 55%. This contrasts with the total body irradiated group in which the level declines drastically to about 20% during the first two days post-irradiation. The number of eosinophils, basophils, and monocytes fluctuates little in the total body irradiated group in comparison to the partially shielded group.

OTHER TISSUES

Introduction

Although the mechanism is unknown, the use of organs to suppress immunity, particularly to a test skin graft, is intriguing. Single or sequential injections of subcellular liver preparations prolong skin allograft survival in mice and kidney allografts and xenografts in rabbits. In pigs, whole orthotopic or heterotopic (accessory) liver allografts extend the survival of simultaneously transplanted skin or kidney from the same donor. There are several common denominators among these diverse animal groups. The prolongation of a test skin allograft in salamanders, mice, and rats is favored by weak antigenic disparities. Strong histocompatibility barriers lead to failure of suppression. A second generality is that transplants of the effector tissues alone survive significantly longer than control skin grafts. This is seen best, for example, in rat kidney and pig liver. Mouse or bird gonadal implants exhibit at least partial long term survival despite a pronounced lymphocytic infiltration. Third, effector grafts that elicit clearly recognizable immune responses exert the least immunosuppression when the test grafts are transplanted at the time that the effector grafts are undergoing a significant rejection episode. Maximal suppression, however, occurs when test grafts are transplanted either three weeks before or three weeks after this critical period. A similar diphasic immunosuppression that alternates between prolonged survival and accelerated rejection follows after implantation in rabbits. This is also similar to earthworms if grafts are performed at 15°C. Such information suggests that an effector transplant establishes opposing, but not mutually exclusive, facets of immune reactivity that are manifested by accelerated second-set type rejection (sensitization) and/or prolonged test graft survival (immune suppression).

Urodele Amphibians

Cohen's group (Baldwin and Cohen 1970) has utilized the salamander *Diemictylus viridescens* to study suppression by allogeneic liver fragments implanted heterotopically. These prolong the survival of skin allografts transplanted orthotopically from the original liver donors. There are at least two advantages in using salmanders. First, because of the chronic graft rejection reaction characteristic of salamanders, any allogeneic tissue, even the liver, can become stablized prior to host immunological destruction. Small liver implants in salamanders undergo no severe ischemic necrosis as do grafts of mammalian liver when implanted subcutaneously. Control allogeneic skin grafts and subcutaneous liver fragment implants are chronically rejected at similar times ranging from four to ten weeks post-transplantation. However, when newts implanted with liver are challenged with test skin grafts from the original donors, survival of both skin and liver is often dramatically prolonged. Whereas first- and accelerated second-set control skin graft median survival times are 42.5 and 21.5 days, median survival times for test grafts transplanted one, three, six, or nine weeks after liver implantations are approximately sixty, eighty, thirty-eight, and fifty days respectively. If the liver implant is removed completely at the time of test skin grafting, immunosuppression is virtually eliminated and the opposite effect, accelerated skin graft rejections, is concomittantly increased.

Anuran Amphibians

It is interesting to compare the results obtained by Ruben's group, using liver suppression in *Xenopus laevis* larvae, with those obtained by Cohen's group in the salamander. Ruben et al. (1972) found that the liver is toxic for *Xenopus* larvae, whereas kidney, spleen, and thymus were not. Larvae always receive a graft of kidney and another from either kidney, thymus, spleen, or liver. The allograft response is defined as an infiltration and accumulation of small lymphocytes in the "test" kidney allograft. The aim was to time the initiation of these events in relation to the type of tissue used for suppression. Larvae of all stages developed allograft responses within one week post-implantation when the test implant was kidney, but implants from spleen and thymus suppressed both the initiation and the subsequent intensity of the response. Spleen was more effective than thymus, and both were more effective in the earlier larval stages. Suppression by tissues and organs in amphibians as well as other animals requires more investigation before any firm conclusions can be drawn about mechanisms.

ORGAN ABLATION

Birds
  Bursectomy

Bursectomy by surgical methods clearly and significantly reduces but does not inhibit the subsequent response of chickens to antigenic stimuli. The bursa of Fabricius develops as an outpouching of the gut endoderm on the fifth day of incubation. At this time, complete inhibition of bursal development and reduction in the thymus and spleen weight can be obtained by administration of 19-nortestosterone. Chicks bursectomized at hatching show reduced antibody production to BSA, *Brucella abortus* antigen, and T_2 coliphage when compared to controls. Chicks hatching from 19-nortestosterone-treated eggs lacking the bursa of Fabricius also show a deficient allograft response to injection of adult homologous spleen cells. This is manifested by characteristics of the graft-vs.-host reaction i.e., splenomegaly, nodular growth of donor cells over the peritoneal cavity, subcutaneous effusions of lymph over the abdominal wall, and weight loss (Papermaster et al. 1962).

The survival of chickens is greatly affected by surgical bursectomy at nineteen days; sham bursectomized birds survive indefinitely. All groups of birds survive equally well until the fifth week after hatching, as revealed in Fig. 15-6. After the

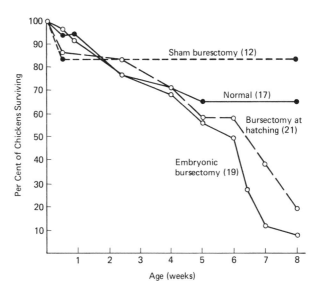

Fig. 15-6 The effect of embryonic (19 days) and post-hatching (21 days) bursectomy on survival of chickens. (*From:* Van Alten, et al., *Nature*, **217**: 358, 1968.)

sixth week there is a sharp decline in survival of both groups of bursectomized chickens. Birds subjected to bursectomy at hatching had depressed antibody responses after primary immunization with SRBC, but they responded as well as controls after a second injection. Birds deprived of their bursae at day 19 of embryonic life had barely detectable primary antibody responses and feeble responses even after secondary immunization (Fig. 15-7). Analysis of circulating immunoglobulin content in

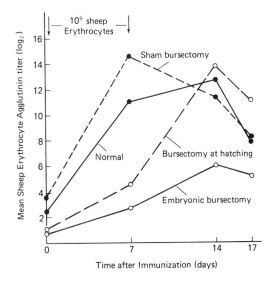

Fig. 15-7 Antibody titers before and after immunization of 4 week old chickens with sheep erythrocytes on day 0 and day 7. The curves show the mean agglutinin titers for the chickens which were bursectomized as embryos (19 days), bursectomized post-hatching, sham bursectomy, and normals. (*From*: Van Alten, et al., *Nature*, **217** : 358, 1968.)

each bird shows a striking reduction of 7S immunoglobulin. However, the 19S immunoglobulin level is normal. Using ϕx bacteriophage as antigen, Ivanyi et al. (1969) found that selective inhibition of IgM or IgG immunoglobulin synthesis occurs with equal frequency in bursectomized chickens. With regard to immunoglobulin structure, Gold and Benedict (1967) found no difference in either the L chain or H chain banding patterns of γG-globulin from bursectomized and normal chickens, indicating that the subunit of γG-globulin is the same for bursectomized and normal chickens.

Apparently, age and genotype influence the bird's response after bursectomy. White Rock and White Leghorn chickens were bursectomized between one and five weeks of age and were challenged with bovine serum albumin at six weeks of age. During this period, the effect of bursectomy on precipitin production is lessened. Bursectomy at four and five weeks of age significantly lowers the response of White Rocks, whereas bursectomy at the same time has no effect on the White Leghorn response. White leghorns bursectomized at one week of age do not exhibit natural antirabbit hemagglutinins until nine weeks of age; those bursectomized at ten days do not begin to show titers until six weeks of age. Controls appear by five weeks of age. Birds bursectomized between two and four weeks are also delayed in attaining the control titer, but did so by nine or twelve weeks of age.

Reversal of Suppression

Surgical removal of the bursa of Fabricius of young chickens prevents the development of normal antibody-producing capacity. This is also achieved by treatment of chick embryos with testosterone and other progestational hormones. In such immunologically deficient chickens the germinal lymphoid centers and plasma cells in the splenic and intestinal lymphoid aggregations are apparently normal, but they have reduced amounts of circulating immunoglobulins. Cooper et al. (1966) bursectomized and irradiated newly hatched chickens. The chickens consistently developed agammaglobulinemia and formed no circulating antibodies. However, if they were treated immediately after operations by intraabdominal injections of unirradiated autologous bursa cells, immunoglobulin production, lymphoid germinal centers, and plasma cells were restored.

Weber and Weidanz (1969) found destruction of lymphoid follicles with lasting lymphocyte depletion when the bursa of Fabricius of day-old chicks is exposed to 1000r doses of x-irradiation on the first and seventh day of post-embryonic life (Figs. 15-8 and 15-9). The bursas from irradiated birds do not reach more than 2%

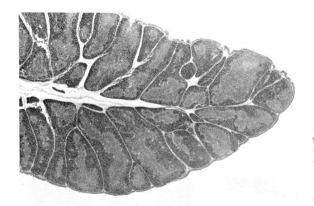

Fig. 15-8 Single bursal fold of a 10-week-old control chicken, showing the normal, characteristic cortico-medullary pattern of bursal follicles. Note that this single bursal fold is larger than the cross-section of the entire bursa from the BI chicken shown in Fig. 15-9. (Hematoxylin and eosin, ×*125*.) (*From*: Weber & Weidanz, *J. Immunol.*, **103**: 536, 1969.)

of the control bursa weights over a ninety-day period. The number of germinal follicles and plasma cells is decreased in the spleens and coecal tonsils of bursa-irradiated chickens. In addition, bursa-irradiated birds show a diminished antibody-producing capability to certain antigens. In fact, several birds showed a transient γG dysgamma-globulinemia (Fig. 15-10). It is interesting that histologic differences between the thymuses of bursa-irradiated and nonirradiated birds were not apparent.

These drastic effects can be curtailed and normal criteria restored by transplanting bursal cells intravenously into surgically bursectomized and bursectomized-irradiated chicks. Toivanen et al. (1972) used $6\frac{1}{2}$ week-old donors isogeneic with recipients at the major histocompatibility locus. The number of chickens producing natural and immune antibodies to SRBC and *Brucella abortus* was approximately two-fold greater

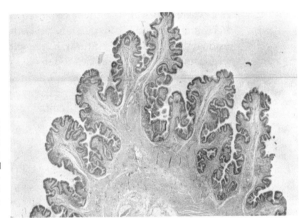

Fig. 15-9 The bursa of Fabricius of a 10-week-old bursa-irradiated (BI) chicken. The bursa had received a 1000r dose of x-radiation on the 1st and 7th day after hatching. There is a complete lack of follicular structures, increased interstitial connective tissue, and extensive epithelial infolding. (Hematoxylin and eosin, ×125.) (*From:* Weber & Weidanz, *J. Immunol.*, **103**: 537, 1969.)

in the transplanted than it was in untransplanted groups. The spleen and coecal tonsils possess germinal centers and plasma cells that parallel the functional evidence for restoration of humoral immunity. Thus, at the time the bursa begins involution bursal stem cells are sufficiently mature to home to other lymphoid organs and to proliferate and develop further without a bursal influence.

If splenic restoration alone is studied the results are somewhat different, still confirming, however, the potential of inoculated bursal cells. Hoshi (1972) used bursectomized and x-irradiated chickens that were given intraperitoneal injections of bursa cells with the aim of restoring the periellipsoidal lymphoid cells of the spleen. It is generally accepted that in the spleen, the development of lymphoid tissue surrounding the arterioles (periarterial lymphoid tissue) is thymus dependent. Germinal center cells and plasma cells are derived from the bursa of Fabricius. Injections of viable autogeneic bursal cells into neonatally bursectomized and x-irradiated chickens produces no recognizable restoration of the bursa-dependent lymphoid elements, i.e., the periellipsoidal lymphoid cells, germinal cells, and plasma cells. There is a slight restorative effect, after inoculations on the eighth and ninth days, of a large number of homologous bursa cells obtained from newly hatched or four-week-old chickens. In chickens that were bursectomized, x-irradiated, and given autologous unirradiated bursa cells at approximately two weeks of age, all the bursa-dependent elements, including the periellipsoidal lymphoid cells, were restored considerably. Perhaps in two-week-old chickens, the periellipsoidal lymphoid cells may be one of the cell lineages stemming from the bursal lymphoid cells.

Thymectomy, Bursectomy, and Splenectomy

To confirm the earlier findings of suppression by thymectomy in rabbits, guinea pigs and, other mammals, Graetzer et al. (1963) thymectomized, bursectomized, or splenectomized separate groups of chickens. Thymectomy of chickens during the first three days of age does not consistently affect precipitin production to BSA when they are challenged at six to nine weeks of age. Actually, in some cases thymectomized groups did not differ in mean peak titer from controls, and in some cases the response is significantly higher. Intact and sham control birds all respond by producing precipitins, whereas 6% of the thymectomized birds gave no detectable response. Higher precipitin titers were often associated with groups that possessed greater amounts of residual thymic tissue. Natural hemagglutinins were not affected by thymectomy. Splenectomy performed at two to ten days of age significantly delayed the appearance of precipitins, but it had no effect on the mean peak titer. Bursectomy at one to two days of age reduced the mean peak precipitin titers and the natural hemagglutinin titers drastically. The results of removing organs are variable.

Drug Effects

Adrenocorticotropic hormone (ACTH) and the corticosteroids are known to interfere with immune responses in several animal species. Immediate hypersensitivity reactions such as anaphylaxis and the Arthus phenomenon are suppressed in sensitized rats, mice, and rabbits, respectively. Furthermore, antibody suppression is also caused in guinea pigs, rats, and mice by administering ACTH. In guinea pigs delayed hypersensitivities and the development of experimental encephalitis are inhibited by ACTH. Cortisone prolongs allograft survival in rabbits, guinea pigs, mice, and chickens; however, it has no appreciable effect in primates or rabbits. Meyer et al. (1964) found that neonatally thymectomized and/or bursectomized White Leghorn chicks treated daily with corticosterone maintain a high percentage of allografts in thymectomized, bursectomized, and intact groups. Such treatment, however, does not appreciably affect circulating antibody production. Cortisone may be acting either through the thymus and/or through its activity as an antiinflammatory agent in maintaining allografts.

Antibody Deficiency in Rabbits

Birds are structurally and functionally divided to give both *T* and *B* immune responses, as measured by events in the thymus and bursa of Fabricius. This is not precisely the case in other vertebrates; thus, birds are unique. However, this structural arrangement has not prevented the search for an equivalent of the avian bursa of Fabricius in mammals. The Peyer's patch type of lymphoid tissue characteristic of the mammalian intestine resembles the avian bursa of Fabricius in several ways. It is gut-associated, lymphoepithelial tissues with follicular organization. In ontogeny these follicles develop like the thymus, but they precede the appearance of germinal centers and plasma cells elsewhere in the body. Lymphoid development in such sites is probably not dependent on antigenic stimulation. The appendix, a Peyer's patch type of tissue, when removed reduces the antibody response in rabbits. If the appendix, sacculus rotundus, and Peyer's patches are removed from rabbits as illustrated in Fig. 15-11, this leads to a pronounced reduction in the levels of circulating immunoglobulins, total numbers of circulating lymphocytes, and the ability to produce antibody to three of four antigens. Furthermore it leads to a marked survival disadvantage (Fig. 15-11). Such operations do not affect development of the capacity to reject skin allografts. Neonatal appendectomy alone results in decreased numbers of circulating lymphocytes and a depression of antibody response to one of four different antigens. Such results may support the theory that the Peyer's patch type of tissue in the rabbit is a functional equivalent of the bursa of Fabricius in the chicken.

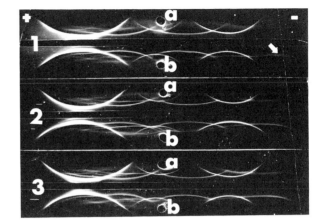

Fig. 15-10 Immunoelectrophoretic patterns of sera from Bl (1 and 2) and normal (3) birds at 6(a) and 9(b) weeks. Arrow indicates γG component which is lacking in 1a. (*From*: Weber & Weidanz, *J. Immunol.*, **103**: 537, 1969.)

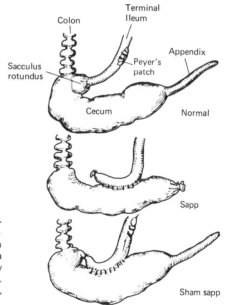

Fig. 15-11 Schematic illustration of the intestinal surgery required for the removal of the organized intestinal lymphoid tissues and the sham surgery designed to simulate the surgical trauma and possible alteration of intestinal physiology without removing organized lymphoid tissue. (*From*: Cooper, et al., *Int. Arch. Allergy*, **33**: 65, 1968.)

Marsupial Mammals
Introduction

Theoretically all organs of the immune system could be removed and thus effectively suppress some aspect of the immune response. In so doing certain cells are selectively removed; still there may be remaining a mixture of different types of immunocytes. For example, thymectomy should primarily remove the thymus-derived lymphocytes, those which evoke cell-mediated responses. Removal of the spleen and lymph nodes, wherein large numbers of B cells are housed, should lead to effective suppression of the antibody synthesizing capacity. Furthermore, this may be combined with other forms of immunosuppression such as irradiation.

Small and medium lymphocytes are first found in the thymus, only later in other lymphoid tissues, and thereafter in the general circulation. The thymus is thought to affect peripheral lymphocytes by migration of thymic lymphocytes to other areas, by a thymic humoral factor, or by both mechanisms. In the neonatal mouse, small and medium lymphocytes appear in the spleen and in the circulation. If mice are thymectomized at birth they eventually show severe lymphoid hypoplasia, but during the first few weeks thereafter it is somewhat difficult to obtain information on the details of thymectomy effects. Does thymectomy at birth influence the origin and initial proliferation of extra thymic lymphocytes, or does it influence the number of lymphocytes that have previously developed by virtue of other mechanisms?

The opossum

Eutherian or placental mammals cannot always provide answers to questions resulting from the effects of thymectomy if performed prior to the origin of extra-thymic lymphoid tissue. By contrast, certain problems are not encountered in less advanced mammals. For example, in the opossum *Didelphys virginiana* a metatherian or marsupial mammal, small numbers of large lymphocytes are found in the thymus on the first day of life and in even larger numbers on the second day. Medium lymphocytes occur in the thymus on the second or third days and small lymphocytes on the fifth or sixth days. Small lymphocytes appear in lymph nodes one or two days after medium lymphocytes. (For further details, refer to Table 7-2 in Chap. 7.)

Thymectomy of opossum pouch "embryos" leads to deranged hemopoiesis. Lymph nodes are clearly deficient in small lymphocytes and show an abnormal

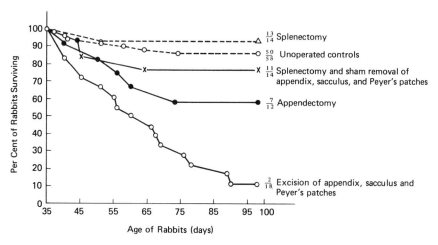

Fig. 15-12   Effect of early removal of organized lymphoid tissues on survival in rabbits. (*From*: Cooper, et al., *Int. Arch. Allergy, 33*: 65, 1968.)

persistence of immature (basophil) erythroblasts and, in most cases, myelocytes. The nodes consist of a framework of reticular tissue with no clear demarcation into cortex and medulla. Only large lymphocytes predominate. In fact, the ratio of basophil erythroblasts to polychromatophil and eosinophil erythroblasts is significantly higher than normal. An abnormal persistence of eosinophil myelocytes is evident, especially around the arterioles and arteriolar capillaries and in the vessel walls. Furthermore, the white pulp, usually evident around the arterioles and arterial capillaries, is absent. Instead, the perivascular areas are occupied either by basophil erythroblasts or, in some cases, by eosinophil myelocytes.

It should be stressed that thymectomy of pouch embryo opossums leads to an abnormal persistance and even increase in myeloid cells, particularly erythroblasts, in the spleen and lymph node. This suggests that the thymus not only plays a role in the origin and maintenance of lymphatic tissue, but it also suppresses myeloid tissue development. According to Miller et al. (1965) the erythroblastic tissue in the spleen and, to some extent in the lymph nodes, increases abnormally. The implication here is a defective type of erythroblast maturation and an ineffective erythropoiesis resembling that seen in certain clinical syndromes such as megaloblastic diseases, di Guglielmo's syndrome, and thalassemia major. The origin of lymphatic tissue (at least in the spleen), the maintenance of lymphatic tissue in lymph nodes, and the suppression of myeloid tissue in lymph nodes and the spleen are all attributable to the thymus in the opossum.

SUMMARY

The immunological competence of any vertebrate animal depends to a large extent on its ability to synthesize antibodies, the specificity of which is ultimately referable to and regulated by nucleic acids. Allograft rejection in fishes and amphibians can be abrogated by two principal external methods. One approach assumes that cells divide after antigenic challenge and, therefore, that certain drugs interfere with nucleic acid or protein synthesis and in so doing prolong allograft survival. Combined drug and temperature therapy similarily prolong scale graft survival. According to the second method, irradiation prolongs the response to an allograft, since immune cells are damaged by irradiation. The organs that produce immunologically competent cells, namely the spleen and thymus, can be removed, leading to suppressed immune reactivity.

BIBLIOGRAPHY

Baldwin, W. M. III and Cohen, N. 1970. Liver-induced immunosuppression of allograft immunity in urodele amphibians. Transplantation 10: 530.

Cooper, E. L., and Schaefer, D. W. 1970. Bone marrow restoration of transplantation immunity in the leopard frog *Rana pipiens*. Proc. Soc. Exptl. Biol. Med. 135: 406.

Cooper, M. D., Schwartz, M. L., and Good, R. A. 1966. Restoration of gamma globulin production in agammaglobulinemic chickens. Science 151: 471.

Gold, E. F., and Benedict, A. A. 1967. Comparison of polypeptide chains of γG-globulin from bursectomized and normal chickens. Proc. Soc. Exp. Biol. Med. 125: 535.

Graetzer, M. A., Wolfe, H. R., Aspinall, R. L., and Meyer, R. K. 1963. Effect of thymectomy and bursectomy on precipitin and natural hemagglutinin production in the chicken. J. Immunol. 90: 878.

Hoshi, H. 1972. Effect of inoculation of bursa cells on the splenic lymphoid tissue of bursectomized and x-irradiated chickens. Tohoku J. Exp. Med. 108: 113.

Ivanyi, J., Marvanova, H., and Skamene, E. 1969. Immunoglobulin syntheses and lymphocyte transformation by anti-immunoglobulin sera in bursectomized chickens. Immunology **17**: 325.

Levy, L. 1963. Effects of drugs on goldfish scale homograft survival. Proc. Soc. Exptl. Biol. Med. **114**: 47.

Meyer, R. K., Aspinall, R. L., Graetzer, M. A., and Wolfe, H. R. 1964. Effect of corticosterone on the skin homograft reaction and on precipitin and hemagglutinin production in thymectomized and bursectomized chickens. J. Immunol. **92**: 446.

Miller, J. F. A. P., Block, M., Rowlands, D. T. Jr., and Kind, P. 1965. Effect of thymectomy on hematopoietic organs of the opossum "embryo." Proc. Soc. Exper. Biol. Med. **118**: 916.

Papermaster, B. W., Friedman, D. I., and Good, R. A. 1962. Relationship of the bursa of Fabricius to immunologic responsiveness and homograft immunity in the chicken. Proc. Soc. Exper. Biol. Med. **110**: 62.

Ruben, L. N., Stevens, J. M., and Kidder, G. M. 1972. Suppression of the allograft response by implants of mature lymphoid tissues in larval *Xenopus laevis*. J. Morphol. **138**: 457.

Stutzman, W. 1967. Combined effects of temperature and immunosuppressive therapy on allograft rejection in goldfish. Transpl. **5**: 1344.

Toivanen, A., Toivanen, P., and Good, R. A. 1972. Transplantation of cells from bursa of Fabricius into surgically bursectomized chicks. Int. Arch. Allergy **43**: 588.

Ugami, N., and Kukita, Y. 1969. X-ray effects on rejection of transplanted fins in the fish. *Oryzias latipes*. Transpl. **8**: 300.

Weber, W. T., and Weidanz, W. P. 1969. Prolonged bursal lymphocyte depletion and suppression of antibody formation following irradiation of the bursa of Fabricius. J. Immunol. **103**: 537.

Chapter 16

Epilogue

INTRODUCTION

The varied modifications which vertebrate immune organs have undergone and the varied immune functions which they have assumed have, of course, come about as the result of evolution. It is impossible to make a comparative study of the vertebrates or the invertebrates without formulating some general concept of the nature of the evolutionary processes. Most structural changes in the organs of the immune system and the functional changes in the immune system were probably adaptive modifications to a variety of environments and modes of life. Clearly there is not sufficient information from functional comparative studies of diverse immune systems to warrant even a hazardous guess as to the nature of the pressures that brought about these evolutionary adaptations.

One might, with humor, compare the vertebrate, particularly the human, immune system to an overly complex bureaucracy. Both are effective and serve their respective constituents; nevertheless there are smaller, less cumbersome immune systems such as those of most invertebrates, just as there are less complicated institutions that also serve their dependents. To argue that five types of immunoglobulin molecules are better than one type or, for that matter, no immunoglobulins at all, is academic. Whatever the animal, each must be viewed as it is, with its own peculiarities and its own environmental niches; then, with that in mind, descriptions can be laid down as to what an animal does to protect itself against detrimental pathogens. Whether these pathogens attack from the exterior or begin as internal parasites or as mutated cells capable of becoming neoplastic, every animal is equipped by nature to handle such potential harm. After all, nature surely has provided all animals with mechanisms for nourishment, respiration, excretion, reproduction, etc. In fact, all physiologists recognize the multiple-organ physiologic systems characteristic of all animals. This book, hopefully, has dispelled the notion that immunity is purely a vertebrate attribute restricted to mammals, particularly humans.

It is unproductive to attempt a classification of immune responses throughout the animal kingdom based, for example, on the environmental niches of particular animals. Such an approach would result in meaningless situations such as comparing the condition of a whale's thymus with a nonexistent thymus in the starfish merely because they both live in the sea; although they do inhabit the ocean, they are totally different animals. Rather than compare incomparable creatures such as apples with oranges, it is more meaningful to recognize that both fruits live in the external

317

world, they both have seeds, fleshy parts, and reproduce their kind. Whales have lymphocytes and react to foreign material just as starfish have coelomocytes and react to foreign material. Thus, instead of standardizing immune systems on the basis of an established criterion such as common environments or presence of vertebrate cells and organs shared by many different animal groups, it seems more appropriate to describe the immune systems of various animals according to particular functions.

As a physiologic event, the immune response, a product of cells, tissues, and organs of the immune system, is unique. It represents a condition found throughout the animal kingdom, but it is probably the least reported of all the functional organ systems, especially in its comparative aspects. Witness its lack of coverage in any biologic textbook from high school primers through to advanced treatises. Respiration, digestion, and reproduction are examples of areas in physiology that are fully treated. Immunity has not been viewed as essential as the other functional qualities of living organisms; thus it is often relegated to specialty-restricted publications.

The immune system is also unique because specificity is one of its chief hallmarks. Where antibody is involved, the response is specific. There are, however, nonspecific immune responses such as phagocytosis that are important in every animal's immunologic armamentarium. Every individual is unique because of its peculiar and specific *self* or antigenic make up. Furthermore every individual, particularly a vertebrate, is amply equipped with cells or their progenitors that are capable of responses to an infinite array of foreign material. Depending on the antigen and the organism, one can expect cell-mediated immune reactions, humoral immune responses, or both responses integrated.

All animals are able to recognize and distinguish between *self* and *not-self* components. At every evolutionary level, the immune response is essential to the well-being of an organism. Without it, each living creature would be preyed upon by a variety of external harmful pathogens, viruses, bacteria and fungi, and by internal parasites. Witness how lymphocytes respond to a parasite (Fig. 16-1). Indeed, cancer, the most potent internal, detrimental threat, is now prominent as a disease that may develop because of a weakened immune system. It is known that the percentage of malignancies is higher in patients with primary immunodeficiencies (Table 16-1). The

Table 16-1

Malignancies in patients with primary immunodeficiency.

Primary disease	Approximate number of malignancies collected	% Cancer
Bruton-type agamma-globulinemia	5 Cases, all leukemic	5–10
Ataxia-telangiectasia	42 Cases, many forms of cancer	10–15
Wiskott-Aldrich syndrome	13 Cases, mostly but not exclusively lymphoreticular malignancies	> 10
Common variable immunodeficiency	More than 30 cases, many forms of cancer	5–10
Severe dual-system immunodeficiency	3 Cases	1–10

From: Axelrod et al. 1973. The Harvey Lectures 1971–1972.

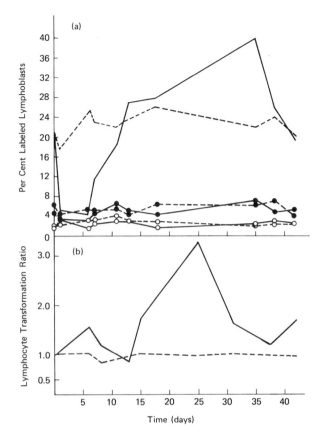

Fig. 16-1 (a) The lymphoblast responses of the spleen: (------, ————) inguinal lymph node; (○----○, ○————○) and cecal lymphoid patches; (●---●, ●————●) in noninfected guinea pigs, and animals infected with 5000 *Trichostrongylus colubriformis*, respectively. (b) *In vitro* lymphocyte transformation ratios of the peripheral lymphocytes of guinea pigs infected with 5000 T. colubriformis (————) and of nonifected animals (------). (*From*: Dobson & Soulsby, *Exp. Parasitol.*, **35**: 16, 1974.)

role of the *immune surveillance system* explained clearly by Burnet (1970) has been extended far beyond the mere development of antibodies to a given antigen. Indeed, this recognition of foreign cells that may become neoplastic is the one feature common to all immune systems regardless of their level of phylogeny. This does not minimize the importance of the antibody synthesizing capacity. Nevertheless, *antibody synthesis*, with its exquisite specificity, is unlike *recognition*; it seems to be purely a vertebrate attribute and is therefore not a common denominator for the immune system as irritability, for example, is for the nervous system.

THE CENTRAL PROBLEM OF ADAPTIVE IMMUNITY

Introduction

It is clear that all animal immune systems are equipped for responding to a variety of antigens. Probably the chief difference between the invertebrate and vertebrate

320   EPILOGUE

responses (if it is indeed a fair comparison) is the limited extent (due to limited knowledge?) to which invertebrates seem to be able to respond. This is important, but it should be acknowledged that the simplest invertebrates cannot respond to a given antigen in the same way that even the advanced invertebrates, and certainly verte-brates, would respond. It will probably emerge that the immune system of advanced invertebrates may not be too remote in functional complexity from that of many vertebrates. Information is scarce because limited research has been done on this subject.

Diversification and Selection

The immune system responds to an infinite number of antigens, many and probably all of which had nothing to do with the evolution of the animal. Haptens (artifically prepared antigens) represent the best example of unnaturally occurring antigens to which animals will respond even though they have never encountered them. According to Smith (1973):

The problem of adaptive immunity thus has two aspects, the problem of antibody diversity and the problem of selection by antigen [Fig. 16-2]. For both of these, the preadaptive nature of immunocompetence poses special difficulties. Preadaptive competence implies that the mechanism by which any particular antigen stimulates the synthesis of only the appropriate antibodies must in general have arisen before it conferred any survival value; this fact imposes constraints on any theory of antigenic selection, which are elegantly met by the clonal selection theory.

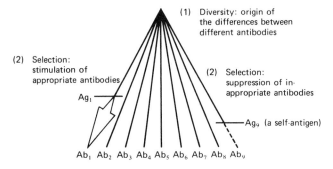

Fig. 16-2 Two central problems of adaptive immunity; that of antibody diversity and that of selection by antigen. (*From*: Smith, 1973, *The Variation and Adaptive Expression of Antibodies.*)

THE IMPACT OF IMMUNOLOGY

Introduction

Immunology is an important discipline today. According to Edelman (1974):

Two major developments have profoundly altered immunological research in the last decade: the theory of clonal selection and the chemical analysis of antibody structure (Cold Spring Harbor Symposium, 1967; Nobel Symposium, 1967). As a result of these developments, it has become clear that the central problem of immunology is to under-stand the mechanisms of selective molecular recognition in a quantitative fashion. Aside from evolution itself, there are few such well-analyzed examples of selective systems in biology or in other fields for that matter. For this reason, the immune system provides a unique opportunity to analyze the problem of selection under defined and experimentally measurable conditions that have so far been hard to achieve in other eukaryotic systems. It is fortunate that the characteristics of the molecules and cells mediating selection in the immune response are known or can be known, and above all, that the time scale of the selective events is well within that required for direct observation and experimentation.

The clonal selection theory of acquired immunity advanced by Burnet (1959) has been widely accepted among immunologists a situation that roughly parallels the degree to which Darwin's theory of natural selection of the species has been accepted among biologists. There is an essential similarity; the two concepts can be equated by substituting the word *lymphocyte* for *species.*

Clonal Selection Theory
  Original statement

In its original form (Burnet 1959) the clonal selection hypothesis

assumes that in the animal there exists clones of mesenchymal cells, each carrying immunologically reactive sites corresponding in appropriate complementary fashion to one (or possibly a small number of) potential antigenic determinants. This provides a popu-lation of cells which, when an appropriate stage of development has been reached, are capable of producing the population of globulin molecules which collectively provide the normal antibodies. When an antigen is introduced it will make contact with a cell of the corresponding clone, presumably a lymphocyte, and by so doing stimulate it to produce in one way or another more globulin molecules of the cell's characteristic type. The obvious way of achieving this is to postulate that stimulation initiates proliferation as soon as the cell in question is taken into an appropriate tissue niche, spleen, lymph node or subacute inflammatory accumulation.

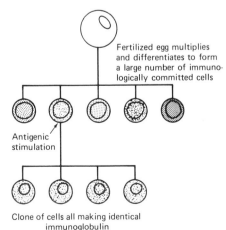

Fertilized egg multiplies and differentiates to form a large number of immuno-logically committed cells

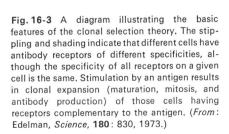

Fig. 16-3 A diagram illustrating the basic features of the clonal selection theory. The stip-pling and shading indicate that different cells have antibody receptors of different specificities, al-though the specificity of all receptors on a given cell is the same. Stimulation by an antigen results in clonal expansion (maturation, mitosis, and antibody production) of those cells having receptors complementary to the antigen. (*From:* Edelman, *Science*, **180**: 830, 1973.)

Antigenic stimulation

Clone of cells all making identical immunoglobulin

Inherent in the theory of clonal selection are the requisites that have brought cellular immunology to where it is today; the theory was followed by an explosion of research (Fig. 16-3). There are, however, some interesting situations in immunology, drawn even from comparative studies, that tend to refute clonal selection. One of particular relevance (reviewed by Jerne 1971) is the work from the laboratory of Simonsen and that of Lafferty involving alloaggression. Graft-vs.-host reactions could be induced in chick embryos with as little as 50–100 cells, a number far below that required for the clonal selection theory, estimated to be approximately 10^4–10^5 cells. Nevertheless the theory is attractive, and it accounts for what should occur in a differentiated organism.

Clonal Selection and Invertebrate Immunology

The clonal selection theory may not be restricted to conditions in the vertebrate animal. Invertebrates by far outnumber the vertebrates and also possess legitimate immune responses; because of this and, most importantly, because they, too, belong to the living world, their immune responses must be brought in line with those of better understood vertebrate responses. After all, no other theory, e.g., that of DNA, restricts its coverage to vertebrates and perhaps the true test of any theory is its extensibility to encompass all life in a unifying manner. To this end Burnet (1974) has contributed to the first major volume on invertebrate immunology. He declares that there is a

> ... similar capacity to recognize the difference between genetically identical and foreign cells or tissues in earthworms and, presumably, many or all coelomate invertebrates. From the point of view of comparative immunology the most interesting future development could be a demonstration that invertebrate hemocytes (or some subgroup of these cells) are capable of differentiation into forms analogous to immunocytes, i.e. multiple clones of cells each with a distinctive pattern or range of patterns of steric reactivity. There are phenomena which hint at specific adaptive immune responses in coelomate invertebrates, but until immunocytes with specific receptors are defined one must remain skeptical.

Surely this skepticism and the lack of knowledge could be dispelled by more intensive research. It should not be forgotten that immunology once consisted of the details of antibody production after vaccination in humans. It is an understatement that the field of immunology is broader than that and it will be even more so.

Minimal requirements in Vertebrates
Somatic differentiation

At the cellular and molecular levels of organization there are at least three requirements focused around cells of the lymphoid system. We must begin with an immunologically competent cell descendent of a stem cell that originated in some generative site such as the bone marrow or its equivalent in animals devoid of marrow. Assuming the T and B cell concept to be valid, such cells should already possess the information for generating antibodies of various specificities in the genome prior to encounter with an antigen. Furthermore, there must be recognition units or receptors on the cell surface to sense these antigens. Once there is interaction between antigen and an antigen-binding cell, clonal expansion is induced. According to Edelman (1973), clonal expansion consists of cellular maturation, cell division, and increased protein synthesis (Fig. 16-4). Simply stated, the clonal selection theory requires

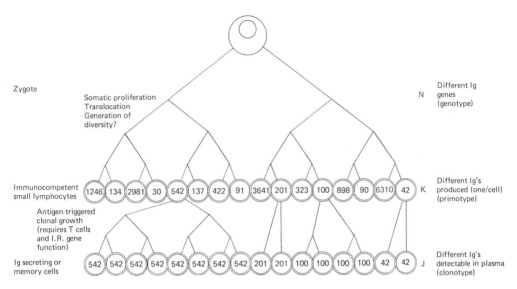

Fig. 16-4 A model of the somatic differentiation of antibody-producing cells according to the clonal selection theory. The number of immunoglobulin genes may increase during somatic growth so that in the immunologically mature animal, different lymphoid cells are formed, each committed to the synthesis of a structurally distinct receptor antibody (indicated by an Arabic numeral). A small proportion of these cells proliferate upon antigenic stimulation to form different clones of cells, each clone producing a different antibody. This model represents bone marrow-derived (B) cells, but with minor modifications it is also applicable to thymusderived (T) cells. (*From*: Edelman, *Soc. Gen. Physiol.*, **29**: 1, 1974.)

A source of diversity among different antibodies and a means of committing a cell or phenotypically restricting it to produce just one of each of the possible kinds of antibody; a means of trapping antigen or favoring encounter with antigen-binding cells; a means by which this encounter is amplified by triggering the cells to divide and produce more antibodies of the same type.

Minimum Elements

Antigen must somehow be recognized by an immunologically competent cell. This is thought to be accomplished by the presence of receptors or recognition units on the surface of the lymphocytes. Receptors are related to the synthesis of immunoglobulin, whose antigen-combining site is specific for the same antigen. Marchalonis et al. (1974) provide direct evidence that immunoglobulin is present on the surfaces of lymphocytes of all classes; the isolated immunoglobulin exhibits binding specificity

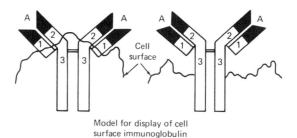

Model for display of cell
surface immunoglobulin

Fig. 16-5 Hypothetical model for the presentation of immunoglobulin upon the lymphocyte surface. The diagram on the left illustrates a situation where the Fc portion of the μ-chain is surrounded by surface components. This condition may obtain for unactivated thymus derived lymphocytes. The dark regions represent the variable regions of the light and heavy polypeptide chains which share the combining site for antigen. 1, constant region of light chain; 2, Fd piece; 3, Fe region of heavy chain; A, combining site for antigen. (*From*: Marchalonis et al., *The Walter & Eliza Hall Inst. Med. Res.*)

for antigen (Fig. 16-5). This takes into account the only situation involving either the *T* or *B* cell. At least a third cell type, the macrophage, a phylogenetic descendant of the invertebrate phagocytic cell, must somehow interact with antigen and the *T* and *B* cells (Fig. 16-6). Finally, Smith (1973) has expressed three fundamental postulates of the clonal selection hypotheses:

> *the antigen receptor site is identical to the antibody combining site whose synthesis it controls . . . cells are specialized . . . for the production of a single molecular species of antibody; . . . cell specialization is inherited . . . [a] specialization [that accounts for] the secondary response. During cell proliferation of the primary response, some of the progeny —each harboring the same specificity which was originally responsible for the stimulation of its progenitor—wait in large numbers for a second contact with the same antigen.*

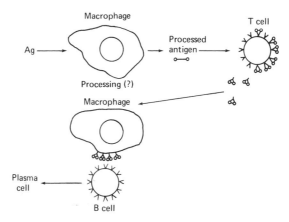

Fig. 16-6 Theoretical shceme for the collaboration of thymus-derived lymphocytes (T-cells) and bone marrow-derived lymphocytes (B-cells). Macrophages play two roles in this scheme. One is to process antigen. The second function is to concentrate the collaborative factor elaborated by T-cells and present it, bound to antigen, to the unstimulated B-cells. (*From*: Marchalonis et al., *The Walter & Eliza Hall Inst. Med. Res.*)

Antibody Structure

Antibody synthesis is an aspect of the immune response apparently unique to vertebrates. Lack of known antibody in invertebrates may be due to its real absence, and if so, recognition is an event universal to the immune responses of all animals; in invertebrates, recognition may be effected by fragments of antibody on the surface of hemocytes, or by other molecular components unrelated to antibody. These components may be in some way relevant to the agglutinins and lysins and other immunosubstances of invertebrate body fluids. Antibody structure is definable away from the cell; this extracellular structure apparently agrees with that found on the surface of certain cells, particularly lymphocytes. Thus, the knowledge of the structure of a cellular recognition unit or receptor for sensing antigen is imminent.

FINAL COMMENT

We may assume that recognition, primordial cell-mediated immunity, and vertebrate immune reactions represent progressions of immunity in the animal kingdom that evolved as protective mechanisms against predation by microorganisms. Unicellular protozoans combine food-getting, recognition, and ultimate sequestration of harmful microorganisms in one system (Burnet 1968). This action occurs by combined chemotaxis and phagocytosis. At this phylogenetic level, *self, not-self* discrimination presumably occurs by means of *protoimmunoglobulins* or other substances. These may act like opsonins, if they exist at all, and are still unknown chemically (Boyden 1960a, b; 1963; 1966). Primitive metazoans exhibiting, as of now, only quasi immunorecognition, may be members of the phylogenetic groups that we should examine for the presence of such cellular recognition units. Nossal (1971) believes that the earthworm coelomocyte may be one model that holds the key to the "molecular ancestor of vertebrate immunoglobulins provided certain blocking and binding studies are exploited to the fullest."

Jerne (1971) proposes that:

> *cell recognition, which must be fundamental in even the most primitive metazoa [as described under quasi immunorecognition—Chap. 2] may require the presence of histocompatibility antigens and of complimentary "antibody" molecules at cell surfaces . . . at some stage of metazoan evolution, an immune system of specialized lymphocytes developed, based on this older recognition system, and that a mechanism evolved for suppressing those lymphocytic stem cells that express v-genes of subset S, (self) [which] produce antibodies against the histocompatibility antigens of the individual. . . . the complimentary subset A (allo) of v-genes determine antibodies directed against all other relevant histocompatibility antigens of [a given] species [absent in a] particular animal . . .*

Another cause for the evolution of recognition of foreignness by cells may be found in Thomas' (1959) theory, later elaborated by Burnet (1970) in his concept of immunologic surveillance. According to this view, the development of neoplasia was a strong force in the evolutionary development of the immune system. Thus we progress phylogenetically from combined food-getting and defense manifested by simple recognition to specific primitive cellular immunity with a memory component effected by cells with definable but unknown receptors, to specific anamnestic immune responses mediated by cells with known receptors (immunoglobulins). The dictum of Haeckal (1891) that "ontogeny recapitulates phylogeny" may be referable to immune responsiveness if we are still to view such dicta as instructive. Indeed, the simplest manifestations of immunity are found throughout the phylogenetic sequence, and each level of metazoan complexity yields species adapted to certain environmental niches. Each level therefore possesses remnants of the steps in their orignal order of appearance, in the development of immunity in both the ontogenetic and phylogenetic development of animal species.

When we deal with the evolution of structure and function we think in terms of *homology* and *analogy*. As an example of homology, we can use the vertebrate forelimb, which has undergone striking modifications in various animals adapted to different environmental niches. In man it is an arm and hand, in birds a wing, and in whales a flipper, to cite several examples. Despite the adaptations, the limb remains basically the same, especially in its ontogenetic development and its later morphological structure. Although the adult structures are superfically different they do possess essentially the same ancestral entities. There is *no* common ancestor of analogous structures; thus, the problem of flight is solved by the development of wings in birds and butterflies. Although these structures are similar (as, analogous) in function and superficial appearance, they are different (not homologous) in development and morphology. Undoubtedly homology and analogy may be found to exist with regard to immune systems when more comparative information is available.

Hopefully the reader has grasped the significance of the universality of immunologic responses. The full array of immune responses in *all* vertebrates, not just the fishes, amphibians, and reptiles, probably arose from certain ancestral invertebrate prototypes. Of the diverse processes necessary for immunity in vertebrates, we recognize among simpler organisms, the same, analogous, or precursors of, such parameters as antigen recognition, phagocytosis, and humoral synthesis of substances that sequester antigen; as examples of cell mediated immunity, cell and tissue transplant destruction also occurs. Invertebrate immune responses are biologic events, worthy of analysis as natural phenomena in their own right.

Invertebrate immune responses were not always interpreted in terms of the equivalent processes in the better-known vertebrates, particularly mammals. Nevertheless the dearth of invertebrate or even poikilothermic vertebrate information forces an association with homiothermic vertebrates, for no other reason than conceptual convenience of the latter as a familiar standard or reference point. Attention is focused on immune adaptation in primitive species: their own methods for solving the problem of threat of extinction by pathogens, the ultimate function of the immune system.

BIBLIOGRAPHY

Boyden, S. V. 1960a. Antibody production. Nature **185**: 724.

———. 1960b. Cellular discrimination between indigenous and foreign matter. J. Theor. Biol. **3**: 123.

———. 1963. Cellular recognition of foreign matter. Int. Rev. Exptl. Pathol. **2**: 311.

———. 1966. Natural antibodies and the immune response. Adv. Immunol. **5**: 1.

Burnet, F. M. 1959. *The Clonal Selection Theory of Acquired Immunity*. Nashville, Tennessee: Vanderbilt University Press.

——. 1968. Evolution of the immune process in vertebrates. Nature **218**: 426.

——. 1970. *Immunological Surveillance*. New York: Pergamon Press.

——. 1974. Invertebrate Precursors to Immune Responses. In *Contemporary Topics in Immunobiology*, ed. E. L. Cooper, IV, 13–24. New York: Plenum Press.

Cold Spring Harbor Symposium Quant. Biol., 1967. **32**: Entire issue.

Edelman, G. M. 1973. Antibody structure and molecular immunology. Science **180**: 830.

——. 1974. Origins and mechanisms of specificity in clonal selection. In *Cellular Selection and Regulation in the Immune Response*, ed. G. M. Edelman, pp. 1–38. New York: Raven Press.

Haeckel, E. 1891. Anthropogenic oder Entwickelungs geschichte des Menschen. Keimes.- und Stamnes-Geschichte. 4th ed. rev. and enl. Leipzig: Wilhalm Engelmann.

Jerne, N. K. 1971. The somatic generation of immune recognition. Eu. J. Immunol. **1**: 1.

Marchalonis, J. J., Cone, R. E., and Atwell, J. L. 1972b. Isolation and partial characterization of lymphocyte surface immunoglobulin. J. Exp. Med. **135**: 956.

Marchalonis, J. J., Cone, R. E., Atwell, J. L., and Rolley, R. T. 1974. Structure and function of lymphocyte surface immunoglobulin. Publication No. 1703, pp. 629–647. Victoria Australia: The Walter and Eliza Hall Institute of Medical Research.

Nobel Symposium. 1967. Ed. J. Killander, Gamma Globulins: Structure and control of biosynthesis. Stockholm: Almquist and Wiksell.

Nossal, G. J. V. 1971. Summary of the Third International Congress of The Transplantation Society: a personal approach. Transplant. Proc. **3**: 967.

Smith, G. P. 1973. *The Variation and Adaptive Expression of Antibodies*. Cambridge, Massachusetts: Harvard University Press.

Thomas, L. 1959. Untitled contribution to the discussion in cellular and humoral aspects of the hypersensitive states, H. S. Lawrence New York: Hoeber Harper. p. 529.

Index

Animal Health Diagnostic Laboratory
P.O. Box 30076   (517) 353-1683
Lansing, MI   48909